Post-treatment Imaging of the Orbit

Daniel Thomas Ginat • Suzanne K. Freitag

Editors

Post-treatment Imaging of the Orbit

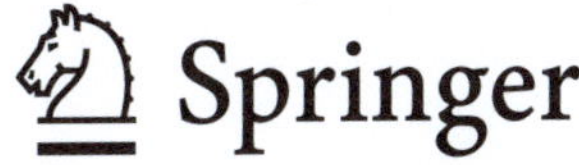

Editors
Daniel Thomas Ginat
Director of Head and Neck Imaging
Department of Radiology
University of Chicago
Chicago, IL
USA

Suzanne K. Freitag
Director, Ophthalmic Plastic Surgery
Service, Department of Ophthalmology
Massachusetts Eye and Ear Infirmary
Harvard Medical School
Boston, MA
USA

ISBN 978-3-662-51130-5   ISBN 978-3-662-44023-0   (eBook)
DOI 10.1007/978-3-662-44023-0
Springer Heidelberg New York Dordrecht London

To my parents, Roselyne and Jonathan, and the wonderful fields of Radiology and Ophthalmology

Daniel Thomas Ginat

To Allison

Suzanne K. Freitag

Foreword I

The management of patients with ophthalmic disorders presents particular-challenges. Ophthalmic disorders are varied and diverse, and so are their treatments. Surgical intervention usually leads to altered anatomy, insertion of metallic or nonmetallic implants, and other devices. More recently, there is a trend towards use of minimally invasive surgical approaches and devices. For all these reasons, there seems to be a need for a resource for ophthalmologists as well as radiologists who may find it challenging to interpret or bital and ocular imaging studies.

Dr Ginat, a Harvard trained radiologist and director of head and neck imaging at the University of Chicago, and Dr Freitag, director of ophthalmic plastic surgery at Massachusetts Eye and Ear Infirmary, have compiled cases from multiple institutions in an easy to use guide that will allow various specialists to understand each other better, to cooperate more efficiently in providing excellent care to their patients, and eventually move the field forward.

The book is comprised of eight chapters, divided by ophthalmic subspecialties, such as cataract surgery, glaucoma surgery, and oculoplastic surgery. Every chapter is authored by a radiologist and an ophthalmologist so as to provide a balanced perspective. Each clinical scenario is illustrated with a clinical summary and correlational multimodality imaging.

It is my sincere hope that readers will find as much pleasure in reading this book as the authors and editors had in writing and editing it.

Cleveland, OH, USA

Arun D. Singh, MD

Foreword II

Radiologists are always a little bit behind the curve. New devices get introduced, new procedures get developed, and new methods are applied to treat familiar diseases. But radiologists may not learn about these innovations until we see them, on the images, affecting our patients. Our colleagues in musculoskeletal imaging are quite familiar with this phenomenon, since orthopedic devices are so frequently updated. But even in head and neck imaging, new prosthetics creep into use, and it is increasingly difficult to remain ahead of the high rate of innovation.

There is another problem that plagues subspecialized radiologists: we need to know as much about these patients' clinical pathways as the surgeons who treat them. We need to speak the same language and use the same terms. But these terms were never taught in medical school; they are unique to the subspecialty. An ophthalmologist will instantly recognize a word like "pseudoaphakia," but it would stump most physicians, including most radiologists. Yet, how can radiologists claim to be contributing to the care of these patients if we cannot even describe what has happened to them?

So, how should we deal with these tough cases? "I'll Google it." The Internet answers all questions, right? Anyone who has tried to use Google images to find the name of a device can attest that it is, to say the least, a nontrivial task. Online lists of prosthetics are usually outdated. You need to at least guess at a possible answer, as a starting point from which to branch out, and you need to know all the old devices so that you can exclude them from your search.

"I'll look it up in the medical record or call the referring doc." That's a great idea, and definitely to be encouraged in times of uncertainty. But you can't sink that kind of time into too many cases, or you'll never get anything done. It's a delicate balance – calling the referring docs often enough to maintain good relationships and solve the truly perplexing cases, but not trampling all over the workflow of two busy physicians.

These are the reasons that books like *Post-Treatment Imaging of the Orbit* are important to practicing radiologists. This is the background knowledge that allows us to ask (and answer) the intelligent questions that demonstrate that we are on the same playing field with our referring clinicians. If we come into the discussion without a basic understanding of the operative procedures and prosthetics, our referring surgeons will (rightly) conclude that our interpretations are not providing value to the patients.

"

I know that this foreword is intended for radiologists, and not everyone who picks up this book will be a radiologist. There will be enterprising surgeons who want to know what their handiwork looks like on imaging. For you, I have only encouragement. I hope that your dedication to learn more about radiology will prompt the radiologists you work with to gain further knowledge about the surgeries that our shared patients undergo.

Pittsburgh, PA, USA   Barton Branstetter, MD

Acknowledgments

Michael Amon, MD Academic Teaching Hospital of St. John, Johannes von Gott Platz, Vienna, Austria

Venkat Avadhanam, MD Royal Sussex County Hospital, Brighton, UK

Karen Capaccioli Massachusetts Eye and Ear Infirmary, Boston, MA, USA

John Christoforidis, MD University of Arizona, Tucson, AZ, USA

Kathryn Colby, MD, PhD Massachusetts Eye and Ear Infirmary, Boston, MA, USA

Ian Francis, MD Moorfields Eye Hospital, London, UK

Dawn DeCastro, MD Massachusetts Eye and Ear Infirmary, Boston, MA, USA

Paul Harasymowycz, MD University of Montreal, Montreal, Quebec, Canada

Lois Hart Massachusetts Eye and Ear Infirmary, Boston, MA, USA

Christopher Liu, MD Royal Sussex County Hospital, Brighton, UK

Susan Loomis REMS, Massachusetts General Hospital, Boston, MA, USA

Sanjay Prabhu, MD Boston Children's Hospital, Boston, MA, USA

Juan Small, MD Lahey Clinic, Burlington, MA, USA

David Tse, MD Bascom Palmer Eye Institute, Miami, FL, USA

Rebecca Tudor, CRA Illinois Eye Institute, Chicago, IL, USA

Demetrios Vavvas, MD Massachusetts Eye and Ear Infirmary, Boston, MA, USA

Contents

Introduction to Approaches and Modalities in Postoperative Orbital Imaging

Daniel Thomas Ginat, Amin Ashrafzadeh, and Suzanne K. Freitag

1.1 Overview

Determining if and when diagnostic imaging is required following ophthalmic and orbital surgery is very much an art. The primary radiological imaging modalities include radiography, computed tomography (CT), magnetic resonance imaging (MRI), and ultrasound. Each of these modalities has certain advantages and disadvantages as described below. Often the different imaging modalities serve complementary roles, and familiarity with each of these is important for optimal management. In many cases, the indications and suitable modalities are similar to those for preoperative imaging, and the *ACR Appropriateness Criteria® orbits, vision and visual loss* offers general guidelines. More detailed information is also provided in the subsequent chapters in this text. Ultimately, familiarity with the basic anatomy of the eye and orbit and the alterations that may result after treatment is critical for interpreting the imaging studies.

1.2 Radiography

Radiographs of the orbits may be helpful in the postoperative setting in particular situations, such as confirming the position of certain punctal plugs and evaluation of eyelid spring function and integrity. Radiographs may be used to screen patients with suspected metal implants from surgery prior to undergoing an MRI (Fig. 1.1). Typically, at least 2 orthogonal views are obtained in order to localize structures, including the occipitomental view (Waters view), which helps to separate the orbits from the maxillary sinuses. Radiographs may also be obtained during dacryocystography procedures, in which contrast material is injected into a canaliculus to assess the lacrimal drainage system patency (Fig. 1.2). Dacryocystography can also be performed in conjunction with CT or MRI to further delineate surrounding anatomy (Fig. 1.3).

D.T. Ginat, MD, MS (✉)
Director of Head and Neck Imaging,
Department of Radiology,
University of Chicago, 5841 S Maryland
Avenue, Chicago, IL 60637, USA
e-mail: ginatd01@gmail.com

A. Ashrafzadeh, MD
Modesto Eye Center, Modesto, CA, USA

S.K. Freitag, MD
Director, Ophthalmic Plastic Surgery Service,
Department of Ophthalmology,
Massachusetts Eye and Ear Infirmary,
Harvard Medical School, Boston, MA, USA

D.T. Ginat, S.K. Freitag (eds.), *Post-treatment Imaging of the Orbit*,
DOI 10.1007/978-3-662-44023-0_1, © Springer-Verlag Berlin Heidelberg 2015

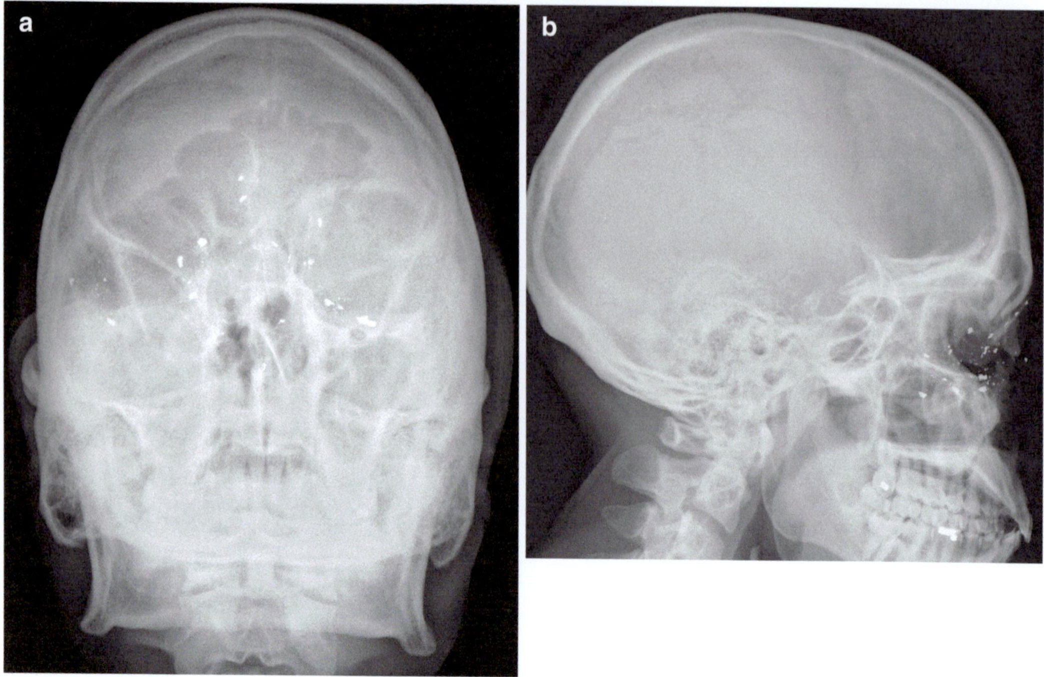

Fig. 1.1 Face radiographs. Waters (**a**) and lateral (**b**) projection radiographs show multiple radiopaque metallic bullet fragments in the bilateral periorbital soft tissues, which remained after orbital and facial reconstructive surgery

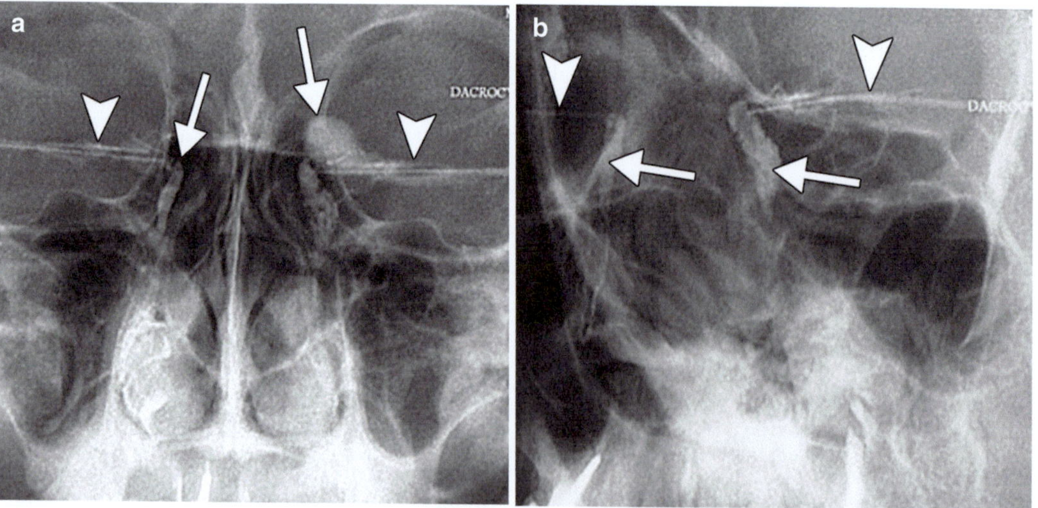

Fig. 1.2 Fluoroscopic dacryocystography. Frontal (**a**) and oblique (**b**) radiographic images show bilateral canalicular catheters (*arrowheads*) and contrast material within the bilateral nasolacrimal system (*arrows*), but no free spillage into the nasal cavity, suggestive of obstruction

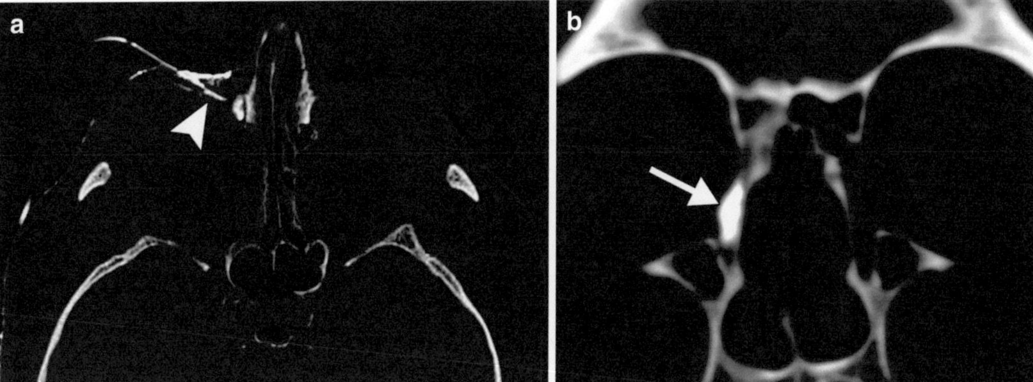

Fig. 1.3 CT dacryocystography. Axial CT image (**a**) shows the catheter and contrast material within the right inferior canaliculus (*arrowhead*). Coronal CT image (**b**) shows contrast within the right lacrimal sac (*arrow*)

1.3 Computed Tomography

Orbital CT is typically acquired with thin axial sections (0.6–1.0 mm) from which coronal and sagittal reformatted images are generated and displayed in both soft tissue and bone algorithms (Fig. 1.4). Thus, CT is well suited for delineating the osseous structures and the positioning of many types of orbital implants in fine detail. 3D surface renderings can be a useful adjunct for visualization of the implants. Except for stainless steel, tantalum, and certain embolization materials, such as Onyx, orbital implants generally do not produce significant streak artifact. In addition, CT is often obtained in emergency situations due to its rapidity, widespread availability, and ability to safely screen for metallic foreign bodies. Administration of iodinated contrast can be useful for evaluating suspected infectious and inflammatory processes and tumors. Contrast is also necessary for performing CTA and CTV, which may be useful for evaluating the status of carotid cavernous fistulas and other vascular lesions after treatment. However, contrast is not necessary for assessing the positioning of implants. Furthermore, in patients with thyroid eye disease, iodinated contrast can aggravate thyroid orbitopathy.

1.4 Magnetic Resonance Imaging

Compared with CT, MRI offers superior soft tissue delineation and no exposure to ionizing radiation, which is particularly important in the pediatric population. Prior to obtaining a scan, it is important that patients are screened for MRI compatibility. A useful reference for determining whether certain implants are MRI compatible can be found at http://www.mrisafety.com/. Other factors that may limit the application of MRI include severe claustrophobia and obesity exceeding table weight limit. The main sequences obtained in orbital MRI are T1-weighted and T2-weighted sequences in multiple planes, including axial, coronal, and sagittal (Fig. 1.5). Administration of gadolinium-based contrast for T1-weighted sequences is useful for defining infectious and inflammatory processes, as well as residual tumors (Fig. 1.6). Implementing fat-suppression techniques with T2 and post-contrast T1-weighted sequences is also helpful for better defining lesions against the hyperintense background of the orbital fat. Many fat-suppression techniques are prone to failure near the air-filled sinonasal cavities due to susceptibility effects, which may lead to misinterpretation. However,

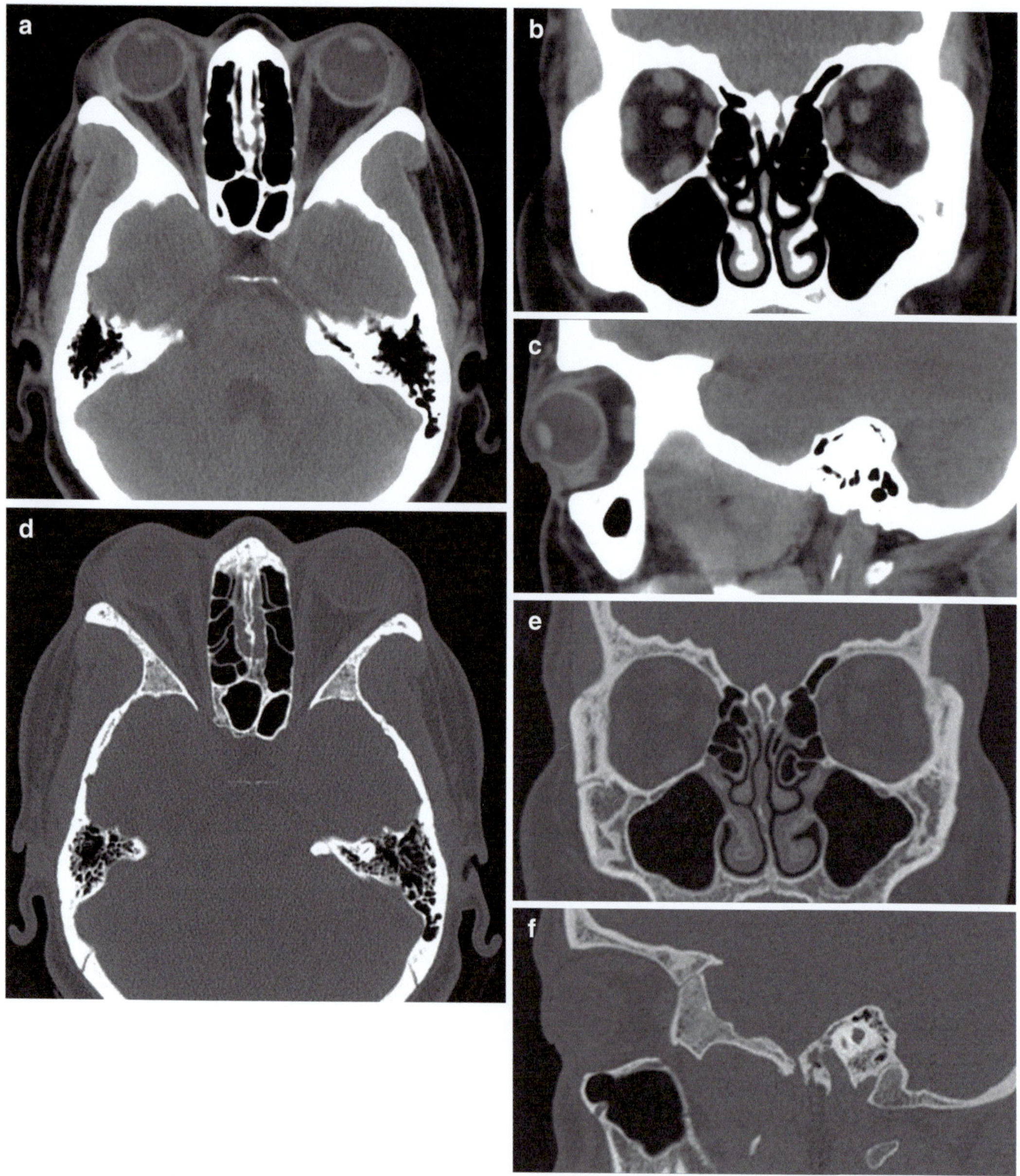

Fig. 1.4 Standard orbit CT images. Selected axial (**a**), coronal (**b**), and sagittal (**c**) soft window images and axial (**d**), coronal (**e**), and sagittal (**f**) bone window images of normal orbits

certain techniques such as Dixon and inversion recovery are less prone to such artifacts. The use of high-resolution microscopy surface coils can yield in-plane resolution of 312 μm and the display pixel dimensions of 156 μm even at 1.5 T. As a result, it is possible to obtain a detailed view of the orbital structures and globe, including Tenon's capsule, tarsal plate, ciliary body, lens zonules, and components of the superior rectus-levator complex. The use of diffusion-weighted imaging in orbital imaging for indications such as monitoring treatment response in tumors remains investigational at the time of this writing. Likewise, the utility of cine (oculodynamic) MRI

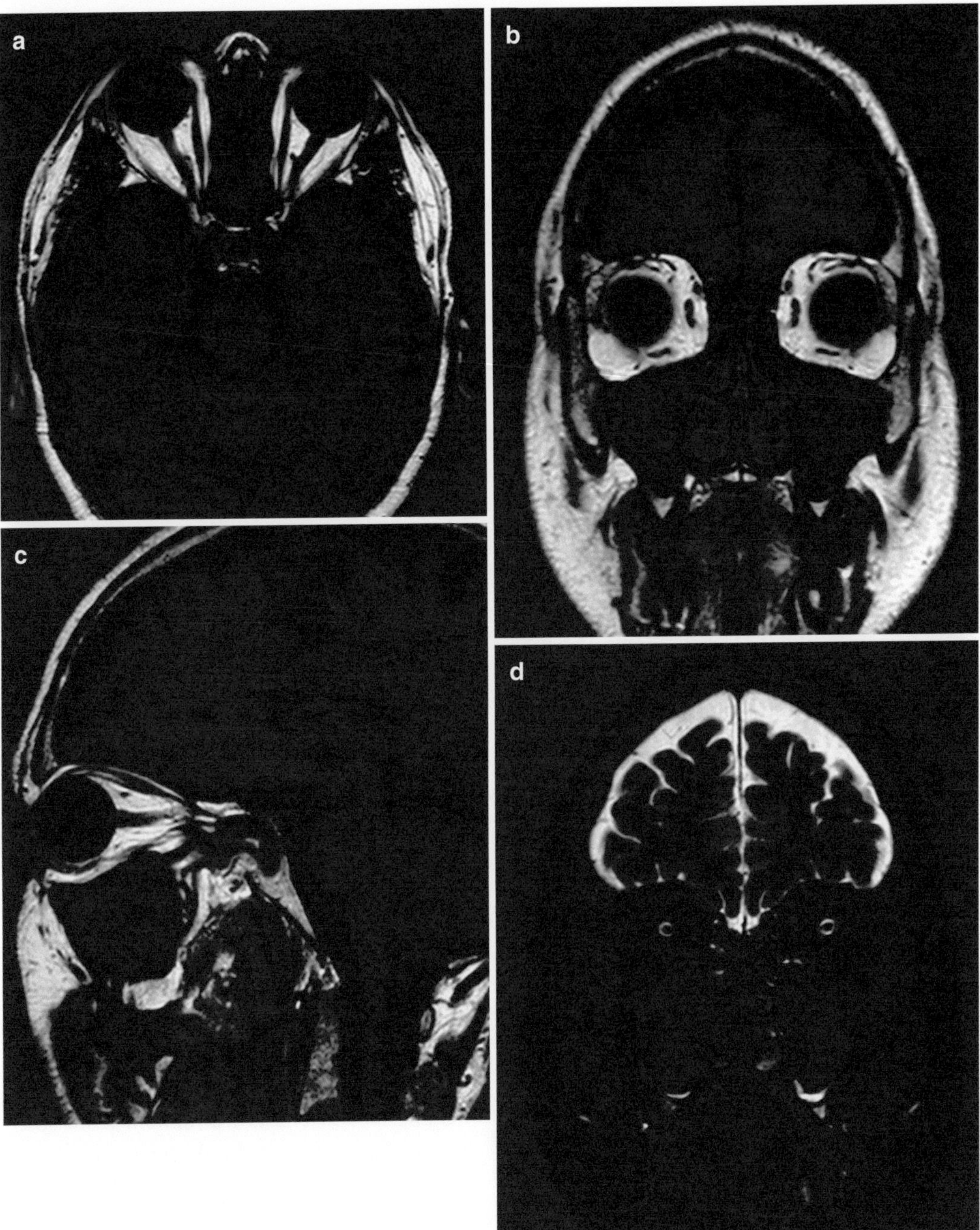

Fig. 1.5 Basic orbit MRI sequences without contrast include axial (**a**), coronal (**b**), and oblique sagittal (**c**) T1-weighted and coronal fat-suppressed T2-weighted (**d**) images

techniques for depicting the motion of the extra-ocular muscles in the postoperative setting is promising, but requires further validation. MRA can be used as a noninvasive method for evaluating patients after stenting and/or embolization of vascular lesions. Time-resolved MRA provides a higher quality imaging of the treated parent vessels compared with time-of-flight imaging.

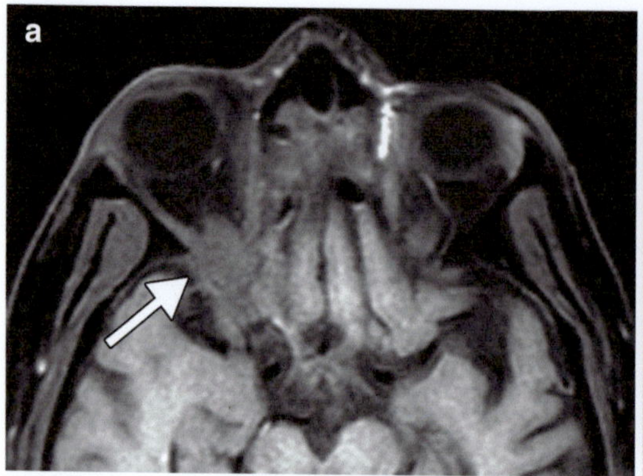

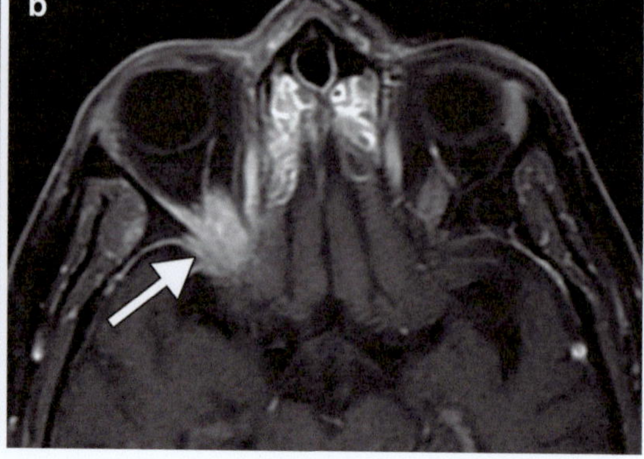

Fig. 1.6 Contrast-enhanced MRI for recurrent tumor assessment. Axial fat-suppressed T1-weighted image (**a**) and post-contrast axial fat-suppressed T1-weighted image (**b**) show an ill-defined, avidly enhancing tumor (squamous cell carcinoma) in the orbital apex (*arrows*)

1.5 Ultrasound

Ultrasound is an important imaging modality that is used for the initial clinical work-up and follow-up of many ophthalmic diseases, as it is relatively inexpensive to perform and readily available to ophthalmologists. The examination entails applying the surface of the probe or transducer to closed eyelids in contact with a gel or immersion fluid. Since a mild amount of pressure is applied to the globe, ultrasound examinations are contraindicated in patients with a possible open globe. Nevertheless, ultrasound is a versatile modality that is particularly well suited toward the evaluation of the intraocular contents, which is a relative limitation of CT and MRI. B-mode ultrasound is commonly performed, which provides a cross-sectional grayscale representation of the globe and surrounding structures in different planes, such as transverse and longitudinal (Fig. 1.7). The aqueous and vitreous are normally nearly anechoic on ultrasound and readily allow passage of the sound waves, while interfaces, such as the eye wall, tend to appear hyperechoic and may even cause shading in some cases. The in-depth spatial resolution that can be achieved with sonography is primarily dependent upon the frequency emitted by the transducer. The use of frequencies of 50 MHz and higher is known as ultrasound biomicroscopy, which can depict

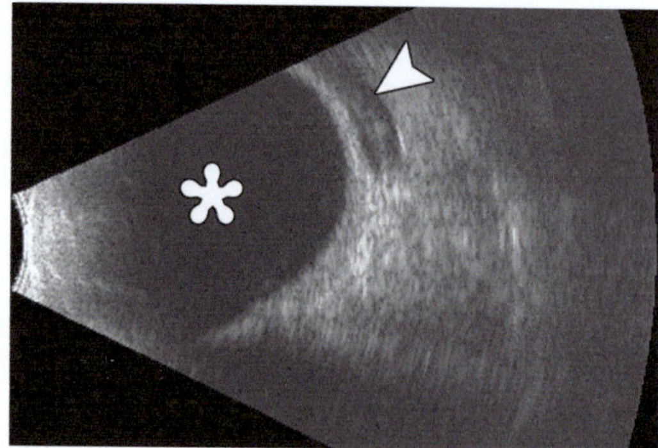

Fig. 1.7 B-mode ultrasound image of a patient with glaucoma drainage device (*arrow*). The vitreous body (*) is anechoic

anatomic structures in exquisite detail, particularly in the anterior chamber and angle (Fig. 1.8). Another ultrasound modality is color Doppler imaging, which consists of simultaneous grayscale imaging of structure and color-coded imaging of blood velocity. This technique enables depiction of moderately small-caliber blood vessels, such as the central retinal artery, from which measures of blood velocity and vascular resistance can be obtained. The use of intravascular contrast agents, such as microbubbles, in orbital imaging is mainly investigational at the time of this writing, although these may have promising and intriguing applications in the realm of molecular diagnosis, therapy, and theranostics.

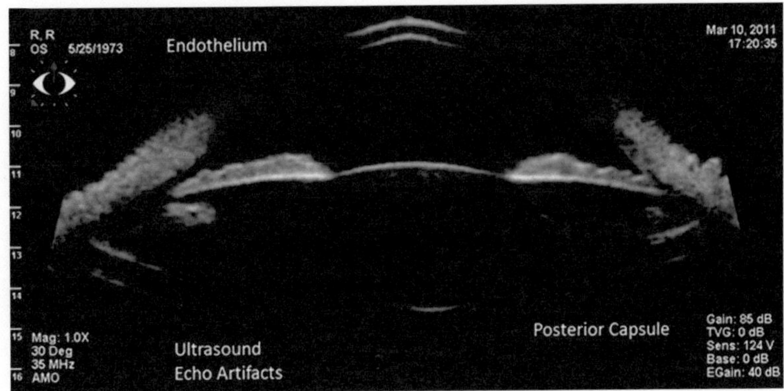

Fig. 1.8 Anterior-segment ultrasound biomicroscopy image depicting normal anatomy

1.6 Optical Coherence Tomography

Optical coherence tomography (OCT) is an optical imaging modality that performs low-coherence interferometry in order to create high-spatial axial resolution, cross-sectional, subsurface tomographic images of tissue microstructure. Thus, OCT is a valuable imaging tool for assessing and guiding the management of surgical complications after such procedures in the anterior chamber and retina. The modality uses infrared light waves for imaging and can provide a spatial resolution on the order of approximately 2–20 μm. OCT can function using time-domain or frequency-domain technology, which has applications in anterior segment as well as vitreoretinal imaging. The first-generation OCT machines used time-domain technology for signal processing allowing for acquisition of approximately 2,000 linear "A-scans" per second. This slow acquisition speed leads to poor resolution and motion artifact. The newer spectral-domain OCTs allow for faster and greater acquisition volume, performing in excess of 30,000 linear "A-scans" per second. These linear scans are then assembled together to create a two-dimensional "B-scan" which are the images seen through this text. Although three-dimensional reconstruction is available, if is of limited clinical utility due to current computer processing

speeds. Nevertheless, this feature is useful when the volume of a lesion is a concern. A 1,310 nm wavelength is the standard light used in the Visante anterior-segment OCT (Carl Zeiss Meditec, Dublin, CA). Most other OCT scanners use 820–840 nm wavelength light. The 820–840 nm wavelength range yields excellent penetration and little absorption by water. This is a desirable feature for the examination of the retina. On the other hand, the 1,310 nm wavelength is subject to greater absorption by water and significantly more scattering. This results in approximately 20-fold reduction in its exposure to the retina, and thus, higher power can be utilized. The high signal intensity allows for faster image acquisition, which is associated with a reduction in motion artifact. Additionally, the 1,310 nm has the capacity to penetrate through partially opaque tissues, such as sclera and opaque cornea. Ultimately, OCT is a versatile imaging modality that is portable and does not require contact with the globe. This modality can provide detailed images of the scleral spur, ciliary body, ciliary sulcus, and even the canal of Schlemm in some cases (Fig. 1.9). In a well-centered cross-sectional scan, the reflection from the anterior vertex of the cornea can saturate the imaging system and produce a vertical flare. This phenomenon helps with the identification of the corneal vertex, from which central corneal thickness measurements and measurements of central graft thickness can

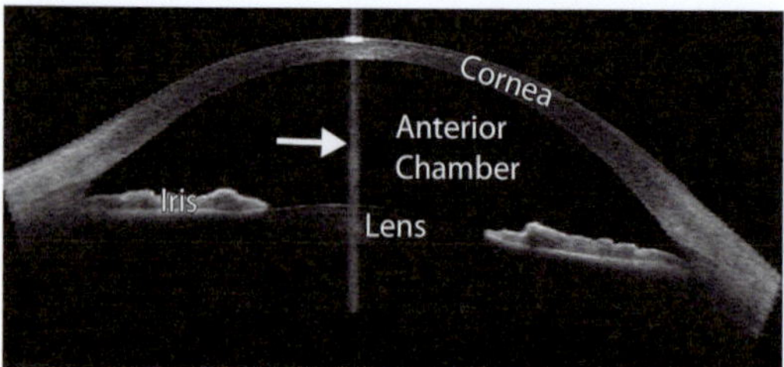

Fig. 1.9 OCT image of the anterior segment depicting normal anatomy. A vertical flare emanating from the apex of a well-centered cornea is present (*arrow*)

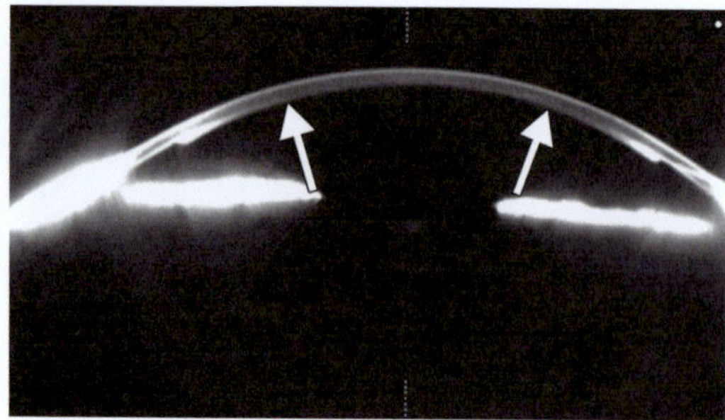

Fig. 1.10 The Scheimpflug image delineates the corneal graft (*arrows*) following successful DSEK operation

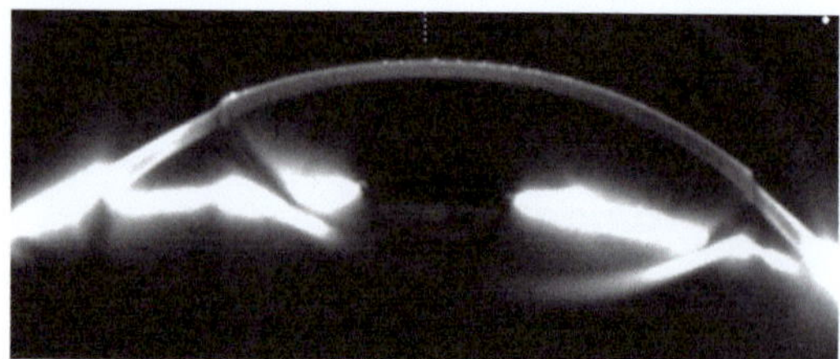

Fig. 1.11 Artifacts with Pentacam-Scheimpflug image of the anterior segment. The image was acquired with a hard contact lens on the cornea. Due to the 45° placement of the camera off the central axis beam of light, the edge of the hard contact lens and the associated optical distortions are evident

be obtained. The OCT images can also be displayed in "rainbow" color in order to visually enhance tissue contrasts. There are several limitations associated with OCT ocular imaging. For example, standardized protocols for image acquisition and quantification are often lacking, assessment of optical density and reflectivity is only qualitative, and there is often insufficient specificity to distinguish among different types of tissues.

1.7 Scheimpflug Optical Imaging

Pentacam-Scheimpflug imaging is a method used for anterior-segment imaging, whereby a central beam of light is shined on the eye. A camera (or two in some devices) placed at 45° angle takes a photograph, and then through ray tracing, the measurements on the image are generated. The slit beam and the camera are on a rotating drum that can produce a tomographic representation of the anterior segment. The commercially available units use an LED of 475 nm blue light. Scheimpflug imaging can produce detailed characterization of anterior-segment structures and can measure net corneal power, a feature particularly useful for cataract patients having undergone previous corneal surgery (Fig. 1.10), as well as provide quantitative information on the geometry of the lens. However, this modality is susceptible to image degradation by opacified tissues, which block or reflect light in the visible spectrum, among other artifacts (Fig. 1.11).

1.8 Summary

- Several imaging modalities are available for the evaluation of the orbit and globe after treatment, including radiographs, dacryocystography, CT, MRI, B-mode ultrasound, ultrasound biomicroscopy, optical coherence tomography, and the Scheimpflug camera.
- Each of these imaging modalities has advantages and disadvantages, and they may sometimes have complementary roles for evaluating certain conditions.
- The posttreatment imaging findings on the various modalities are reviewed and depicted in the subsequent chapters.

Further Reading

Bailey CC, Kabala J, Laitt R, Weston M, Goddard P, Hoh HB, Potts MJ, Harrad RA. Cine magnetic resonance imaging of eye movements. Eye (Lond). 1993;7(Pt 5):691–3.

Bedi DG, Gombos DS, Ng CS, Singh S. Sonography of the eye. AJR Am J Roentgenol. 2006;187(4):1061–72.

Belden CJ, Zinreich SJ. Orbital imaging techniques. Semin Ultrasound CT MR. 1997;18(6):413–22.

Berg I, Palmowski-Wolfe A, Schwenzer-Zimmerer K, Kober C, Radue EW, Zeilhofer HF, Scheffler K, Kunz C, Buitrago-Tellez C. Near-real time oculodynamic MRI: a feasibility study for evaluation of diplopia in comparison with clinical testing. Eur Radiol. 2012;22(2):358–63.

Chen J, Lee L. Clinical applications and new developments of optical coherence tomography: an evidence-based review. Clin Exp Optom. 2007;90(5):317–35.

Fledelius HC. Ultrasound in ophthalmology. Ultrasound Med Biol. 1997;23(3):365–75.

Francisco FC, Carvalho AC, Francisco VF, Francisco MC, Neto GT. Evaluation of 1000 lacrimal ducts by dacryocystography. Br J Ophthalmol. 2007;91(1):43–6.

Freitag SK, Sergott RC. Color Doppler imaging in ophthalmology. In: Tasman W, Jaeger EA, editors. Foundations of clinical ophthalmology. Philadelphia: Lippincott-Raven; 2000.

Georgouli T, Chang B, Nelson M, James T, Tanner S, Shelley D, Saldana M, McGonagle D. Use of high-resolution microscopy coil MRI for depicting orbital anatomy. Orbit. 2008;27(2):107–14.

Goh PS, Gi MT, Charlton A, Tan C, GangadharaSundar JK, Amrith S. Review of orbital imaging. Eur J Radiol. 2008;66(3):387–95.

ACR Appropriateness Criteria® orbits, vision and visual loss. http://www.guideline.gov/content.aspx?id=37934. Accessed on 20 August 2014.

http://www.mrisafety.com/. Accessed on 20 August 2014.

Huang LL, Hirose T. Portable optical coherence tomography in management of vitreoretinal diseases: current developments, indications, and implications. Semin Ophthalmol. 2012;27(5–6):213–20.

Kiessling F, Fokong S, Koczera P, Lederle W, Lammers T. Ultrasound microbubbles for molecular diagnosis, therapy, and theranostics. J Nucl Med. 2012;53(3): 345–8.

Konstantopoulos A, Hossain P, Anderson DF. Recent advances in ophthalmic anterior segment imaging: a new era for ophthalmic diagnosis? Br J Ophthalmol. 2007;91(4):551–7.

Lee AG, Brazis PW, Garrity JA, White M. Imaging for neuro-ophthalmic and orbital disease. Am J Ophthalmol. 2004;138(5):852–62.

Lee AG, Johnson MC, Policeni BA, Smoker WR. Imaging for neuro-ophthalmic and orbital disease – a review. Clin Experiment Ophthalmol. 2009;37(1):30–53.

Lieb WE. Color Doppler imaging of the eye and orbit. Radiol Clin North Am. 1998;36(6):1059–71.

Liebmann JM, Ritch R. Ultrasound biomicroscopy of the anterior segment. J Am Optom Assoc. 1996;67(8): 469–79.

Nesi TT, Leite DA, Rocha FM, Tanure MA, Reis PP, Rodrigues EB, Campos MS. Indications of optical coherence tomography in keratoplasties: literature review. J Ophthalmol. 2012;2012:989063.

Testoni PA. Optical coherence tomography. Sci World J. 2007;7:87–108.

Williamson TH, Harris A. Color Doppler ultrasound imaging of the eye and orbit. Surv Ophthalmol. 1996; 40(4):255–67.

Wu AY, Jebodhsingh K, Le T, Law C, Tucker NA, DeAngelis DD, Oestreicher JH, Harvey JT. Indications for orbital imaging by the oculoplastic surgeon. Ophthal Plast Reconstr Surg. 2011;27(4):260–2.

Zysk AM, Nguyen FT, Oldenburg AL, Marks DL, Boppart SA. Optical coherence tomography: a review of clinical development from bench to bedside. J Biomed Opt. 2007;12(5):051403.

Imaging After Cornea Surgery

2

Sotiria Palioura, Amin Ashrafzadeh,
Daniel Thomas Ginat, and James Chodosh

2.1 Overview

The cornea is an avascular tissue in the anterior portion of the globe that consists of six layers, including the epithelium, basement membrane, Bowman's layer, stroma, Descemet's membrane, and endothelium. The cornea measures approximately 500 μm in thickness centrally and features an intrinsic convex outward curvature, which provides light refraction. Corneal opacification is the second most common cause of blindness worldwide. In fact, according to the World Health Organization, glaucoma, age-related macular degeneration, and diabetic retinopathy are less common causes. Corneal opacification can result from postinfectious corneal scars, trauma, cicatrizing disorders (e.g., trachoma), nutritional deficiencies (e.g., vitamin A deficiency), and inherited disorders. Treatment options for corneal opacification include corneal transplantation, either penetrating (full-thickness) or lamellar (partial-thickness), or a corneal prosthetic device (keratoprosthesis). Cross-sectional imaging after keratoplasty is obtained when the cornea is opaque – from edema and graft failure or rejection, for example – and direct visualization of the anterior chamber and the fundus is not possible. Ultrasound biomicroscopy (UBM) is used to assess the anterior chamber and the drainage angle of the eye and B-scan ultrasound to evaluate the status of the vitreous and retina. Occasionally diagnostic imaging is performed to evaluate for postoperative complications. Otherwise, normal post-keratoplasty changes observed on CT or MRI can be incidental findings on diagnostic imaging performed for unrelated reasons. Imaging with CT or MRI is done after keratoprosthesis implantation to evaluate rare orbital complications of the procedure or to assess for tooth resorption in the case of the osteo-odonto-keratoprosthesis (OOKP). Corneal surgery can also be performed for correcting refractive errors of the eye, such as myopia, hyperopia, astigmatism, and presbyopia, usually with the goal of eliminating the need for glasses or contact lenses. This field is known as refractive surgery and encompasses numerous types of procedures. Laser-assisted in situ keratomileusis (LASIK) is the most widely performed method of refractive surgery. Other corneal refractive surgical procedures include laser thermal keratoplasty (LTK) and intrastromal corneal ring segments (Intacs). Complications after refractive cornea surgeries are generally diagnosed clinically; anterior

S. Palioura, MD, PhD • J. Chodosh, MD, MPH
Department of Ophthalmology, Massachusetts
Eye and Ear Infirmary, Boston, MA, USA

A. Ashrafzadeh, MD
Modesto Eye Center, Modesto, CA, USA

D.T. Ginat, MD, MS (✉)
Director of Head and Neck Imaging,
Department of Radiology, University of Chicago,
5841 S Maryland Avenue, Chicago, IL 60637, USA
e-mail: ginatd01@gmail.com

D.T. Ginat, S.K. Freitag (eds.), *Post-treatment Imaging of the Orbit*,
DOI 10.1007/978-3-662-44023-0_2, © Springer-Verlag Berlin Heidelberg 2015

segment optical coherence tomography (OCT) can serve as an adjunctive to diagnosis and planning for possible further interventions.

2.2 Penetrating Keratoplasty (PKP)

In penetrating keratoplasty, full-thickness diseased or damaged host corneal tissue is replaced with healthy donor corneal tissue. In contrast to cataract surgery, which can be performed under topical anesthesia, adequate anesthesia for cornea transplantation is achieved with a peribulbar or retrobulbar block. The cornea is removed using circular blade trephines or femtosecond laser ablation from both the host and the donor and placed into position and secured using very fine sutures (typically 10–0 nylon). On the OCT, the incision site appears as a small disruption at the graft–host junction (Fig. 2.1). The sutures can also be evident as curvilinear hyperreflective structures.

Femtosecond laser technology has recently enabled femtosecond-assisted penetrating keratoplasty (FAKP). The femtosecond laser is a type of laser that can produce pulses of light of extremely short duration. The application of femtosecond laser in surgery results in no thermal effect or shock wave, so that this laser is unlikely to cause tissue injuries outside the irradiation area of the laser beam. The femtosecond laser is ablative and utilized to perform incision with varying size and shape of the cuts of the corneal tissue. The laser can be used to accurately cut a more complex shape of both the donor tissue and the host tissue, such as a top hat, mushroom, Christmas tree, or zigzag configurations using software products, such as the IntraLase (AMO, Inc, Santa Ana, CA, USA), which is otherwise known as IntraLase-enabled keratoplasty (IEK). These arrangements provide better fixation of the corneal graft. The graft interfaces are readily visible on OCT, but residual host corneal tissue can reflect light and create "noise" that degrades anatomic detail on Pentacam-Scheimpflug imaging (Fig. 2.2).

A rare but potentially vision-threatening complication of a retrobulbar or peribulbar block performed prior to corneal transplant surgery is intraorbital hemorrhage. Expanding proptosis, pain, ophthalmoplegia, and decreased vision are the immediate signs of a retrobulbar hemorrhage. An orbit CT without contrast can be obtained to confirm and localize the hemorrhage, which appears as hyperattenuating collections in the acute setting (Fig. 2.3). An emergent lateral canthotomy and inferior cantholysis may

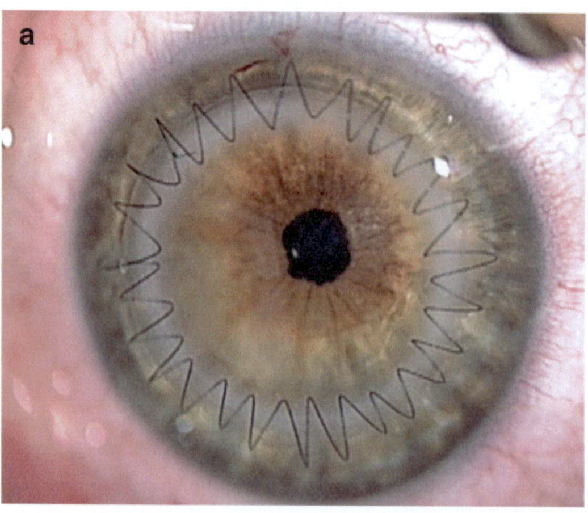

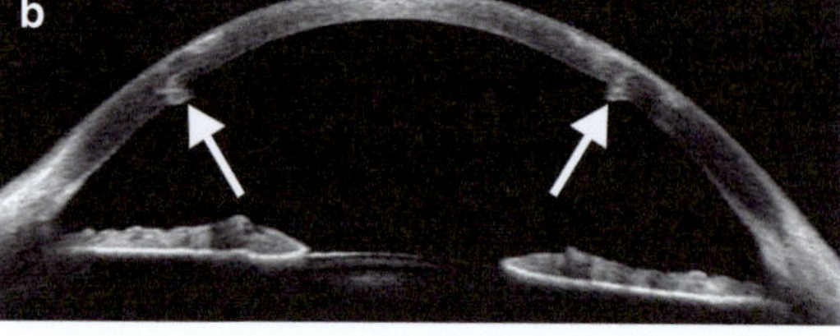

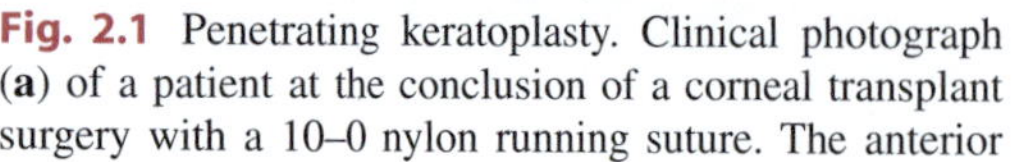

Fig. 2.1 Penetrating keratoplasty. Clinical photograph (**a**) of a patient at the conclusion of a corneal transplant surgery with a 10–0 nylon running suture. The anterior segment OCT image (**b**) of an eye with healed corneal transplant shows the graft–host junction (*arrows*)

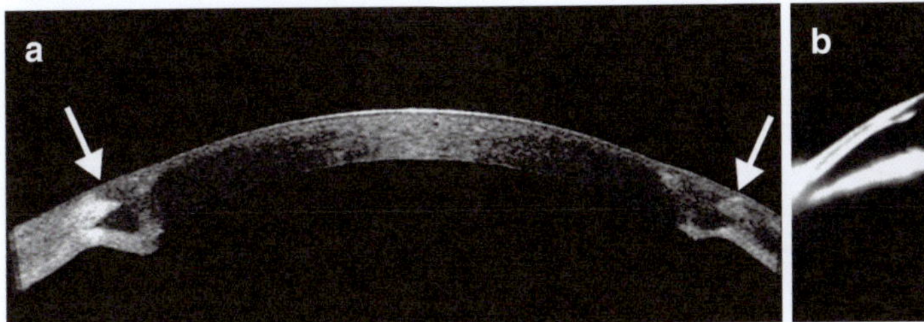

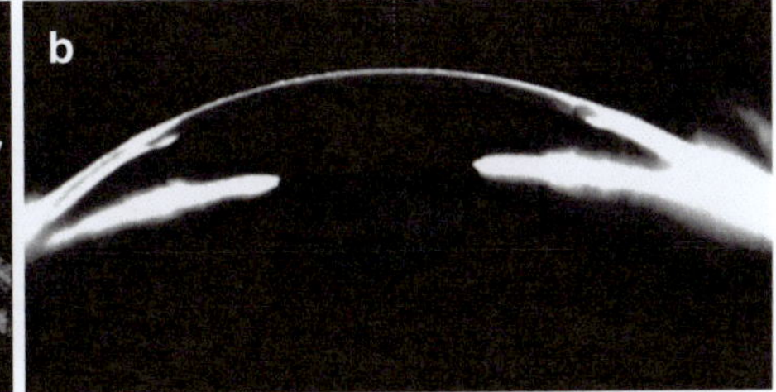

Fig. 2.2 FAKP with zigzag IEK. Anterior segment OCT image (**a**) shows the graft–host junctions are clearly depicted as zigzag patterns between the donor and the host matching at the peripheral edge of the graft (*arrows*). The Pentacam-Scheimpflug image (**b**) of the same eye shows that the remaining host corneal tissue reflects light and creates "noise" in the image and loss of anatomic detail

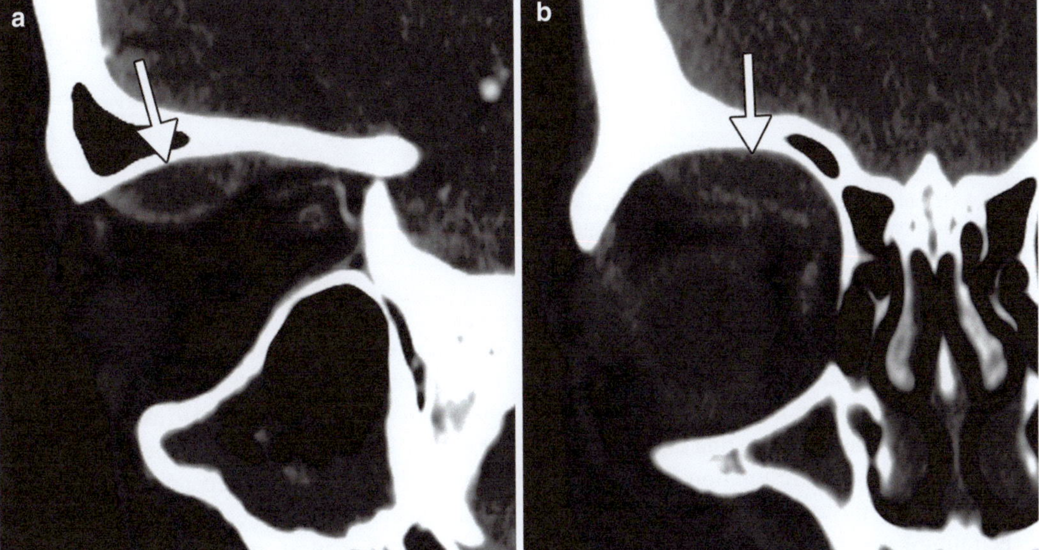

Fig. 2.3 Intraorbital hemorrhage secondary to retrobulbar block. Sagittal (**a**) and coronal (**b**) CT images show a subperiosteal hematoma in the right superior orbit (*arrows*)

be required to decompress the orbit and prevent an ischemic optic neuropathy or a central retinal artery occlusion.

One of the most dreaded complications of penetrating keratoplasty is expulsive suprachoroidal hemorrhage. This occurs due to spontaneous bleeding of a choroidal blood vessel after decompression of the globe and has an incidence of approximately 0.5–1.1 % of corneal transplantation cases. After phacoemulsification and foldable IOL implantation, UBM typically reveals shifting of the iris posteriorly, and deepening of the anterior chamber by 850 micrometers on average. Risk factors for suprachoroidal hemorrhage include older age, a history of glaucoma or myopia, hypertension, diabetes mellitus, generalized atherosclerosis, and Valsalva maneuver in the context of an open eye, such as sudden coughing during the surgery. Preventative measures include proper positioning of the patient, adequate anesthesia, best possible control of blood pressure, and reducing the intraocular pressure prior to surgery with medication, such as intravenous mannitol. Postoperatively, a noncontrast CT of the orbit can be obtained to demonstrate the extent of the hemorrhage, which can project

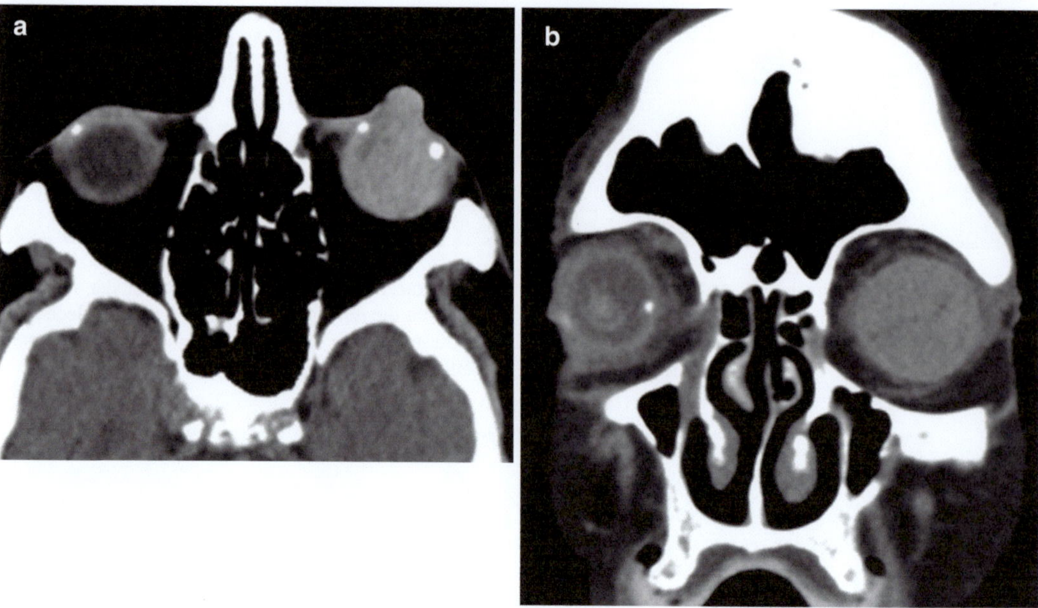

Fig. 2.4 Expulsive hemorrhage following penetrating keratoplasty. Axial (**a**) and coronal (**b**) CT images show diffuse hyperattenuation within the left globe with protrusion through the corneal dehiscence

beyond the margins of the globe through the corneal incision (Fig. 2.4). Otherwise, B-scan ultrasound is the imaging modality of choice for assessing the status of the retina and evaluating the potential for visual restoration.

Other early postoperative complications of penetrating keratoplasty include wound leakage and hypotony, persistent epithelial defect, infection, elevated intraocular pressure, and primary graft failure, that is, failure of the donor graft to achieve optical clarity. The most devastating complication is endophthalmitis (Fig. 2.5), and its incidence after penetrating keratoplasty ranges from 0.2 to 2.0 %. The source of infection is usually the patient's periocular flora or a contaminated donor tissue. Risk factors for the development of endophthalmitis include concomitant vitrectomy, aphakia, history of previous surgery or inflammation, and corticosteroid use. Endophthalmitis is a clinical diagnosis and a view to the retina is usually precluded by the presence of intense vitritis. Thus, although B-scan ultrasound is not diagnostic of endophthalmitis, it can show the status of the retina and choroid prior to any surgical intervention. Orbital signs and symptoms (painful proptosis,

ophthalmoplegia) suggest spread of the infection to the orbit and panophthalmitis. In such cases, orbital CT or MRI is indicated to assess the extent of orbital involvement and rule out the presence of an abscess. Treatment depends on the severity of the infection but generally includes removal of the graft, repeat penetrating keratoplasty, intravitreal injections of antibiotics, and, sometimes, pars plana vitrectomy. The main differential diagnosis for infectious endophthalmitis is toxic anterior segment syndrome. Toxic anterior segment syndrome is a sterile postoperative inflammatory reaction caused by a noninfectious substance that enters the anterior segment. The process typically begins 12–48 h after anterior segment surgery, is Gram stain and culture negative, and often responds to steroid treatment.

Corneal melt (keratolysis) consists of a breakdown of the cornea with expansion of the anterior chamber, which can occur as a complication of corneal transplant surgery. Inflammation at the limbus appears to be a causative factor for postoperative corneal melting. Damage to the limbal stem cells predisposes to invasion of conjunctival epithelium onto the corneal surface, which in turn leads to an irregular and unstable epithelium,

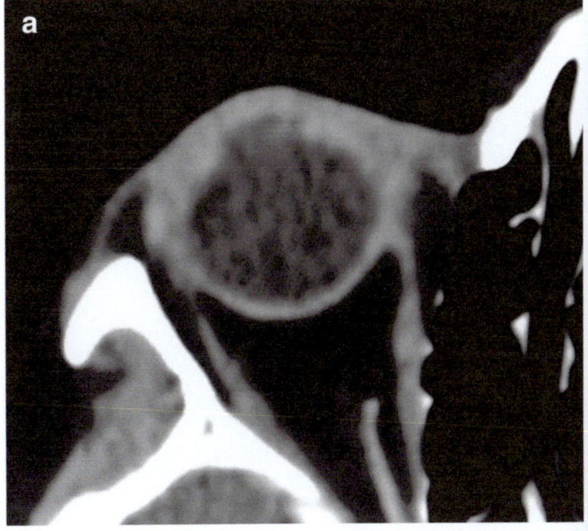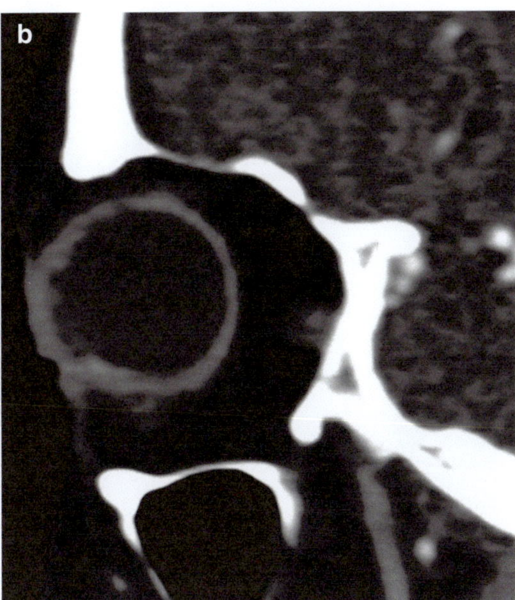

Fig. 2.5 Endophthalmitis following penetrating kerato-plasty. Axial (**a**) and sagittal (**b**) contrast-enhanced CT images show irregularity of the right cornea as well as diffuse intraocular hyperdensity, uveoscleral thickening, and preseptal edema. The patient was subsequently treated via removal of the corneal graft, repeat penetrating kerato-plasty, and intravitreal injections of voriconazole and vancomycin

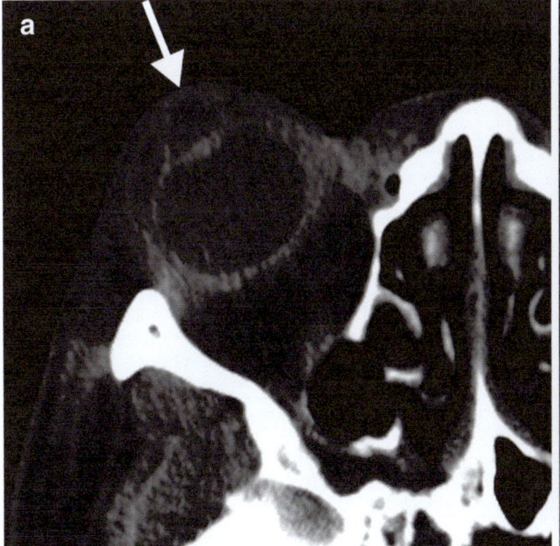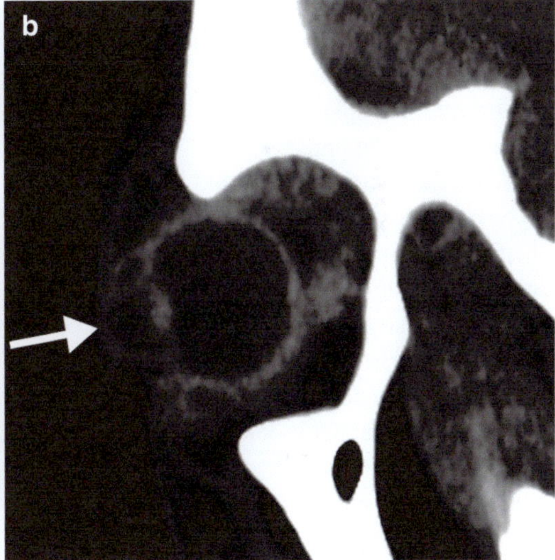

Fig. 2.6 Corneal melt. Axial (**a**) and sagittal (**b**) CT images show a considerably enlarged anterior chamber (*arrows*) of the right eye. There are diffuse preseptal and postseptal inflammatory changes related to concomitant panophthalmitis. The lens is in a normal position

with corneal ulceration. Since the cornea forms the anterior wall of the eye, loss of structural integrity leads to enlargement of the anterior chamber. This produces a characteristic appearance on CT, in which the distended anterior chamber is filled with material of a similar attenuation to the vitreous chamber (Fig. 2.6). In addition, there may be accompanying inflammatory or infectious changes that are apparent on imaging. Corneal melt can be treated using a

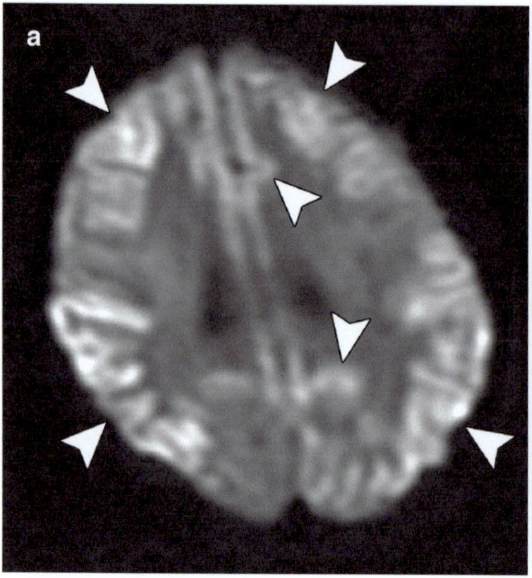
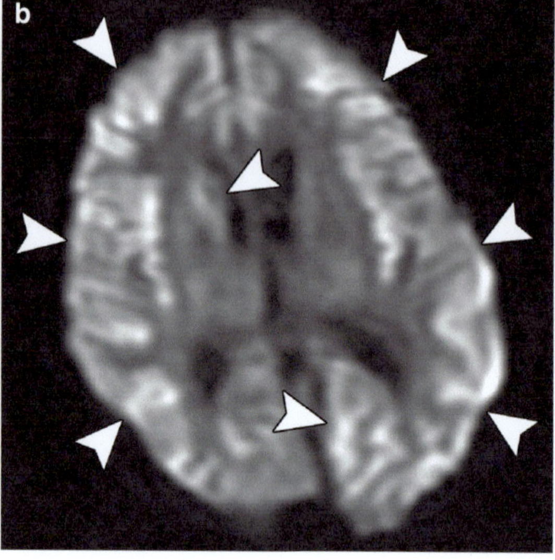

Fig. 2.7 Creutzfeldt–Jakob disease presumed to be associated with corneal transplantation. Axial diffusion-weighted images (**a, b**) of the brain demonstrate diffuse areas of restricted diffusion in the cortex and portions of the basal ganglia (*arrowheads*). The images are degraded by patient motion artifact

full-thickness corneal button denuded of endothelium in conjunction with temporary tarsorrhaphy and systemic steroids.

Corneal transplant donors are routinely screened for the presence of various infectious diseases, such as HIV and hepatitis B and C. Nevertheless, there have been rare instances of prion transmission from corneal transplantation, resulting in Creutzfeldt–Jakob disease. Patients typically present with a rapidly progressive dementia. Brain MRI, particularly diffusion-weighted imaging, can be very helpful in the diagnosis of Creutzfeldt–Jakob disease, in which diffusion abnormalities involving the cortex and deep gray matter nuclei can be observed (Fig. 2.7).

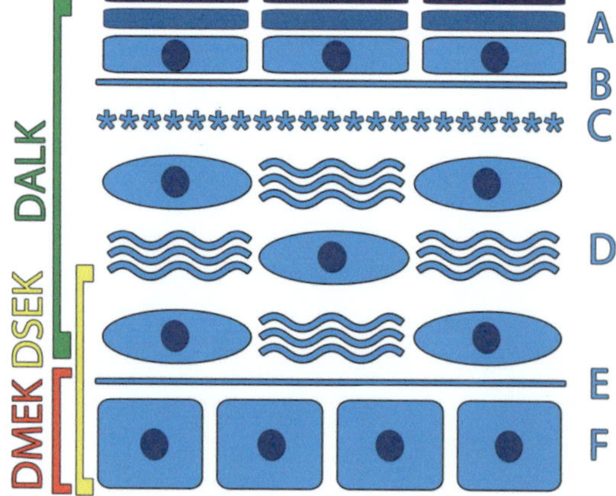

Fig. 2.8 Schematic of the corneal layers removed during the DLEK, DSEK, and DMEK procedures. *A* epithelium, *B* basement layer, *C* Bowman's layer, *D* stroma, *E* Descemet's layer, *F* endothelium

2.3 Lamellar Keratoplasty

Lamellar keratoplasty aims at replacing only the diseased corneal tissue while leaving the healthy tissue intact. The most common keratoplasty techniques in widespread use currently are deep anterior lamellar keratoplasty (DALK), Descemet's stripping endothelial keratoplasty (DSEK) or Descemet's stripping automated endothelial keratoplasty (DSAEK), and Descemet's membrane–endothelial keratoplasty (DMEK). Each of these procedures entails replacement of different layers of the cornea (Fig. 2.8).

DALK replaces both the epithelium and most of the stroma with the donor tissue and is indicated when the corneal disease spares the posterior stroma, Descemet's membrane, and endothelium (e.g., postinfectious stromal corneal scars, keratoconus). Since the host endothelium remains intact, the incidence of graft rejection is less with DALK than with penetrating keratoplasty. Smoothness of the stromal interface correlates with visual outcome.

DSEK/DSAEK aims at replacing a diseased endothelium (e.g., in pseudophakic bullous keratopathy or Fuchs' endothelial dystrophy) while leaving most of the host stroma intact. Compared to full-thickness grafts, EK provides a better visual outcome by minimizing the postoperative astigmatism that is inherent to the tissue warpage, surface mismatches, and multiple corneal sutures in a penetrating keratoplasty, and it also ensures a globe that is tectonically stable to trauma and less prone to suture-related infections. Endothelial keratoplasty is a reliable surgical technique for Fuchs' endothelial dystrophy and pseudophakic bullous keratopathy. The procedure consists of selective replacement of a patient's diseased or dysfunctional endothelium with a graft of the posterior stroma and endothelium from a donor cornea. In DSAEK, the donor corneal dissection is changed from a manual approach to an automated, microkeratome-assisted procedure. Hence, the stromal interface is smoother and more uniform in shape in DSAEK as compared to DSEK.

DMEK is a more recent procedure that is indicated for patients with endothelial dysfunction. The procedure consists of stripping the host corneal Descemet's membrane and endothelium and replacing it with harvested tissue from a healthy donor cornea (Descemet's membrane–endothelial cell graft or lenticule). The thin Descemet's membrane–endothelial cell graft measures only a few microns in thickness and is transplanted through a small (~3 mm) corneal incision, via a transfer device (such as a glass pipette) and then unrolled and adhered to proper location.

Anterior segment OCT may be considered the cross-sectional imaging modality of choice for depicting the layers of the cornea after ante-

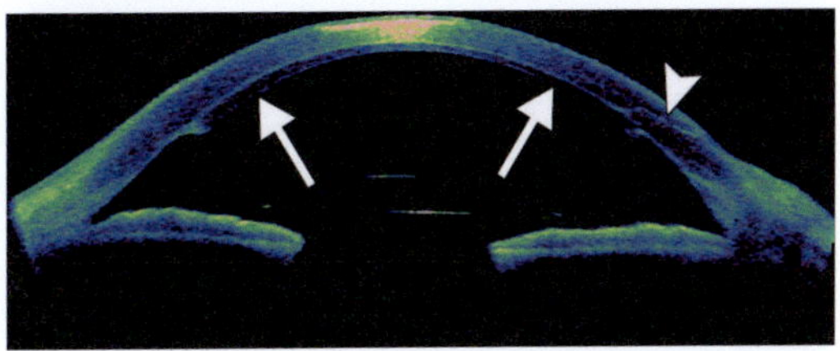

Fig. 2.9 DSEK. The anterior segment "rainbow" color OCT image shows the thin layer of donor posterior stromal tissue along with Descemet's membrane and endothelium applied to the native host tissue (*arrows*). The graft–host interface appears as thin hyperreflective line. The clear corneal incision is also visible (*arrowhead*)

rior and posterior lamellar keratoplasty procedures. It is indicated in the follow-up of corneal deturgescence, in the evaluation of the donor disk and recipient stroma adhesion and apposition, and for the study of donor tissue thickness and its regularity, which may influence the final visual acuity and refractional changes after surgery. The grafts should be flush against the host tissue and the graft–host junction normally appears as a thin, smooth, hyperreflective line (Fig. 2.9). Furthermore, OCT is useful for evaluating postoperative complications, such as graft detachment, posterior lamellar dislocation, primary graft failure, and anterior chamber crowding with consequent chamber angle encroachment and pupillary block after Descemet's stripping automated endothelial keratoplasty (DSAEK).

Graft detachment is the most common complication during the early postoperative period. Anterior segment OCT is very useful for diagnosing and delineating graft detachment, particularly when graft stromal edema obscures direct visualization (Fig. 2.10). Graft detachment can produce the appearance with "double anterior chamber formation" due to the hyporeflective space between the graft and the host cornea. Furthermore, anterior segment OCT can monitor Descemet's detachments at precise topographic regions and allows appropriate clinical decisions to be made for surgical intervention, which may involve graft reshaping, repositioning, or rebubbling. Indeed, OCT is useful for evaluating the graft for potential factors that predispose to this complication, such as the presence of stromal tags (Fig. 2.11). Another notable, but uncommon, complication is interface epithelial ingrowth or downgrowth, which can undermine the results of endothelial keratoplasty by causing corneal clouding and potentially resulting in graft detachment. The sheet of proliferating epithelial cells deep in the corneal flap is clearly visible on anterior segment OCT as a highly reflective layer (Fig. 2.12). The use of shorter wavelength scanners in particular can delineate the lesion with great detail. However, penetration of the short wavelength light beyond the lesion is relatively limited.

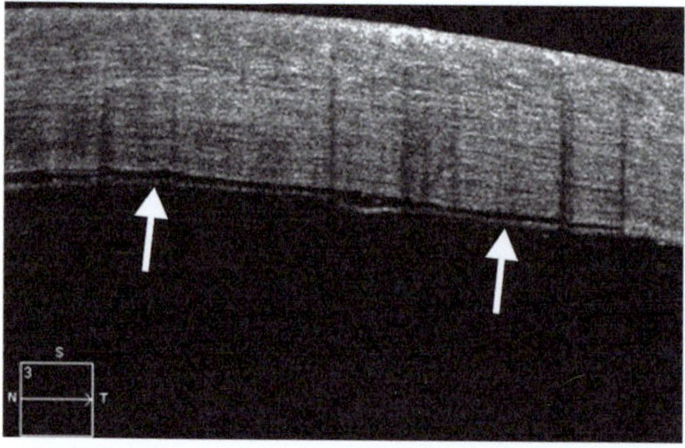

Fig. 2.10 Graft detachment following DMEK. Anterior segment OCT image shows the Descemet's membrane–endothelial layer (*arrows*) is not fully adhered to the stromal tissue. There is a thin hyporeflective gap between the graft and the host cornea

2.4 Keratoprosthesis

The success rate of penetrating keratoplasty is as high as 90 % after 1 year for patients with corneal scarring due to trauma, keratoconus, and corneal dystrophies and degenerations. However, corneal graft survival is poor in cases of autoimmune ocular surface disorders, such as Stevens–Johnson syndrome/toxic epidermal necrolysis and mucous membrane pemphigoid, after severe chemical burns and severe keratoconjunctivitis sicca, or in the presence of corneal vascularization from other causes. In such cases of complicated corneal blindness, the implantation of a keratoprosthesis may be the only option for visual rehabilitation.

The Boston keratoprosthesis (KPro), previously known as the Dohlman-Doane keratoprosthesis, is the most commonly used keratoprosthesis worldwide and comes in two forms. More than 10,000 of these devices have been implanted since approval for marketing by the US Food and Drug Administration in 1992. The type I device is a collar button-shaped device composed of a polymethyl methacrylate (PMMA) front plate and its stem and a PMMA or titanium back plate (Fig. 2.13). The type II device has an additional anterior nub that allows for through-the-lid implantation (Fig. 2.14). A corneal donor graft is sandwiched between the front and the back plates; the titanium back plate locks the device in place. The assembled keratoprosthesis and

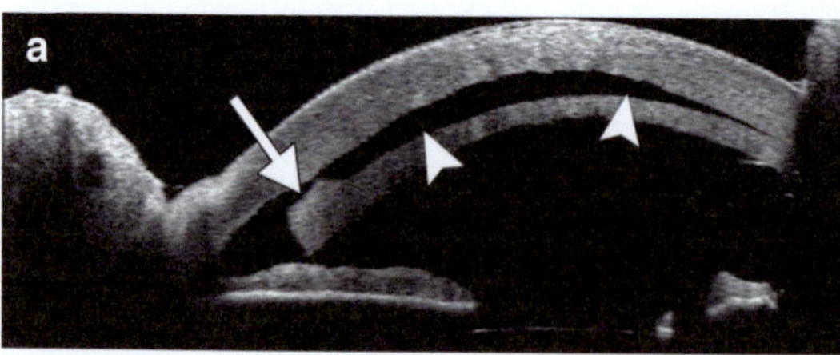

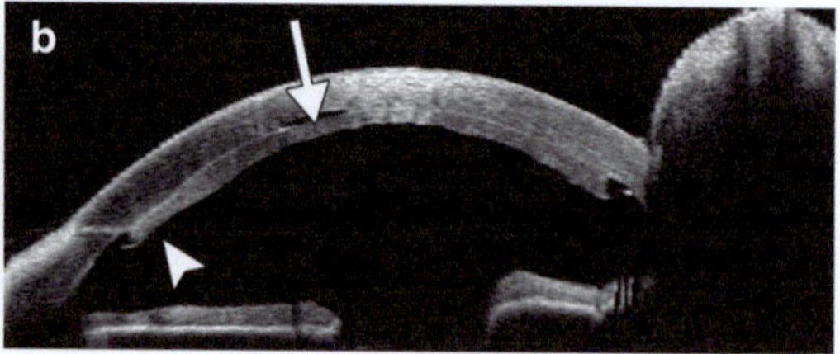

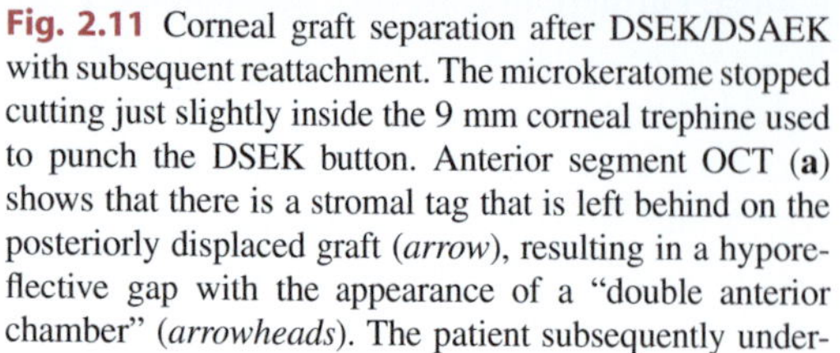

Fig. 2.11 Corneal graft separation after DSEK/DSAEK with subsequent reattachment. The microkeratome stopped cutting just slightly inside the 9 mm corneal trephine used to punch the DSEK button. Anterior segment OCT (**a**) shows that there is a stromal tag that is left behind on the posteriorly displaced graft (*arrow*), resulting in a hyporeflective gap with the appearance of a "double anterior chamber" (*arrowheads*). The patient subsequently underwent explant of the corneal graft, which was trimmed using fine scissors and then reinserted. Anterior segment OCT obtained after the revision surgery (**b**) shows that there is a small air bubble trapped within the interface (*arrow*), which is otherwise markedly improved, and that the graft is slightly thinner where the stromal tag was previously located (*arrowhead*)

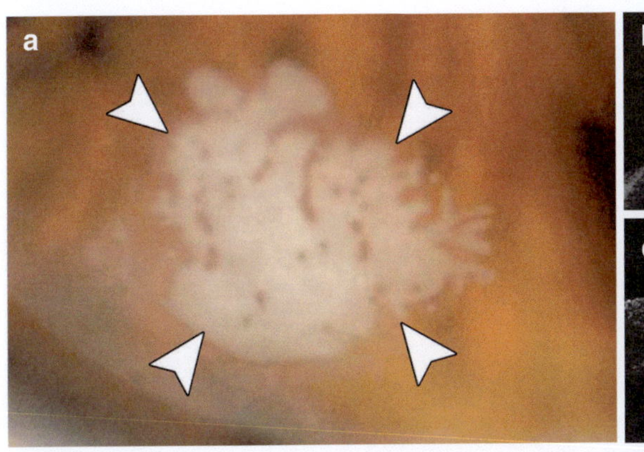
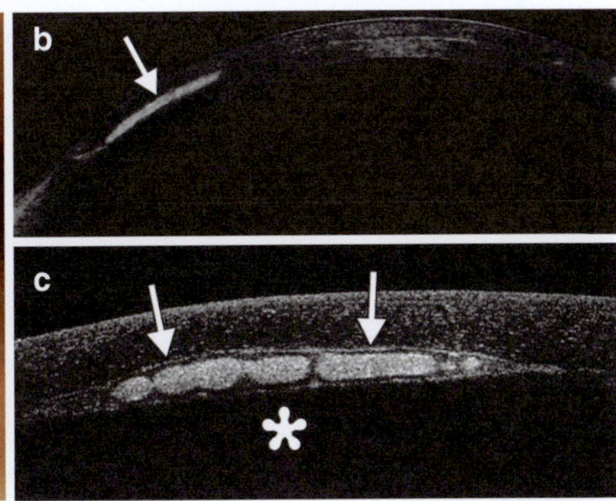

Fig. 2.12 Epithelial ingrowth after IntraLase-enabled DALK. The patient presented 19 months after surgery with a patch of epithelial ingrowth at the graft–host interface (*arrowheads*), as demonstrated on the clinical photograph (**a**). Anterior segment OCT image obtained using 1,310 nm wavelength light (**b**) shows the hyperreflective epithelial ingrowth (*arrow*) situated within the interface of the graft and the native cornea. Anterior segment OCT image obtained using 840 nm wavelength light (**c**) shows exquisite, higher-resolution detail of the epithelial ingrowth (*arrows*), but the corneal stroma posterior to the lesion is obscured (*) due to the relatively weaker penetration of the shorter wavelength light

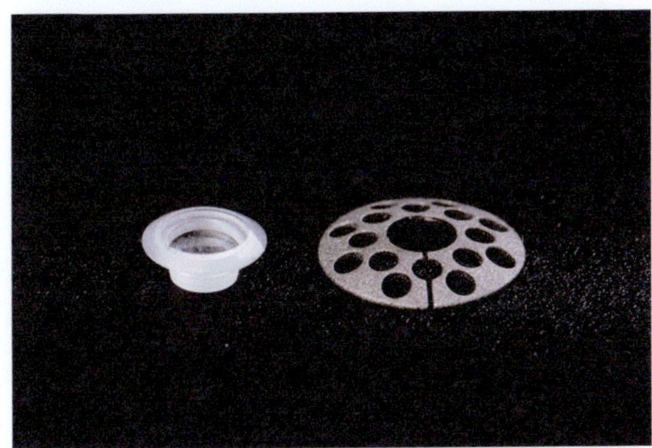

Fig. 2.13 Photomicrograph of FDA-approved version of the Boston keratoprosthesis type I device, prior to assembly

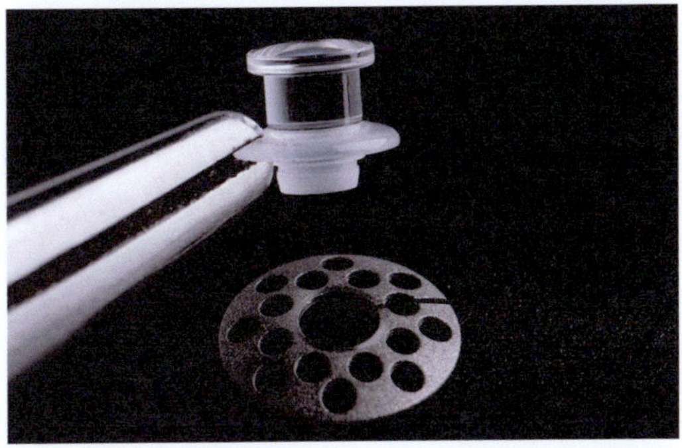

Fig. 2.14 Photomicrograph of FDA-approved version of the Boston keratoprosthesis type II device, prior to assembly

corneal donor graft are sutured in place in a fashion similar to standard penetrating keratoplasty.

On CT, both the type 1 and 2 Boston keratoprostheses are discernible, in which the PMMA components appear as soft tissue attenuation alongside the higher attenuation titanium plates (Figs. 2.15 and 2.16). CT can also depict the surrounding orbital contents rather well, without significant artifacts from the keratoprostheses. On the other hand, the Boston keratoprostheses are MRI conditional, since the implants produce artifact. UBM can grossly depict the major components of the keratoprostheses and surrounding anatomy (Fig. 2.17). Fourier-domain anterior segment OCT is also a useful imaging technique in patients with a KPro and provides the ability to identify changes that are sometimes difficult to appreciate by clinical evaluation. The higher spatial resolution Fourier-domain systems may aid in the clinical diagnosis and management of pathology that might not be imaged with instruments of lower resolution. Anterior segment OCT has the potential for monitoring the anatomic stability of an implanted KPro and may also help to monitor for complications. Moreover, high spatial resolution imaging may enhance our understanding of periprosthetic anatomy.

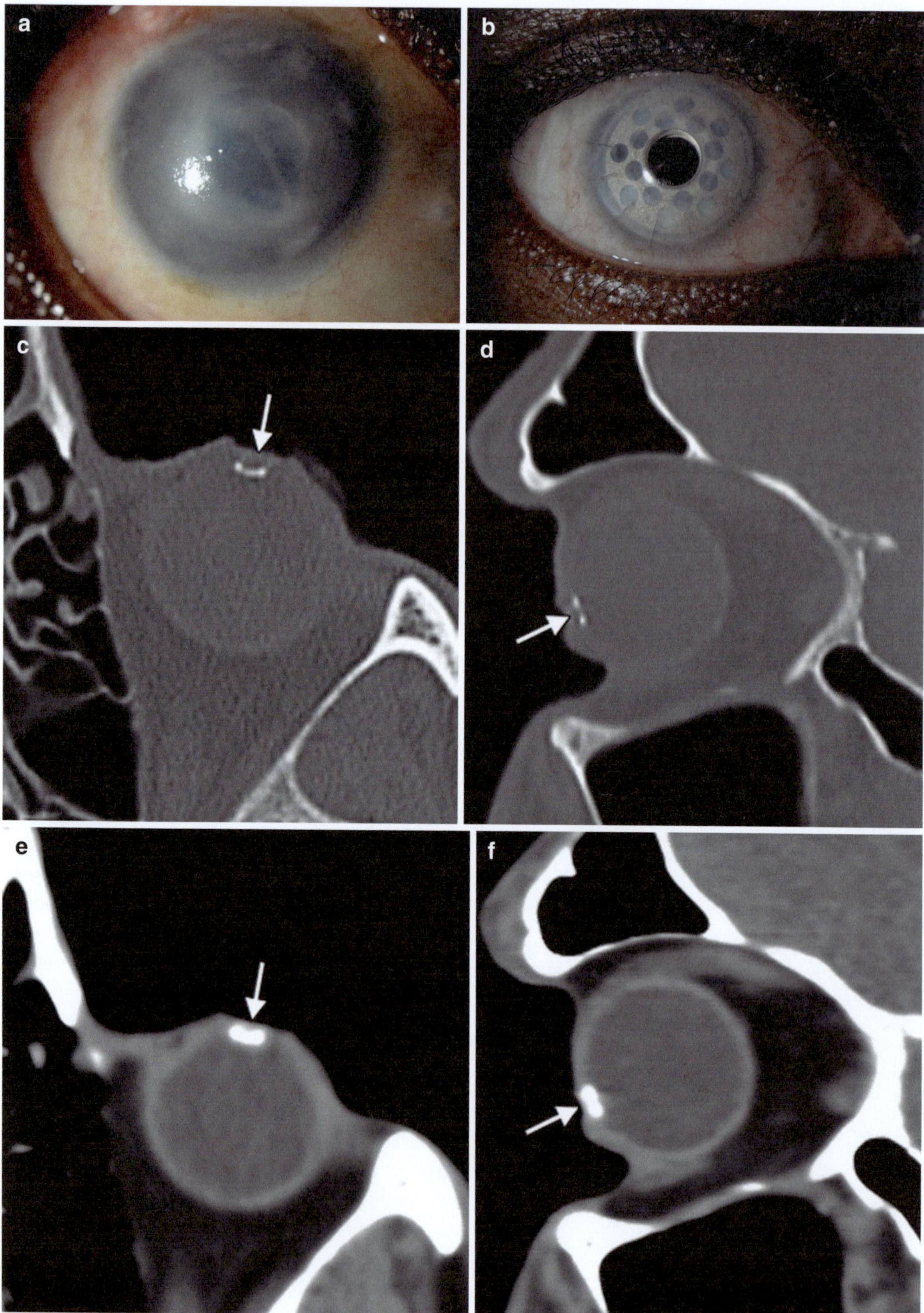

Fig. 2.15 Boston keratoprosthesis type I. Preoperative (**a**) and 1-year postoperative (**b**) clinical photographs of the right eye of a patient with history of chronic uveitis, glaucoma, and corneal opacity. Axial and sagittal CT images (**c–f**) in bone windows and soft tissue show a titanium component (*arrows*) within the anterior chamber of the globe. The other portions of the prosthesis are not well delineated

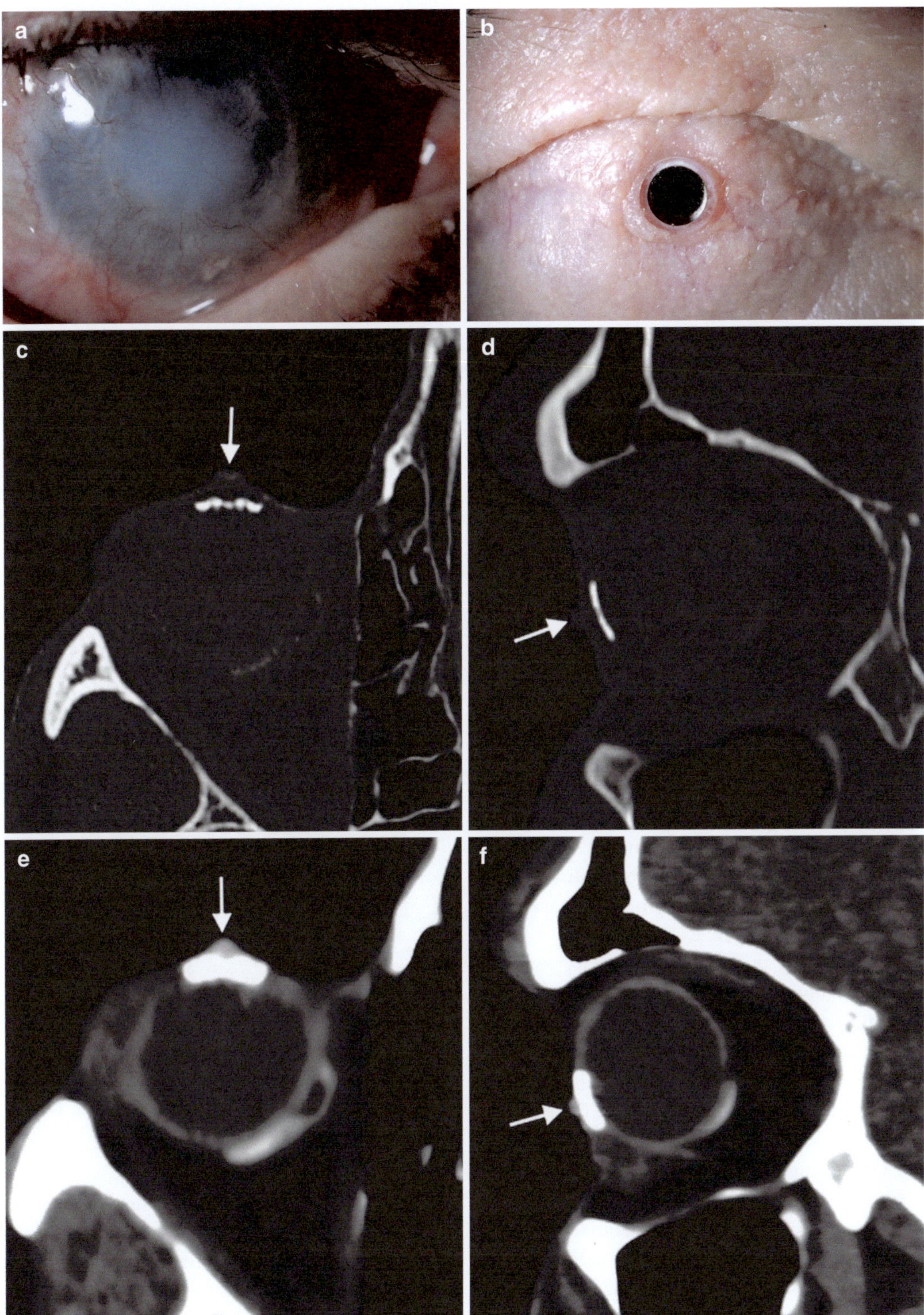

Fig. 2.16 Boston keratoprosthesis type II. Preoperative (**a**) and 1-year postoperative (**b**) clinical photographs of the right eye of a patient with history of Stevens–Johnson syndrome, symblephara, and multiple failed penetrating keratoplasty surgeries. The type II device is similar to the type I except for an additional anterior extension that allows for implantation through surgically closed eyelids. Axial and sagittal CT images (**c–f**) in the bone windows and soft tissue show the titanium component and anterior cylinder (*arrows*), which protrudes through the closed eyelids

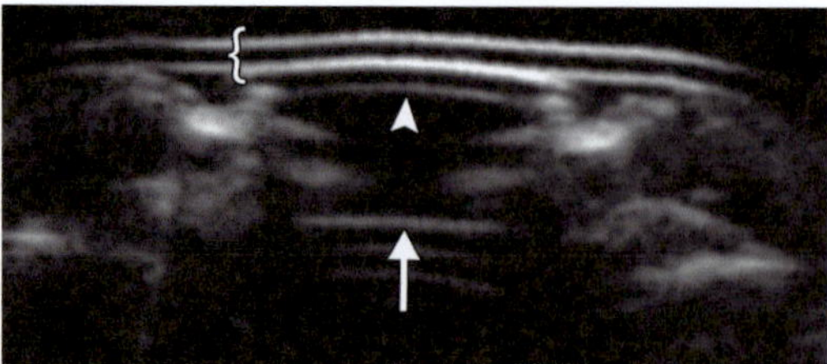

Fig. 2.17 Boston keratoprosthesis type I depicted on UBM. The front plate (*arrowhead*) and back plate (*arrow*), which appear as echogenic lines. The prosthesis is covered by a bandage contact lens (*bracket*) (Courtesy of Kathryn Colby MD, PhD and Demetrios Vavvas MD)

Osteo-odonto-keratoprosthesis (OOKP) is another type of keratoprosthesis that consists of an optical polymethacrylate cylinder mounted on a tooth–alveolar bone complex that is covered by a buccal mucosa graft and embedded in the host cornea. The OOKP is an option for patients with end-stage corneal blindness not amenable to penetrating keratoplasty. The prosthesis is relatively stable in the setting of dry keratinized eyes resulting from severe Stevens–Johnson syndrome, ocular cicatricial pemphigoid, trachoma, and chemical injury. The rigid optical cylinder of the OOKP provides excellent vision. Multidetector CT is a useful modality for characterizing the OOKP, whereby the components of the implant can be delineated (Fig. 2.18). The tooth–alveolar bone complex should maintain its original high attenuation appearance, except centrally through which a slot is drilled for the mildly hyperattenuating optical cylinder. The buccal mucosa graft may appear as a thin soft tissue attenuation layer overlying the prosthesis. Furthermore, the high-resolution multidetector CT enables 3D reconstructions to be generated, which enable accurate linear and volumetric measurements of the OOKP lamina to be obtained.

Postoperative complications related to keratoprosthesis surgery include glaucoma, retinal or choroidal detachment, infectious endophthalmitis, tissue necrosis, device extrusion, retroprosthetic membrane, and sterile vitritis. Glaucoma progression is a major cause of visual decline post-KPro, which is why a glaucoma drainage device is often implanted before or at the time of

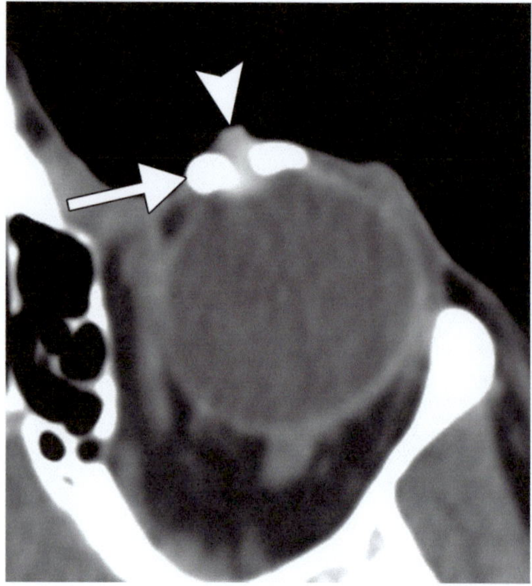

Fig. 2.18 Osteo-odonto-keratoprosthesis (OOKP). Axial CT image shows the tooth (*arrow*) in the anterior segment with a slot for the optic cylinder (*arrowhead*) (Courtesy of Venkat Avadhanam MD, Ian Francis MD, and Christopher Liu MD)

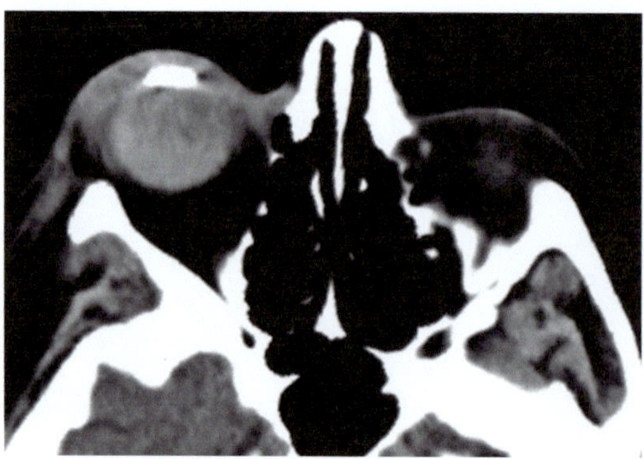

Fig. 2.19 Vitreous hemorrhage after keratoprosthesis insertion. Axial CT shows hyperattenuation within the right globe with the keratoprosthesis in position. There is also preseptal swelling

surgery in carefully selected patients. Vitreous hemorrhage can occur postoperatively either in association with a retinal detachment or as a complication of a concomitant vitrectomy during the original surgery (Fig. 2.19). B-scan ultrasound is the imaging method of choice to assess the integrity of the retina in such cases. A rare complication after keratoprosthesis type II

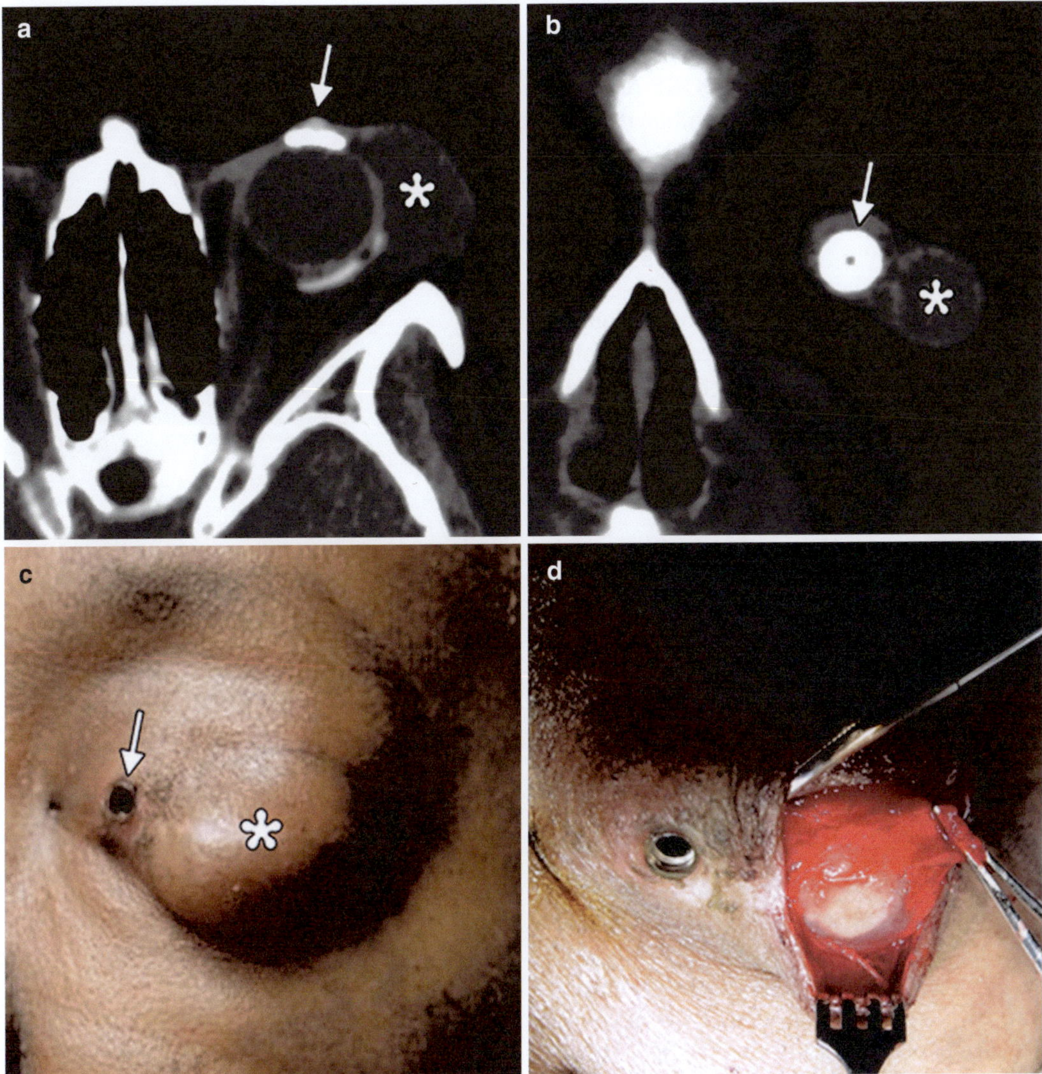

Fig. 2.20 Inclusion cyst after Boston keratoprosthesis type II implantation. Axial (**a**) and coronal (**b**) CT images show a fluid attenuation lesion (*) in the left eyelid lateral to the prosthesis (*arrow*). The lesion was separate from the glaucoma drainage device bleb. Clinical photograph (**c**) shows bulging of the eyelid (*) lateral to the prosthesis (*arrow*). Intraoperative photograph (**d**) shows the decompressed cyst remnant

implantation is the formation of an inclusion cyst beneath the surgically closed eyelids (Fig. 2.20). The main differential diagnosis in a case of encystment in a type II KPro patient is dacryocele, which is a cystic dilatation of the lacrimal "gland" due to distal obstruction, versus a giant bleb associated with an adjacent glaucoma device. Extensive dissection and delicate removal of all ocular surface epithelium is the most important measure to prevent encystment.

A complication specific to the OOKP is dissolution of the osteodental lamina, making close follow-up mandatory. Since ultrasound biomicroscopy cannot be used in these cases, CT with 3D reconstruction is a suitable alternative diagnostic modality. Although a minor reduction of the lamina, mainly in the anterior and inferior part, occurs in virtually all cases without loss of stability and integrity of the lamina cylinder complex, the presence of complete resorption of the inferior half of the osteodental lamina or a "moth-eaten" dissolution of dentine and bone tissue may be more problematic. On CT, OOKP resorption appears are areas of lucency within the tooth component and decrease in size of the prosthesis and can be responsible for extrusion. Long-term follow-up is recommended in order to detect and treat complications. Regular imaging with CT can help detect bone and dentine loss in the OOKP. Indeed, CT evidence of resorption precedes clinical exam findings. Once this complication is identified, treatment using bisphosphonates may prevent further progression.

2.5 Laser-Assisted In Situ Keratomileusis (LASIK), Photorefractive Keratectomy (PRK), and Laser Subepithelial Keratomileusis (LASEK)

LASIK surgery consists of cutting a thin layer of tissue from the top surface of the cornea (the flap) using a metal blade or laser microkeratome. Once the flap is reflected away, the underneath surface is exposed, and an ultraviolet excimer laser is used to reshape the stroma of the cornea. The flap is then returned to position. The flaps are generally thicker along the periphery than at the center and have a smooth transition at the edge. The boundary between the stromal bed and flap normally appears as a thin dark line on OCT (Fig. 2.21). Precise measurements of the corneal thickness after surgery can be made using anterior segment OCT, particularly using spectral-domain technique, which provides greater anatomic detail, as compared to time-domain OCT (Fig. 2.22). These LASIK flaps are typically thicker in the periphery and thinner in the center, as compared to the uniform thickness of IntraLase flaps. The flap may also have some capacity to move and form wrinkles (striae).

Postoperative complications associated with LASIK include flap dislocation, diffuse lamellar keratitis, infectious keratitis, epithelial ingrowth, and corneal ectasia. They are diagnosed upon slit-lamp biomicroscopy. Diffuse lamellar keratitis is

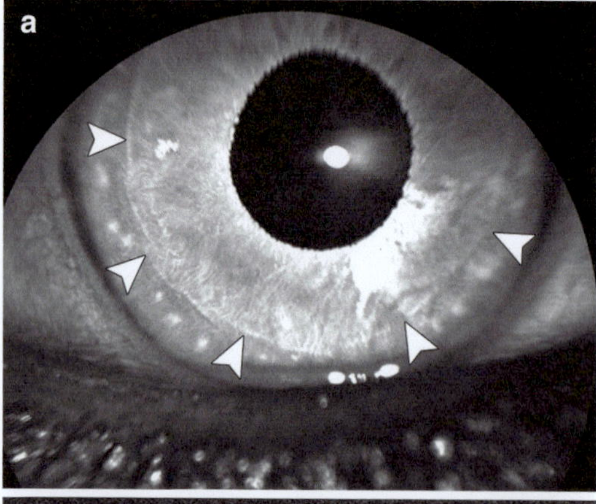

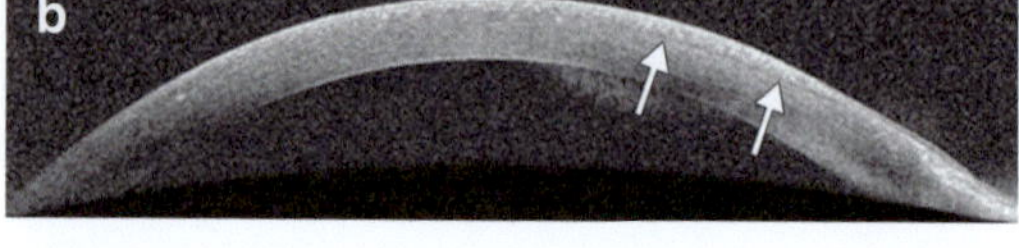

Fig. 2.21 LASIK. Clinical photograph (**a**) shows the margin of the flap (*arrowheads*). Anterior segment OCT image (**b**) shows the dark line in the stroma (*arrows*) that corresponds to the boundary between the stromal bed and flap (Courtesy of Lili Farrokh-Siar MD and Fatoumata Yanoga MD)

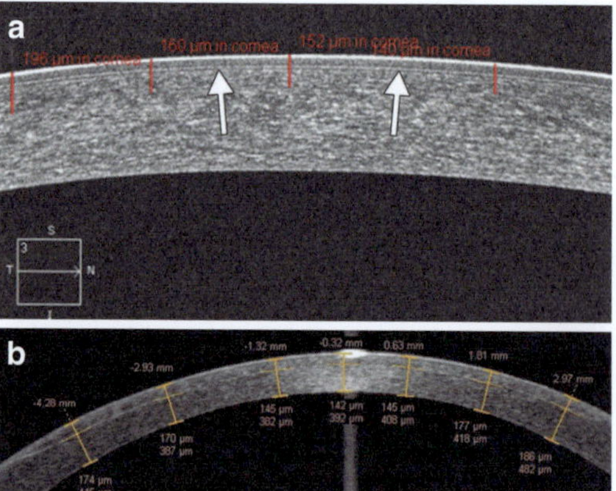

Fig. 2.22 Spectral- versus time-domain OCT for post-LASIK evaluation. The OCT image obtained using 840 nm light scanner (Cirrus) after a blade microkeratome LASIK surgery shows that Bowman's layer (*arrows*) under the epithelium is fully preserved (**a**). However, with 840 nm light, the flap, which is demarcated by the edge of the red caliper markers, is not as conspicuous as it is on the OCT image obtained using 1,310 nm light (**b**). The greater detail depicted using 840 nm light OCT scanner is attributable to spectral-domain technique, as compared to 1,310 nm (Visante), which is time-domain OCT. Anterior segment OCT shows multiple calipers marking the thickness of the flap and the cornea overall. It can be noted that the flap is thicker in the periphery and thinner in the center

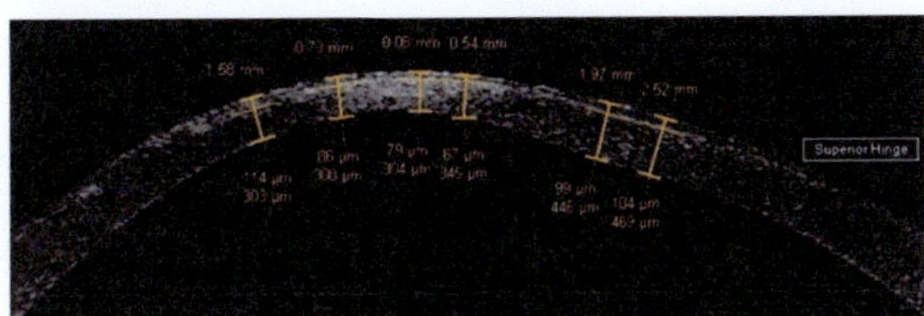

Fig. 2.23 Post-LASIK ectasia. The patient underwent LASIK followed by two enhancement procedures for correction of residual refraction. The OCT image demonstrates that despite the residual stromal tissue of at least 300 μm, the thinner portion of the cornea bulges anteriorly. The patient subsequently underwent corneal transplant surgery

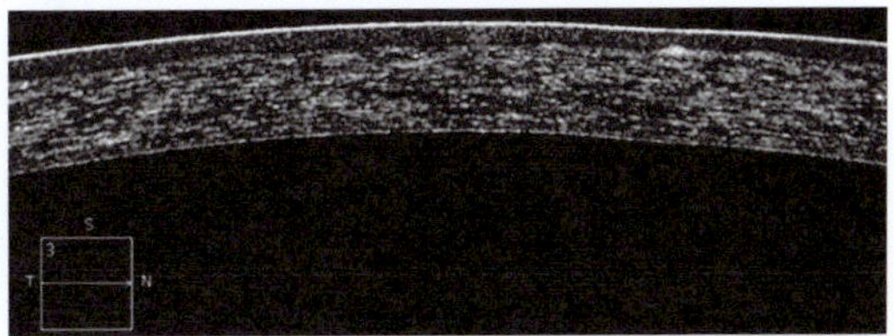

Fig. 2.24 Expected findings after PRK. Anterior segment OCT image shows absence of the Bowman's membrane resulting from excimer laser delivery

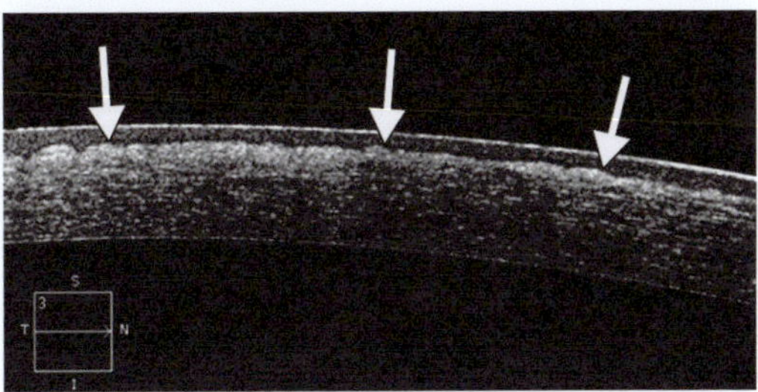

Fig. 2.25 Stromal scarring after PRK. Anterior segment OCT image shows that the Bowman's membrane no longer exists, but there are anterior stromal opacities that represent moderate scar tissue formation (*arrows*)

a noninfectious condition that is characterized by the presence of multiple grainy corneal infiltrates under the corneal flap. They typically resolve after intense corticosteroid therapy, and corneal clarity is restored. Epithelial ingrowth results from proliferation of corneal epithelial cells under the LASIK flap. Clinically, it is seen as an irregular haze between the flap and the underlying stroma. If this is present in the visual axis, flap lifting, scraping, and repositioning can improve the final visual acuity. One of the most devastating consequences of LASIK eye surgery is the development of ectasia. As the laser removes corneal tissue, it can either cause or hasten the natural progression of a patient's cornea to bulge. Thus, it is generally accepted that when LASIK is performed, a minimum of 250 μm of stromal tissue must remain. Nevertheless, the incidence of post-LASIK ectasia or "lectasia" is approximately 0.05–0.25 %. Topographic measurements that can be obtained using anterior segment OCT can be useful for quantifying the degree of postoperative ectasia, which appears as focal areas of thinning and bulging tissue (Fig. 2.23).

Photorefractive keratectomy (PRK) is analogous to LASIK but consists of delivering laser energy to the stromal surface, at Bowman's membrane. PRK is an excellent option for mild to moderate corrections, particularly for cases with thin corneas, recurrent erosions, or a predisposition for trauma. The main but often subtle finding on OCT following successful PRK is the absence of the Bowman's membrane and preservation of

the cornea (Fig. 2.24). Laser subepithelial keratomileusis (LASEK) is a recent modification of PRK and consists of creating an epithelial flap, which is replaced after laser ablation. Corneal scarring and haze formation are particularly a concern after PRK due to removal of Bowman's layer, which plays an important role in corneal homeostasis. Scar tissue formation appears as a hyperreflective material at the flap interface (Fig. 2.25).

2.6 Laser Thermal Keratoplasty (LTK)

Laser thermal keratoplasty can be performed using a noncontact holmium:YAG (Ho:YAG) laser for the treatment of hyperopia. LTK alters the curvature of the cornea via heat-induced shrinkage of collagen fibers. This produces a cinching effect in the peripheral cornea to induce myopia in the treated eye. The sequela of LTK can be observed as foci of hyperreflectivity on OCT (Fig. 2.26). Imaging can be useful for

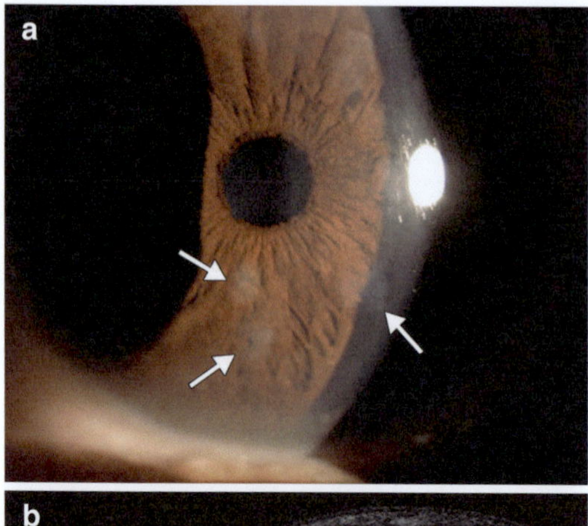

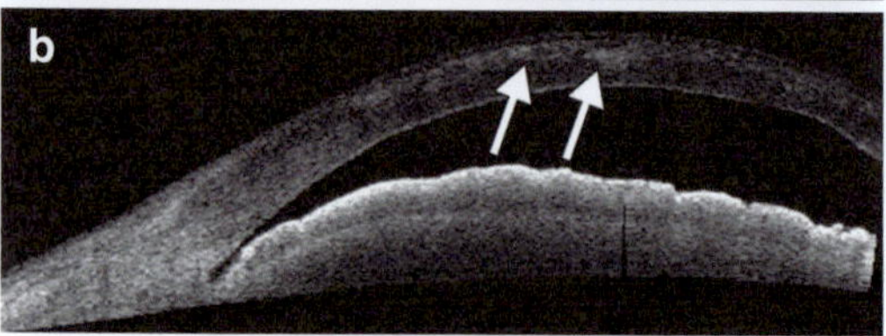

Fig. 2.26 Laser thermal keratoplasty for hyperopic correction. Slit-lamp photograph (**a**) shows areas of corneal opacification resulting from the laser burns (*arrows*). The corresponding anterior segment OCT (**b**) shows hyperreflective foci that represent the laser burns (*arrows*) (Courtesy of Lili Farrokh-Siar MD and Fatoumata Yanoga MD)

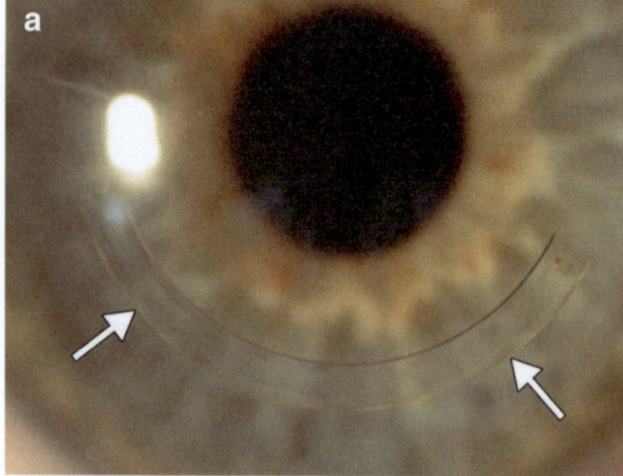

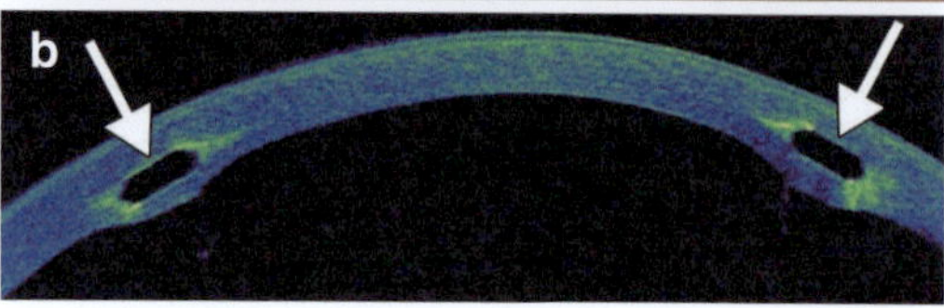

Fig. 2.27 Intrastromal corneal ring segment. Clinical photograph (**a**) of an Intacs ring segment device. Anterior segment "rainbow" color OCT image (**b**) shows the position of the hyporeflective device rings (*arrows*) within the stroma of the cornea

evaluating the configuration of the cornea in patients who underwent LTK and who may require additional treatment via LASIK.

2.7 Intrastromal Corneal Ring Segments (Intacs)

Another form of corneal refractive surgery that does not involve use of the excimer laser is the insertion of intrastromal corneal ring segments (Intacs). This treatment is FDA approved for the correction of low degrees of myopia but is also used in patients with keratoconus and post-LASIK ectasia. Intacs are composed of polymethyl methacrylate (PMMA) and are implanted in the deep corneal stroma in order to modify the corneal curvature. Postoperatively, the position of Intacs within the corneal stroma can be delineated both clinically and by anterior segment OCT. On OCT, the device appears as a hyporeflective structure embedded within the periphery of the corneal stroma (Fig. 2.27).

2.8 Summary

- There is truly an alphabet soup of procedures that can be performed and implants that can be used for corneal transplantation and refractive surgery (PKP, FAPK, IEK, DALK, DSEK, DSAEK, DMEK, KPro, OOKP, LASIK, PRK, LASEK, and Intacs), and these are in constant evolution.
- CT may be indicated for evaluating gross complications after cornea surgery, such as hemorrhage, orbital infection, and epidermal cyst formation. It is also useful for follow-up of OOKP laminar resorption. Otherwise, the various corneal implants may be encountered incidentally on CT and should be appropriately recognized.
- MRI of the brain is the imaging modality of choice for evaluating patients with suspected Creutzfeldt–Jakob disease, which may rarely result from prions transmitted during corneal transplantation. Otherwise, the utility of MRI for direct evaluation of corneal surgeries is limited and the modality is considered conditional for patients with KPro implants.

- Anterior segment OCT provides high-resolution cross-sectional images that allow for a qualitative and quantitative appraisal of the anatomy after lamellar surgery and to screen for postoperative complications, particularly in cases of corneal edema, which limits direct visual inspection.
- It is sometimes necessary to quantify the thickness of the cornea after refractive surgery, and anterior segment OCT can provide precise measurements.

Further Reading

Aiello LP, Javitt JC, Canner JK. National outcomes of penetrating keratoplasty. Risks of endophthalmitis and retinal detachment. Arch Ophthalmol. 1993;111(4):509–13.

Ambrósio Jr R, Wilson S. LASIK vs LASEK vs PRK: advantages and indications. Semin Ophthalmol. 2003;18(1):2–10.

Bluestone A, Ackert J, Som PM. The CT appearance of a corneal melt: report of 2 cases. AJNR Am J Neuroradiol. 2012;33(5):E72–3.

Cameron JA, Antonios SR, Cotter JB, Habash NR. Endophthalmitis from contaminated donor corneas following penetrating keratoplasty. Arch Ophthalmol. 1991;109(1):54–9.

Chen SH, Pineda 2nd R. Epithelial and fibrous downgrowth: mechanisms of disease. Ophthalmol Clin North Am. 2002;15(1):41–8.

Chen MC, Cortés DE, Harocopos G, Mannis MJ. Epithelial downgrowth after penetrating keratoplasty: imaging by high-resolution optical coherence tomography and in vivo confocal microscopy. Cornea. 2013;32(11):1505–8.

DelMonte DW, Kim T. Anatomy and physiology of the cornea. J Cataract Refract Surg. 2011;37(3):588–98.

Guss RB, Koenig S, De La Pena W, Marx M, Kaufman HE. Endophthalmitis after penetrating keratoplasty. Am J Ophthalmol. 1983;95(5):651–8.

Higashiura R, Maeda N, Nakagawa T, Fuchihata M, Koh S, Hori Y, Inoue T, Nishida K. Corneal topographic analysis by 3-dimensional anterior segment optical coherence tomography after endothelial keratoplasty. Invest Ophthalmol Vis Sci. 2012;53(7):3286–95.

Hill JC. Treatment of simple hyperopia: comparison of laser in situ keratomileusis and laser thermal keratoplasty. J Cataract Refract Surg. 2003;29(5):912–7.

Hirano K, Ito Y, Suzuki T, Kojima T, Kachi S, Miyake Y. Optical coherence tomography for the noninvasive evaluation of the cornea. Cornea. 2001;20(3):281–9.

Hou P, Lu Y, Ye F, Lan W, Huang Z. Application of femtosecond laser in ocular surgery. Eye Sci. 2013;28(2):103–7.

Ingraham HJ, Donnenfeld ED, Perry HD. Massive suprachoroidal hemorrhage in penetrating keratoplasty. Am J Ophthalmol. 1989;108(6):670–5.

Ivarsen A, Hjortdal J. Seven-year changes in corneal power and aberrations after PRK or LASIK. Invest Ophthalmol Vis Sci. 2012;53(10):6011–6.

Kaluzny BJ, Szkulmowski M, Bukowska DM, Wojtkowski M. Spectral OCT with speckle contrast reduction for evaluation of the healing process after PRK and transepithelial PRK. Biomed Opt Express. 2014;5(4):1089–98.

Kamyar R, Weizer JS, de Paula FH, Stein JD, Moroi SE, John D, Musch DC, Mian SI. Glaucoma associated with Boston type I keratoprosthesis. Cornea. 2012;31(2):134–9.

Kang JJ, Allemann N, Vajaranant T, de la Cruz J, Cortina MS. Anterior segment optical coherence tomography for the quantitative evaluation of the anterior segment following Boston keratoprosthesis. PLoS One. 2013; 8(8):e70673.

Khan B, Dudenhoefer EJ, Dohlman CH. Keratoprosthesis: an update. Curr Opin Ophthalmol. 2001;12(4):282–7.

Leveille AS, McMullan FD, Cavanagh HD. Endophthalmitis following penetrating keratoplasty. Ophthalmology. 1983;90(1):38–9.

Lim LS, Aung HT, Aung T, Tan DT. Corneal imaging with anterior segment optical coherence tomography for lamellar keratoplasty procedures. Am J Ophthalmol. 2008;145(1):81–90.

Lim LS, Ang CL, Wong E, Wong DW, Tan DT. Vitreoretinal complications and vitreoretinal surgery in osteo-odonto-keratoprosthesis surgery. Am J Ophthalmol. 2014;157(2):349–54.

Linebarger EJ, Hardten DR, Lindstrom RL. Diffuse lamellar keratitis: diagnosis and management. J Cataract Refract Surg. 2000;26(7):1072–7.

Liu C, Paul B, Tandon R, Lee E, Fong K, Mavrikakis I, Herold J, Thorp S, Brittain P, Francis I, Ferrett C, Hull C, Lloyd A, Green D, Franklin V, Tighe B, Fukuda M, Hamada S. The osteo-odonto-keratoprosthesis (OOKP). Semin Ophthalmol. 2005;20(2):113–28.

Maddox RA, Belay ED, Curns AT, Zou WQ, Nowicki S, Lembach RG, Geschwind MD, Haman A, Shinozaki N, Nakamura Y, Borer MJ, Schonberger LB. Creutzfeldt-Jakob disease in recipients of corneal transplants. Cornea. 2008;27(7):851–4.

Mamalis N, Edelhauser HF, Dawson DG, Chew J, LeBoyer RM, Werner L. Toxic anterior segment syndrome. J Cataract Refract Surg. 2006;32(2):324–33.

Melki SA, Azar DT. LASIK complications: etiology, management, and prevention. Surv Ophthalmol. 2001;46(2):95–116.

Moshfeghi DM, Kim BY, Kaiser PK, Sears JE, Smith SD. Appositional suprachoroidal hemorrhage: a case-control study. Am J Ophthalmol. 2004;138(6):959–63.

Moshirfar M, Smedley JG, Muthappan V, Jarsted A, Ostler EM. Rate of ectasia and incidence of irregular topography in patients with unidentified preoperative risk factors undergoing femtosecond laser-assisted LASIK. Clin Ophthalmol. 2014;8:35–42.

Nesi TT, Leite DA, Rocha FM, Tanure MA, Reis PP, Rodrigues EB, Campos MS. Indications of optical coherence tomography in keratoplasties: literature review. J Ophthalmol. 2012;2012:989063.

Niederkorn JY. Mechanisms of corneal graft rejection: the sixth annual Thygeson Lecture, presented at the Ocular Microbiology and Immunology Group meeting, October 21, 2000. Cornea. 2001;20(7):675–9.

Park CY, Ji YH, Chung ES. Changes in keratometric corneal power and refractive error after laser thermal keratoplasty. J Cataract Refract Surg. 2004;30(4):867–72.

Price Jr FW, Whitson WE, Ahad KA, Tavakkoli H. Suprachoroidal hemorrhage in penetrating keratoplasty. Ophthalmic Surg. 1994;25(8):521–5.

Priglinger SG, Neubauer AS, May CA, Alge CS, Wolf AH, Mueller A, Ludwig K, Kampik A, Welge-Luessen U. Optical coherence tomography for the detection of laser in situ keratomileusis in donor corneas. Cornea. 2003;22(1):46–50.

Purcell Jr JJ, Krachmer JH, Doughman DJ, Bourne WM. Expulsive hemorrhage in penetrating keratoplasty. Ophthalmology. 1982;89(1):41–3.

Rabinstein AA, Whiteman ML, Shebert RT. Abnormal diffusion-weighted magnetic resonance imaging in Creutzfeldt-Jakob disease following corneal transplantations. Arch Neurol. 2002;59(4):637–9.

Rahman I, Carley F, Hillarby C, Brahma A, Tullo AB. Penetrating keratoplasty: indications, outcomes, and complications. Eye (Lond). 2009;23(6):1288–94.

Robert MC, Pomerleau V, Harissi-Dagher M. Complications associated with Boston keratoprosthesis type 1 and glaucoma drainage devices. Br J Ophthalmol. 2013;97(5):573–7.

Schechter BA, Rand WJ, Nagler RS, Estrin I, Arnold SS, Villate N, Velazquez GE. Corneal melt after amniotic membrane transplant. Cornea. 2005;24(1):106–7.

Shapiro BL, Cortés DE, Chin EK, Li JY, Werner JS, Redenbo E, Mannis MJ. High-resolution spectral domain anterior segment optical coherence tomography in type 1 Boston keratoprosthesis. Cornea. 2013;32(7): 951–5.

Shehadeh Mashor R, Bahar I, Rootman DB, Kumar NL, Singal N, Slomovic AR, Rootman DS. Zig Zag versus Top Hat configuration in IntraLase-enabled penetrating keratoplasty. Br J Ophthalmol. 2014;98:756–9.

Sipkova Z, Lam FC, Francis I, Herold J, Liu C. Serial 3-dimensional computed tomography and a novel method of volumetric analysis for the evaluation of the osteo-odonto-keratoprosthesis. Cornea. 2013;32(4): 401–6.

Speaker MG, Guerriero PN, Met JA, Coad CT, Berger A, Marmor M. A case-control study of risk factors for intraoperative suprachoroidal expulsive hemorrhage. Ophthalmology. 1991;98(2):202–9.

Stoiber J, Forstner R, Csáky D, Ruckhofer J, Grabner G. Evaluation of bone reduction in osteo-odontokeratoprosthesis (OOKP) by three-dimensional computed tomography. Cornea. 2003;22(2):126–30.

Suh LH, Yoo SH, Deobhakta A, Donaldson KE, Alfonso EC, Culbertson WW, O'Brien TP. Complications of Descemet's stripping with automated endothelial keratoplasty: survey of 118 eyes at One Institute. Ophthalmology. 2008;115(9):1517–24.

Taneri S, Zieske JD, Azar DT. Evolution, techniques, clinical outcomes, and pathophysiology of LASEK: review of the literature. Surv Ophthalmol. 2004;49(6): 576–602.

Torquetti L, Berbel RF, Ferrara P. Long-term follow-up of intrastromal corneal ring segments in keratoconus. J Cataract Refract Surg. 2009;35(10):1768–73.

Tugal-Tutkun I, Akova YA, Foster CS. Penetrating keratoplasty in cicatrizing conjunctival diseases. Ophthalmology. 1995;102(4):576–85.

Ustundag C, Bahcecioglu H, Ozdamar A, Aras C, Yildirim R, Ozkan S. Optical coherence tomography for evaluation of anatomical changes in the cornea after laser in situ keratomileusis. J Cataract Refract Surg. 2000;26(10): 1458–62.

Vargas LG, Vroman DT, Solomon KD, Holzer MP, Escobar-Gomez M, Schmidbauer JM, Apple DJ. Epithelial downgrowth after clear cornea phacoemulsification: report of two cases and review of the literature. Ophthalmology. 2002;109(12):2331–5.

Wang MY, Maloney RK. Epithelial ingrowth after laser in situ keratomileusis. Am J Ophthalmol. 2000;129(6): 746–51.

Zhang Y, Chen YG, Xia YJ. Comparison of corneal flap morphology using AS-OCT in LASIK with the WaveLight FS200 femtosecond laser versus a mechanical microkeratome. J Refract Surg. 2013;29(5):320–4.

Imaging After Cataract and Intraocular Lens Implant Surgery

3

Sotiria Palioura, Lili Farrokh-Siar,
Fatoumata Yanoga, Daniel Thomas Ginat,
and James Chodosh

3.1 Overview

The intraocular (crystalline) lens is a biconvex structure that serves to refract the incident light in conjunction with the cornea. The crystalline lens is comprised of the lens capsule (which completely surrounds the lens anteriorly and posteriorly), the lens epithelium, and lens fibers (which includes the cortex). Cataracts consist of opacification of the normally transparent intraocular lens and collectively represent the most common cause of vision loss. There are several etiologies for the development of cataracts, which can be congenital or more commonly acquired as a result of age-related degeneration, trauma, intraocular inflammation, exposure to ionizing radiation, and through the use of certain systemic or topical medications, such as corticosteroids.

S. Palioura, MD, PhD • J. Chodosh, MD, MPH
Department of Ophthalmology, Massachusetts
Eye and Ear Infirmary, Boston, MA, USA

L. Farrokh-Siar, MD
Department of Ophthalmology, Illinois
Glaucoma Center, Chicago, IL, USA

F. Yanoga, MD
Department of Ophthalmology, University
of Chicago, Chicago, IL, USA

D.T. Ginat, MD, MS (✉)
Director of Head and Neck Imaging,
Department of Radiology, University of Chicago,
5841 S Maryland Avenue, Chicago, IL 60637, USA
e-mail: ginatd01@gmail.com

Cataract surgery is generally performed when the decrease in visual acuity or the presence of progressive glare limits a patient's activities of daily life. Surgical options for treating cataracts include lensectomy with aphakia and lensectomy with artificial intraocular lens implantation (pseudophakia). Intraocular lens implants are also used in the treatment of myopia (phakic intraocular lens implantation) and for hyperopic eyes that require a high power lens after cataract removal (piggyback intraocular lens implantation). Imaging after cataract surgery and phakic intraocular lens implantation is indicated for the evaluation of potential complications in cases of intraocular hemorrhage or corneal edema that obscures the clinical view to the fundus. The modalities of choice include B-mode ultrasound, UBM, and OCT. Otherwise, sequelae of cataract surgery and phakic intraocular lens implantation can be encountered as incidental findings on CT and MRI that include the orbits. The corresponding imaging findings of cataract surgery and associated complications are reviewed in the subsequent sections.

3.2 Lensectomy with Aphakia

Cataracts are most commonly extracted via phacoemulsification, which consists of ultrasonic fragmentation, and aspiration of the native crystalline lens. The diseased lens can be accessed via a clear corneal approach or via a scleral tunnel into the cornea. The incision in the

D.T. Ginat, S.K. Freitag (eds.), *Post-treatment Imaging of the Orbit*,
DOI 10.1007/978-3-662-44023-0_3, © Springer-Verlag Berlin Heidelberg 2015

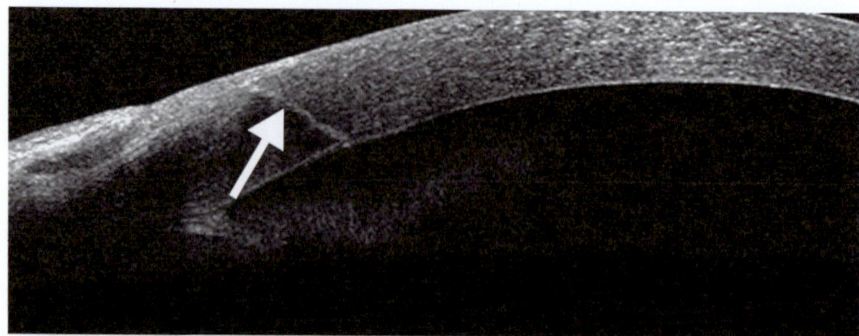

Fig. 3.1 Clear cornea incision. Anterior segment OCT shows the scar (*arrow*) from a clear cornea incision in a patient who underwent cataract extraction with phacoemulsification

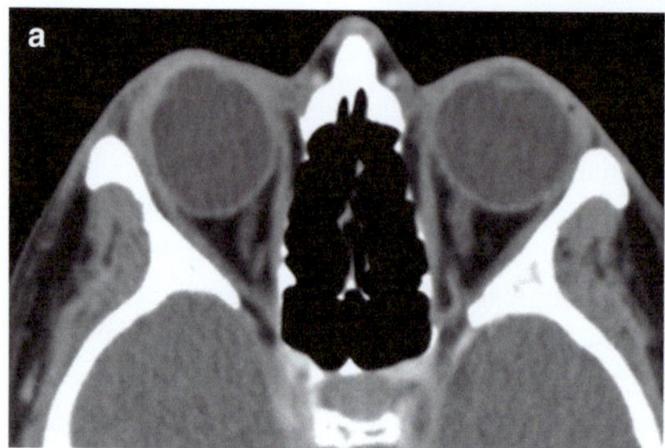

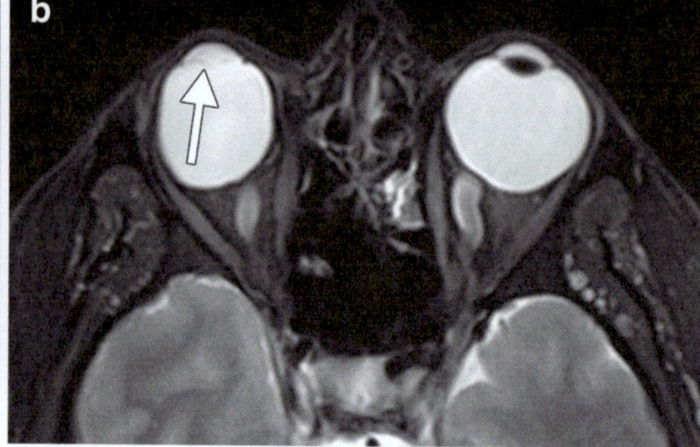

Fig. 3.2 Lensectomy. The patient has a history of congenital cataract. Axial CT image (**a**) and axial T2-weighted MRI (**b**) show absence of the right crystalline lens, but intact left lens. Faint linear hypointense strands at the lensectomy site may represent residual portions of the capsular bag (*arrow*). There is staphylomatous deformity of both globes

cornea can be visible postoperatively on high-resolution imaging, such as OCT (Fig. 3.1). Lensectomy with aphakia used to be performed for the treatment of cataracts when artificial intraocular lens implants were not yet available. Alternatively, intraoperative complications may preclude the safe insertion of a lens implant at the time of surgery, thereby mandating temporary aphakia. Occasionally, infants with congenital cataracts are treated with lens extraction without immediate artificial intraocular lens insertion. In such cases, these patients are fitted with a contact lens, and intraocular lens implantation is undertaken 1 or 2 years later. Traditionally, the anterior lens capsule is removed (capsulorhexis) in order to facilitate extraction of all the lens material and minimize the occurrence of an inflammatory response. Regardless of the reason for aphakia, the result of lensectomy appears as a gap between the anterior chamber and vitreous cavity on diagnostic imaging (Fig. 3.2). Lensectomy can also be performed

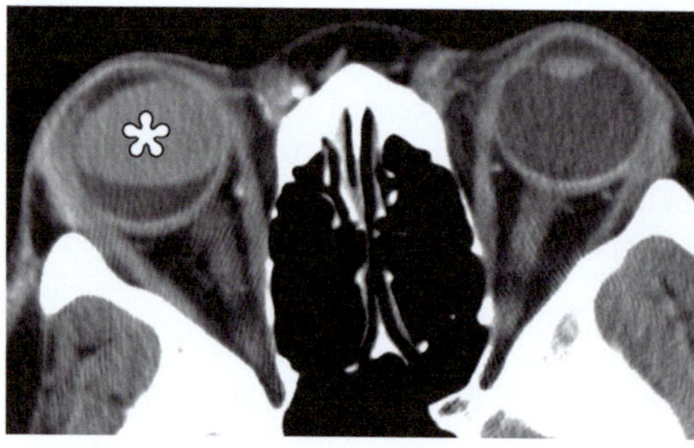

Fig. 3.3 Combined lensectomy, vitrectomy, and silicone oil injection. Axial CT image shows the hyperattenuating silicone oil floating within the left globe (*) and absence of the intraocular lens

in conjunction with vitrectomy and silicone oil injection for the treatment of retinal detachment (Fig. 3.3). In such cases, it can be beneficial to preserve the lens capsule, while removing the rest of the lens tissue in order to prevent migration of silicone oil into the anterior chamber and facilitate eventual intraocular lens implantation.

3.3 Lensectomy with Intraocular Lens Implant (Pseudophakia)

Cataract extraction with implantation of an artificial intraocular lens (IOL) implant is the currently accepted treatment for symptomatic cataracts, other than the situations delineated in the previous section. Although there are several different designs that are commercially available, the basic components of an IOL implant include the central optic portion and two haptics that hold the device in position (Fig. 3.4). The haptics can be configured as open versus closed loops. IOL implants are composed of polymethyl methacrylate (PMMA), polypropylene (Prolene), silicone, water-compatible polyhydroxyethyl methacrylate (hydrogel), or polyethylene (Dacron). Most rigid IOL optics are composed of PMMA, and the haptics are composed of either PMMA or Prolene, while flexible (foldable) IOLs are composed of either silicone or polyhydroxyethylmethacrylate (PHEMA). Following lens extraction, an IOL can be inserted either into the anterior chamber or the posterior chamber. Posterior chamber IOL insertion is now performed much more commonly than anterior chamber insertion for cataract surgery. The optic and haptics of posterior chamber IOL implants are located behind the iris and are supported by the residual capsule of the lens or by haptics positioned in the ciliary sulcus, just anterior to the ciliary process. The haptic loops maintain the position of the IOL and prevent the lens from dislocating and eventually become encased and secured by fibrous tissue. Anterior chamber IOL surgery is technically more straightforward than posterior chamber implantation, but has been associated with a relatively high complication rate, particularly when rigid IOLs were used. Nevertheless, indications for anterior chamber IOL include lens dislocation, loss of posterior capsular support during surgery, and selected cases of secondary implantation. After phacoemulsification and foldable IOL implantation, UBM typically reveals shifting of the iris posteriorly, deepening of the anterior chamber, and widening of its angle by approximately 10°.

Only the optic component of the IOL implant is perceptible on CT or MRI. In fact, cross-sectional diagnostic imaging of cases with IOLs can be mistaken for aphakia if the section thickness is not small enough, such that partial volume averaging obscures the pupillary opening. Otherwise, the optic portion of an IOL appears as a thin linear hyperattenuating structure in the anterior portion of the globe on CT (Fig. 3.5). IOL implants are MRI

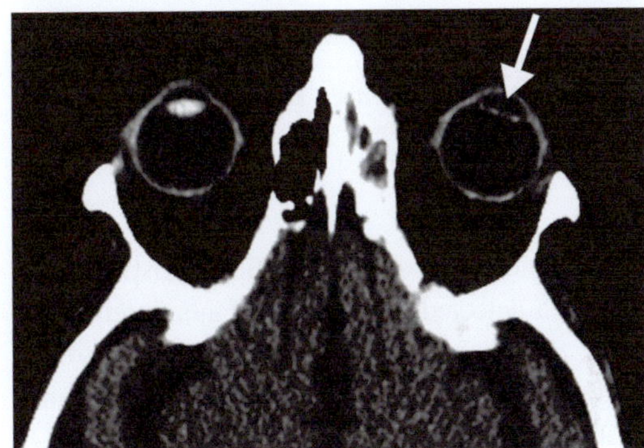

Fig. 3.5 Posterior chamber IOL implant depicted on CT. Axial CT image shows a hyperattenuating linear IOL implant (*arrow*) situated posterior to the expected plane of the iris. Compare the IOL implant to the normal native right lens

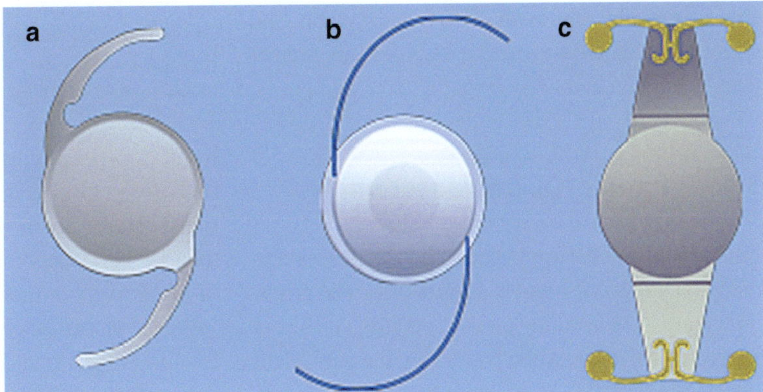

Fig. 3.4 Schematic of different types of intraocular lens implants, including Technis IOL (**a**), ReZoom (**b**), and Crytalens (**c**)

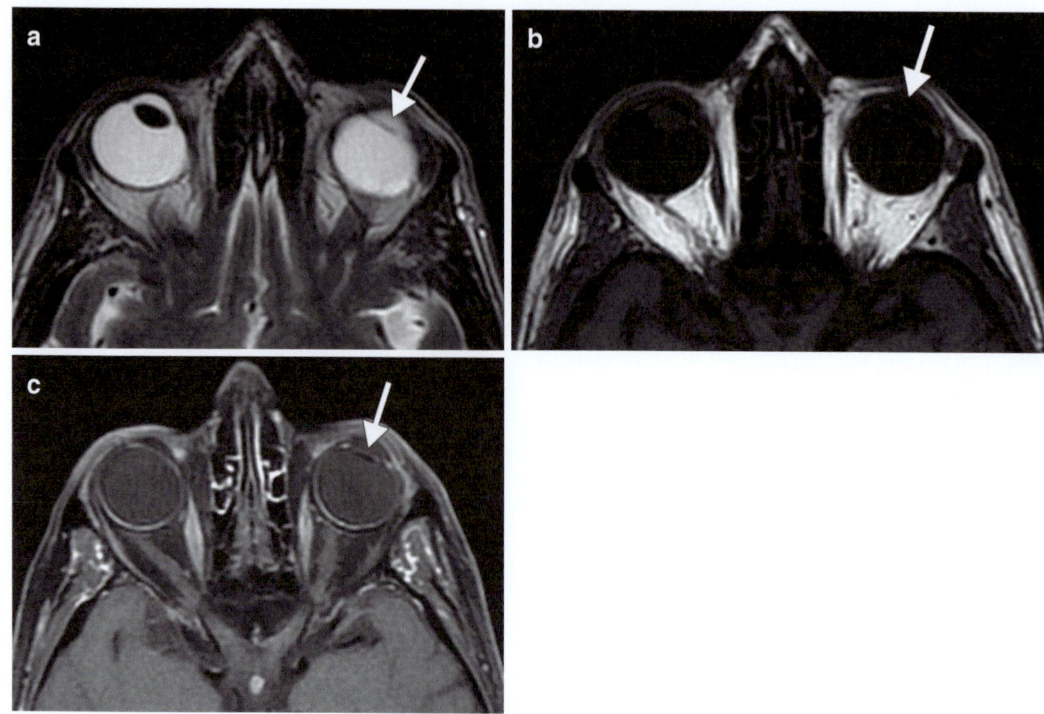

Fig. 3.6 Posterior chamber IOL implant depicted on MRI. Axial T2-weighted (**a**), T1-weighted (**b**), and fat-suppressed post-contrast T1-weighted (**c**) MR images show the non-enhancing hypointense implant (*arrows*). Compare the IOL implant to the normal right native lens, which is also hypointense

compatible. Indeed, no significant displacement has been detected with IOL implants tested at 7 T MRI. However, magnetic susceptibility artifact may be observed with IOL implants that contain a platinum component (Worst Platinum Clip IOL implant) at high field strengths. The optic portion of IOL implants can be delineated on MRI as hypointense linear structures and is most conspicuous on T2-weighted sequences (Fig. 3.6). IOL implants do not enhance since they are impermeable to vascular ingrowth. The IOL implants and surrounding anatomy can be depicted in greater detail on UBM and OCT (Fig. 3.7).

3.4 Phakic IOL Implantation

Phakic IOL (PIOL) implantation is effective for correcting myopia and myopic astigmatism. The procedure consists of securing an IOL, such as Veriflex or Verisyse, to the iris, while preserving the native lens intact. The anterior chamber IOL implant and its

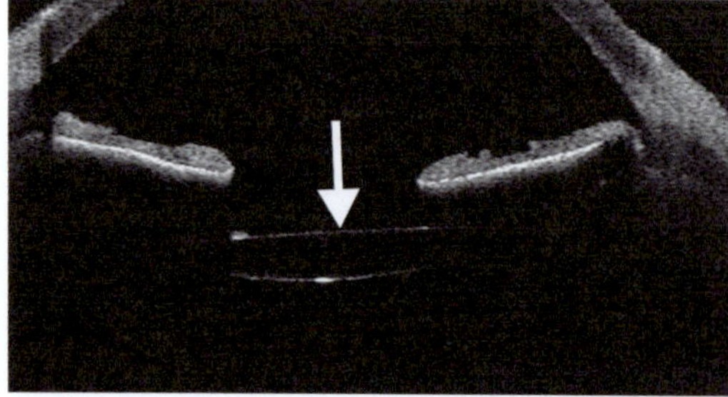

Fig. 3.7 Posterior chamber IOL implant depicted on OCT. The anterior chamber OCT image shows an IOL implant (*arrow*) that appears as a hyperreflective line located posterior to the iris

insertion site onto the iris can be readily delineated on UBM or OCT (Fig. 3.8), which can provide additional details about the anterior segment anatomy than slit lamp examination. In cases of high myopia of −8 diopters or more, PIOL implants can provide superior visual outcome compared with keratorefractive surgeries and a lower risk of complications than refractive lens exchange. Nevertheless, long-

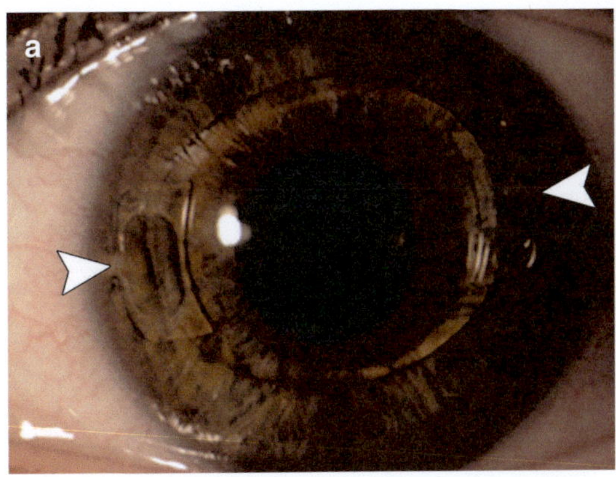
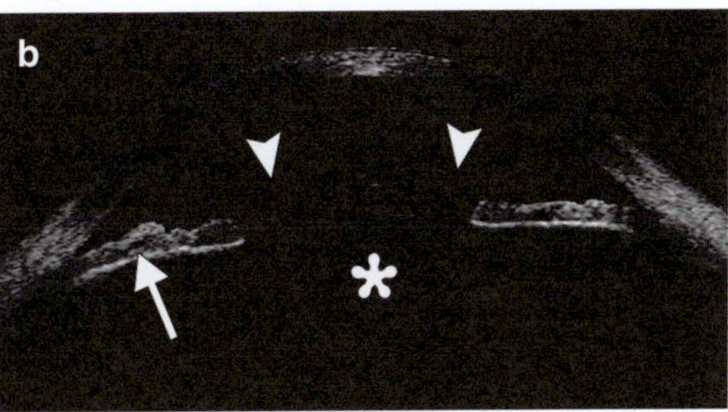

Fig. 3.8 PIOL implant. The patient has a history of high myopia treated with a Veriflex PIOL. Slit lamp photograph (**a**) shows the anterior chamber IOL implant with closed haptic loops that are fixated to the iris at approximately 3 and 9 o'clock positions (*arrowheads*). Anterior chamber OCT (**b**) shows the anterior chamber IOL implant (*arrowheads*), the insertion of the IOL in the iris (*arrow*), and the natural crystalline lens (*) (Courtesy of Rebecca Tudor)

term postoperative follow-up examinations, including imaging with OCT or UBM, are useful to monitor for and prevent complications.

3.5 Piggyback Intraocular Lens Implantation (Polypseudophakia)

The piggyback technique was first described by Gayton in 1993 and consists of implanting two or sometimes more intraocular lenses in one eye. The implants can be inserted together into the capsular bag, or the addition IOL implant can be positioned in the ciliary sulcus. The piggyback technique is indicated to treat high hyperopia (in which a single high-power IOL implant would not have provided sufficient power), pseudophakic refractive errors (using minus-power IOL implants, the technique can benefit even myopic pseudophakia), and to correct the often high refractive errors of pseudophakic-penetrating keratoplasty patients, for whom lens exchange presents even more risk. The increased depth of focus provided by piggyback IOL implants is attributable to a contact zone between the lenses. A unique complication of the piggyback IOL implants is interlenticular cellular growth with resultant hyperopic shift, opacification, and loss of vision. This tends to be a late complication

associated with IOL implants located together within the lens capsular bag and implants that are composed of hydrophobic acrylic. OCT, UBM, and Pentacam-Scheimpflug imaging can adequately delineate the components of piggyback IOL implants (Fig. 3.9).

3.6 Complications

Several complications related to cataract surgery and IOL implantation can be depicted on the various diagnostic imaging modalities. These include the presence of retained lens fragments, IOL implant dislocation, formation of dystrophic calcifications associated with IOL implants, and bullous keratopathy. Some of these complications can lead to additional morbidity and prompt diagnosis through the use of imaging, and clinical examination can optimize patient outcome.

3.6.1 Retained Lens Fragments

Although the lens nucleus is readily fragmented and aspirated using modern phacoemulsification technique, complete removal of the lens cortex can be difficult in certain patients without undue complications (e.g., rupture of the posterior capsular bag and vitreous loss). Retained lens fragments

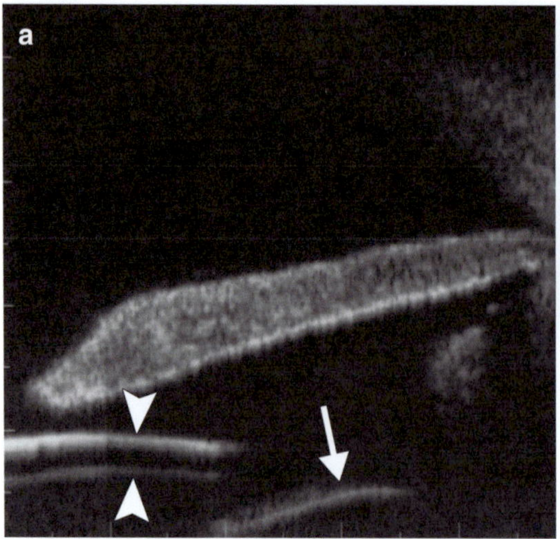

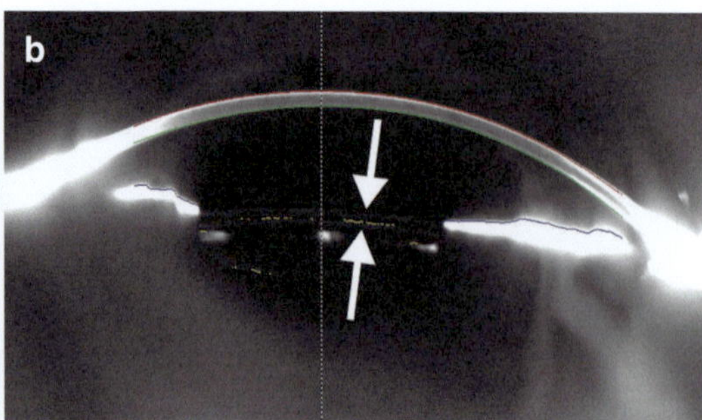

Fig. 3.9 Piggyback intraocular lens implantation. UBM image (**a**) shows two stacked IOL implants within the ciliary sulcus (*arrowheads*). The capsular bag (*arrow*) is located posterior to the implants. Pentacam-Scheimpflug image (**b**) also shows the two piggyback IOL implants in position (*arrows*) (Courtesy of Michael Amon MD)

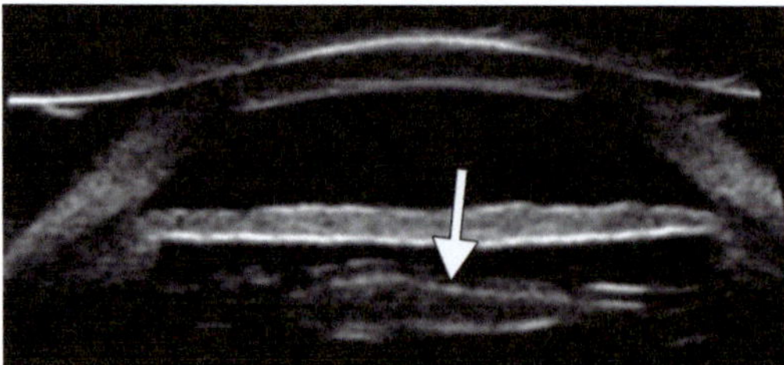

Fig. 3.10 Residual lens cortex in the anterior segment. UBM image of residual echogenic lens cortex peripherally (*arrow*) under the iris (Courtesy of Karen Capaccioli and Lois Hart)

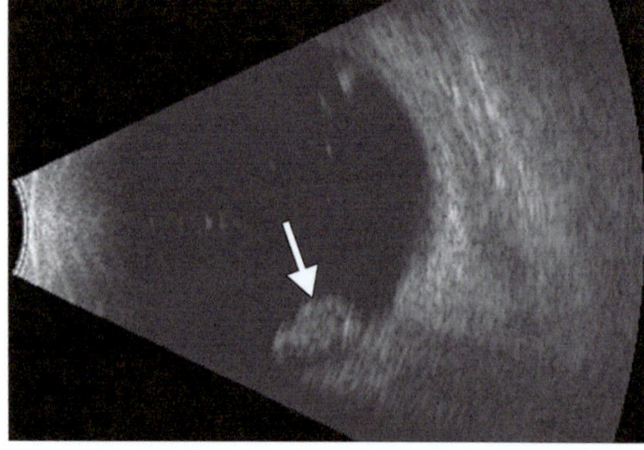

Fig. 3.11 Residual lens cortex in the vitreous body. B-scan ultrasound image demonstrates the detached echogenic residual lens cortex in the vitreous cavity (*arrow*) (Courtesy of Karen Capaccioli and Lois Hart)

in the peripheral anterior segment can result in inflammation and glaucoma and are best delineated via OCT or UBM (Fig. 3.10). In patients that do not respond to topical or oral medications, additional anterior segment surgery to remove retained lens fragments may be necessary. If a rupture of the posterior capsule occurs, then nuclear or cortical fragments may fall into the vitreous cavity. This phenomenon can often be adequately depicted on B-mode ultrasound, in which there is echogenic material present within the otherwise anechoic or hypoechoic vitreous (Fig. 3.11). The incidence of posteriorly displaced lens fragments ranges between 0.3 and 1.1 %. These fragments can be removed with pars plana vitrectomy.

3.6.2 IOL Implant Dislocation

Implant dislocation may occur in the absence of appropriate capsular or zonular support or following traumatic injury to anterior ocular tissues and can be characterized as either in the bag or out of the bag, with correspondingly different etiologies. The most common in-the-bag etiologies are pseudoexfoliation and prior vitreoretinal surgery. The most common out-of-the-bag etiology is capsular rupture during cataract surgery.

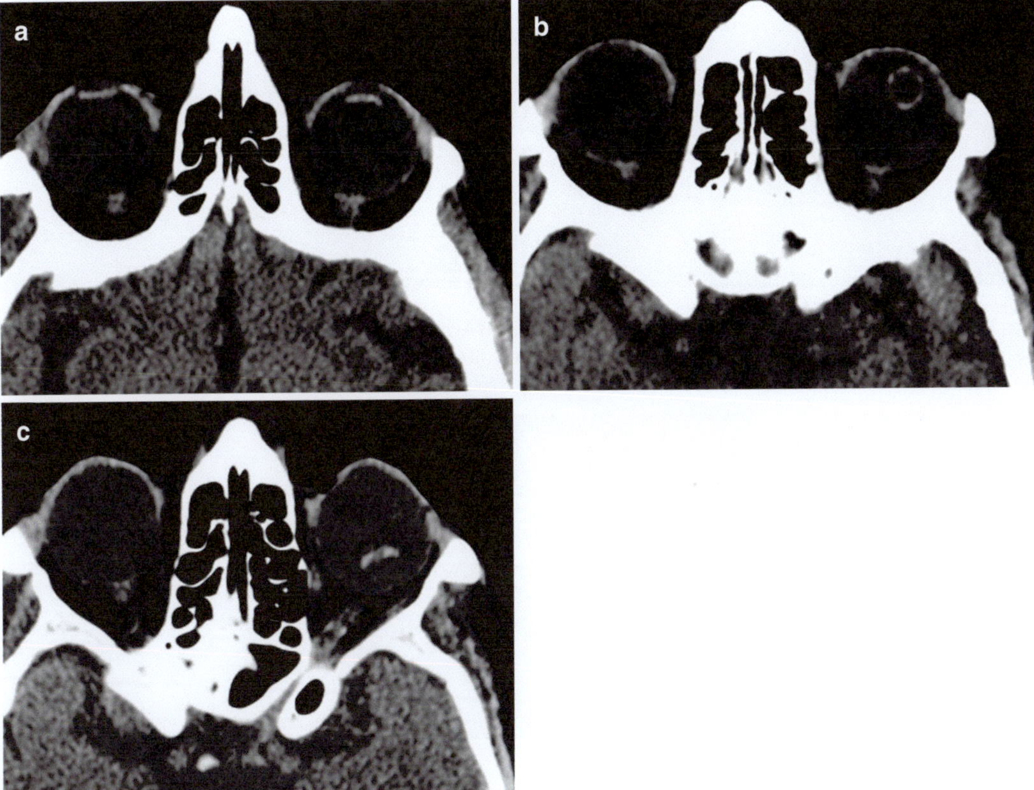

Fig. 3.12 IOL implant dislocation depicted on CT. Sequential axial CT images show initial slight tilting of the left lens implant within the anterior segment (**a**), followed by partial detachment and subluxation into the vitreous cavity with presumed residual fixation by one of the haptics (**b**), and finally complete posterior dislocation dependently into the vitreous (**c**)

Retinal detachment is an important comorbidity associated with dislocated IOLs, affecting approximately 6 % of cases. Both MRI and CT scan depict gross displacement of the dislocated IOL implant (Fig. 3.12). These modalities may be obtained to rule out etiologies for patients who present with "vision changes" that are not necessarily related to the IOL implant, such as stroke or tumor along the visual pathway, and implant dislocation may be incidentally discovered on these exams. However B-mode ultrasound may be more appropriate for dedicated evaluation of distant out-of-the-bag implant dislocation and the condition of the retina (Fig. 3.13). UBM and OCT are valuable tools for more subtle changes in implant positioning in the anterior segment,

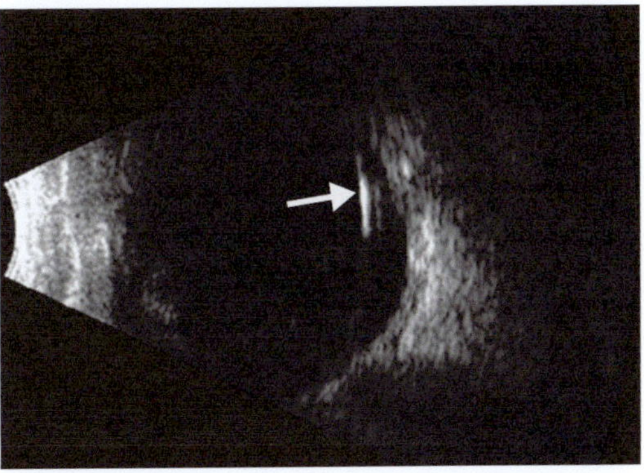

Fig. 3.13 Intraocular lens implant dislocation depicted on ultrasound. The B-scan ultrasound shows the dislocated IOL (*arrow*) in the vitreous cavity, adjacent to the retina

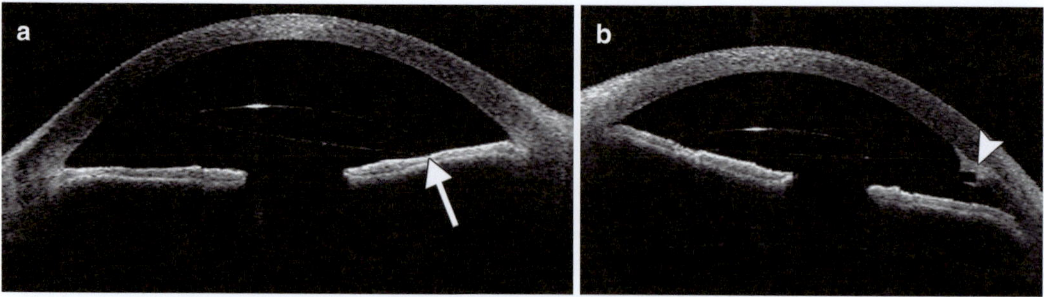

Fig. 3.14 Anterior segment OCT images (**a**, **b**) showing a tilted ACIOL with one haptic rubbing against the iris nasally (*arrow*), and the other haptic fibrosed in the cornea temporally (*arrowhead*)

Fig. 3.15 IOL eroding the iris. Anterior OCT image shows the haptic of a three-piece intraocular lens has penetrated through the iris (*arrow*) from the ciliary sulcus

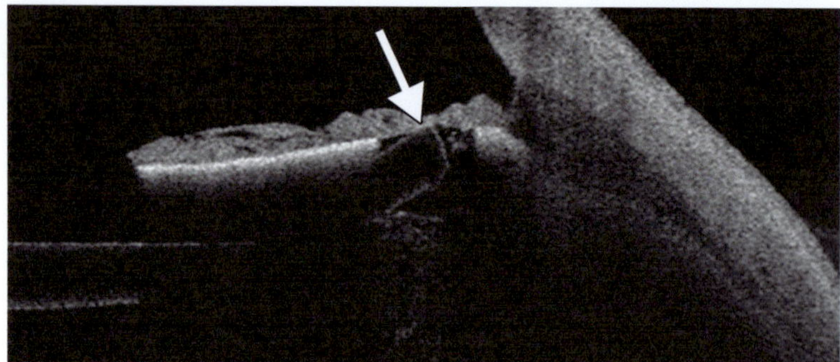

providing the necessary visualization of the errant optic and haptic components and affected surrounding soft tissues. For example, slightly subluxated or tilted implants within the anterior segment can cause inflammation and even perforation of the iris as well as scarring of the cornea if these structures are chronically impacted by the implant. These changes can be depicted on UBM and OCT (Figs. 3.14 and 3.15). Furthermore, UBM and OCT are useful for confirming the presence of haptic-induced uveitis-glaucoma-hyphema syndrome, which can otherwise be difficult to evaluate on direct slit lamp evaluation due to opacification of the anterior chamber (Fig. 3.16). In particular, the offending haptic can be in contact with the iris pigment epithelium, the pars plicata, or have prolapsed into the angle recess near a filtration bleb internal ostium. Alternatively, while the haptic portion of the implant may not be obviously in contact with the affected iris or cornea at the moment of imaging, the presence of malalignment may serve as sufficient evidence, since the implant may still be freely mobile.

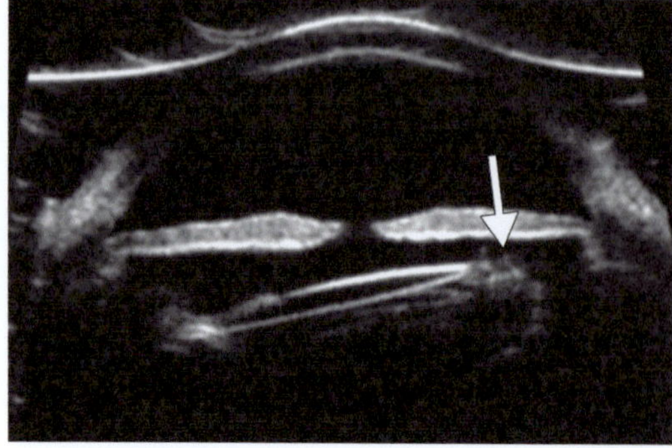

Fig. 3.16 Haptic-induced uveitis-glaucoma-hyphema syndrome. UBM shows a tilted posterior chamber IOL implant. The patient presented with recurrent hyphema due to rubbing of the lens haptic against the posterior surface of the iris (*arrow*), although no hyphema is apparent on the scan (Courtesy of Karen Capaccioli and Lois Hart)

3.6.3 Dystrophic IOL Implant Calcifications

Deposition of calcium hydroxyapatite crystals on IOL implants is a potential early or late complication of phakic cataract surgery, including

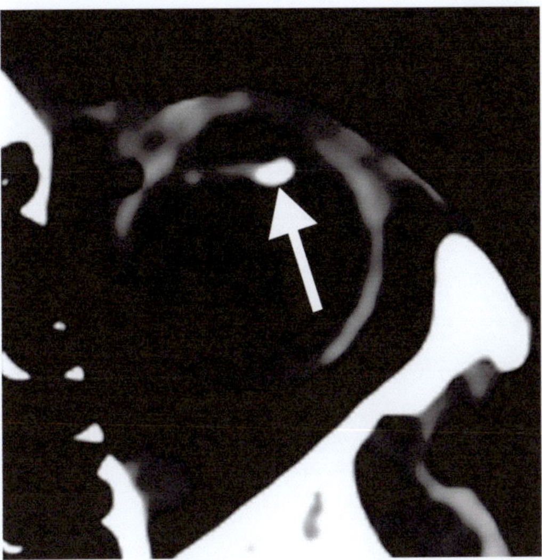

Fig. 3.17 Intraocular lens implant dystrophic calcification. Axial CT image shows a hyperattenuating focus attached to the surface of the left IOL implant (*arrow*)

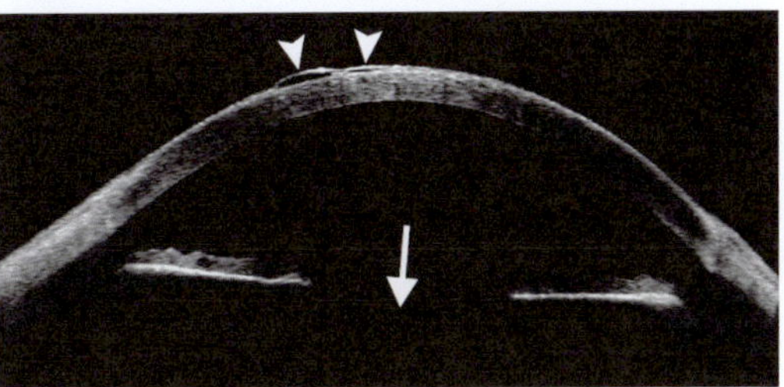

Fig. 3.18 Pseudophakic bullous keratopathy. Anterior segment OCT image shows that the bullous changes on the surface of the cornea appear as hyporeflective areas with minimal distortion (*arrowheads*). The anterior surface of the posterior chamber IOL is clearly depicted (*arrow*) (Courtesy of Amin Ashrafzadeh MD)

plastic and hydrogel implants. The calcifications can form on the surface of any or all portions of the IOL implants. When the granules are sufficiently large, these can be detected on orbital CT as punctate or linear hyperattenuating foci associated with the IOL implant (Fig. 3.17). The deposits can be sequestered by the posterior capsule and can undermine visual acuity. Although the exact mechanism of calcification remains elusive, there is histopathologic and transmission electron microscopic evidence that cell-mediated dystrophic calcification and the phosphate components used in the viscoelastic preparations to buffer the solution may be responsible.

3.6.4 Pseudophakic Bullous Keratopathy

The older closed-loop anterior chamber lenses are associated with a high incidence of bullous keratopathy due to corneal endothelial dysfunction and decompensation. UBM and OCT can demonstrate corneal thickening due to the presence of edema and bullae (Fig. 3.18). Ulcerative keratitis develops in approximately 5 % of patients with bullous keratopathy, which may require corneal transplantation. The newer

open-loop lenses have a much lower incidence of these complications.

3.6.5 Anterior Capsular Contraction Syndrome

Anterior capsular (capsulorrhexis) contraction syndrome is characterized by a progressive reduction in the diameter of the anterior capsulotomy after intraocular lens implantation surgery that results from fibrosis and phimosis. The complication is associated with small diameter capsulorrhexis and can lead to displacement or dislocation of the intraocular lens implants and decreased visual acuity. On ultrasound, the fibrous tissue responsible for anterior capsular contraction syndrome appears as a mildly echogenic membrane along the anterior aspect of the implant (Fig. 3.19). B-mode ultrasound is also useful for measuring the decrease in continuous curvilinear capsulorrhexis size and demonstrating changes in the intraocular lens implant position.

3.7 Summary

- Cataract surgery is commonly performed, and the resulting changes are often encountered on the various diagnostic imaging modalities.
- Likewise, intraocular lens implants are routinely used in the treatment of cataracts or to treat refractive disorders.

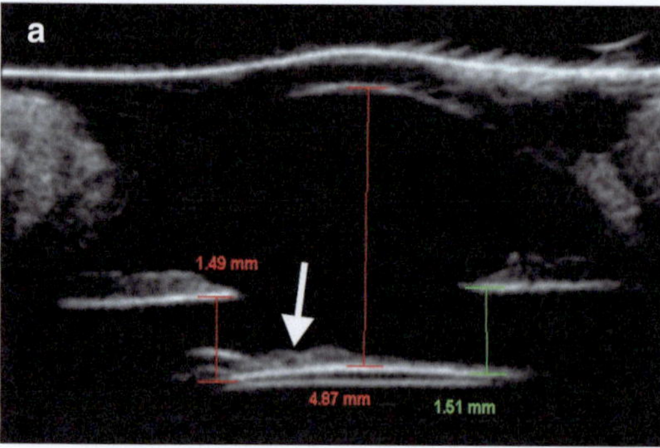

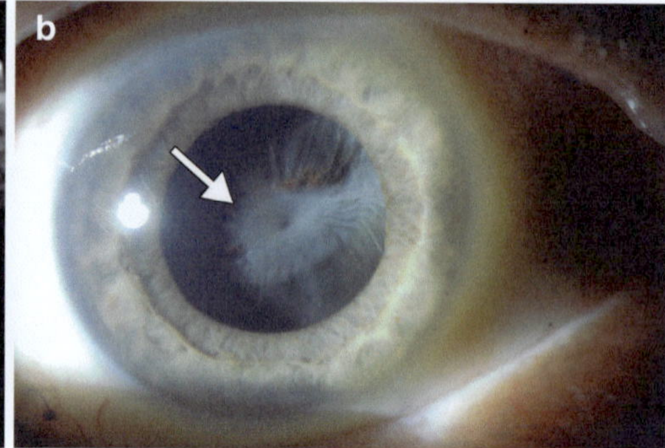

Fig. 3.19 Anterior capsular contraction syndrome. B-mode ultrasound image (**a**) shows a mildly echogenic membrane along the anterior surface of a portion of the intraocular lens implant (*arrow*) with associated slight tilting of the implant. Clinical photograph (**b**) shows the anterior capsule has contracted over the lens, resulting in a streaky opacity (*arrow*)

- Familiarity with the various procedures and corresponding diagnostic imaging findings pertaining to intraocular lens removal and implantation is important, whether they are incidental or specifically intended for guiding management.
- Although the effects of lens extraction and implantation are grossly discernable on CT and MRI, high-resolution imaging techniques such as UBM and OCT are best suited for more precise and dedicated postoperative assessment.

Further Reading

Aksoy FG, Gomori JM, Halpert M. CT and MR imaging of contact lenses and intraocular lens implants. Comput Med Imaging Graph. 1999;23(4):205–8.

Amon M. Enhancement of refractive results after cataract surgery and IOL-implantation with a supplementary IOL implanted in the ciliary sulcus. Oftalmologia. 2009;53(4):91–5.

Bergman M, Laatikainen L. Long-term evaluation of primary anterior chamber intraocular lens implantation in complicated cataract surgery. Int Ophthalmol. 1996–1997;20(6):295–9.

Bucher PJ, Büchi ER, Daicker BC. Dystrophic calcification of an implanted hydroxyethylmethacrylate intraocular lens. Arch Ophthalmol. 1995;113(11):1431–5.

Calladine D, Evans JR, Shah S, Leyland M. Multifocal versus monofocal intraocular lenses after cataract extraction. Cochrane Database Syst Rev. 2012;9, CD003169.

Campo RV, Chung KD, Oyakwa RT. Pars plana vitrectomy in the management of dislocated posterior chamber lenses. Am J Ophthalmol. 1989;108:529–33.

Carlson AN, Stewart WC, Tso PC. Intraocular lens complications requiring removal or exchange. Surv Ophthalmol. 1998;42(5):417–40.

Chan CK, Agarwal A, Agarwal S, Agarwal A. Management of dislocated intraocular implants. Ophthalmol Clin North Am. 2001;14(4):681–93.

Chang SH, Lim G. Secondary pigmentary glaucoma associated with piggyback intraocular lens implantation. J Cataract Refract Surg. 2004;30(10):2219–22.

Dick HB, Budo C, Malecaze F, Güell JL, Marinho AA, Nuijts RM, Luyten GP, Menezo JL, Kohnen T. Foldable Artiflex phakic intraocular lens for the correction of myopia: two-year follow-up results of a prospective European multicenter study. Ophthalmology. 2009;116(4):671–7.

Douglas MJ, Scott IU, Flynn Jr HW. Pars plana lensectomy, pars plana vitrectomy, and silicone oil tamponade as initial management of cataract and combined traction/rhegmatogenous retinal detachment involving the macula associated with severe proliferative diabetic retinopathy. Ophthalmic Surg Lasers Imaging. 2003;34(4):270–8.

Fenzl RE, Gills 3rd JP, Gills JP. Piggyback intraocular lens implantation. Curr Opin Ophthalmol. 2000;11(1):73–6.

Fernando GT, Crayford BB. Visually significant calcification of hydrogel intraocular lenses necessitating explantation. Clin Experiment Ophthalmol. 2000;28(4):280–6.

Garner A. Complications of prosthetic intraocular lens implantation: a histopathological study. Br J Ophthalmol. 1989;73(12):940–5.

Gui JM, Jia L, Liu L, Liu JD. Vitrectomy, lensectomy and silicone oil tamponade in the management of retinal detachment associated with choroidal detachment. Int J Ophthalmol. 2013;6(3):337–41.

Hayashi K, Hayashi H, Nakao F, Hayashi F. Anterior capsule contraction and intraocular lens decentration and tilt after hydrogel lens implantation. Br J Ophthalmol. 2001;85(11):1294–7.

Hayashi K, Hirata A, Hayashi H. Possible predisposing factors for in-the-bag and out-of-the-bag intraocular lens dislocation and outcomes of intraocular lens exchange surgery. Ophthalmology. 2007;114:969–75.

Health Quality Ontario. Phakic intraocular lenses for the treatment of refractive errors: an evidence-based analysis. Ont Health Technol Assess Ser. 2009;9(14):1–120. Epub 2009 Oct 1.

Huang D, Schallhorn SC, Sugar A, Farjo AA, Majmudar PA, Trattler WB, Tanzer DJ. Phakic intraocular lens implantation for the correction of myopia: a report by the American Academy of Ophthalmology. Ophthalmology. 2009;116(11):2244–58.

Izak AM, Werner L, Pandey SK, Apple DJ. Calcification of modern foldable hydrogel intraocular lens designs. Eye (Lond). 2003;17(3):393–406.

Kuo MD, Hayman LA, Lee AG, Mayo GL, Diaz-Marchan PJ. In vivo CT and MR appearance of prosthetic intraocular lens. AJNR Am J Neuroradiol. 1998;19(4):749–53.

Kurosaka D, Ando I, Kato K, Oshima T, Kurosaka H, Yoshino M, Nagamoto T, Ando N. Fibrous membrane formation at the capsular margin in capsule contraction syndrome. J Cataract Refract Surg. 1999;25(7):930–5.

Lima BR, Pichi F, Hayden BC, Lowder CY. Ultrasound biomicroscopy in chronic pseudophakic ocular inflammation associated with misplaced intraocular lens haptics. Am J Ophthalmol. 2014;157(4):813–817.e1.

Liu T, Xu Y, Sun D, Xie L. Histological evaluation of corneal scar formation in pseudophakic bullous keratopathy. PLoS One. 2012;7(6):e39201.

MacCumber MW, Packo KH, Civantos JM, Greenberg JB. Preservation of anterior capsule during vitrectomy and lensectomy for retinal detachment with proliferative vitreoretinopathy. Ophthalmology. 2002;109(2):329–33.

Mittra RA, Connor TB, Han DP, Koenig SB, Mieler WF, Pulido JS. Removal of dislocated intraocular lenses using pars plana vitrectomy with placement of an open-loop, flexible anterior chamber lens. Ophthalmology. 1998;105(6):1011–4.

Pereira FA, Cronemberger S. Ultrasound biomicroscopic study of anterior segment changes after phacoemulsification and foldable intraocular lens implantation. Ophthalmology. 2003;110(9):1799–806.

Piette S, Canlas OA, Tran HV, Ishikawa H, Liebmann JM, Ritch R. Ultrasound biomicroscopy in uveitis-glaucoma-hyphema syndrome. Am J Ophthalmol. 2002;133(6):839–41.

Pueringer SL, Hodge DO, Erie JC. Risk of late intraocular lens dislocation after cataract surgery, 1980–2009: a population-based study. Am J Ophthalmol. 2011;152(4):618–23.

Rosales P, Marcos S. Pentacam Scheimpflug quantitative imaging of the crystalline lens and intraocular lens. J Refract Surg. 2009;25(5):421–8.

Schaal S, Barr CC. Management of retained lens fragments after cataract surgery with and without pars plana vitrectomy. J Cataract Refract Surg. 2009;35(5):863–7.

Tahzib NG, Nuijts RM, Wu WY, Budo CJ. Long-term study of Artisan phakic intraocular lens implantation for the correction of moderate to high myopia: ten-year follow-up results. Ophthalmology. 2007;114:1133–42.

Taravati P, Lam DL, Leveque T, Van Gelder RN. Postcataract surgical inflammation. Curr Opin Ophthalmol. 2012;23(1):12–8.

The Infant Aphakia Treatment Study Group, Lambert SR, Lynn MJ, Hartmann EE, Dubois L, Drews-Botsch C, Freedman SF, Plager DA, Buckley EG, Wilson ME. Comparison of contact lens and intraocular lens correction of monocular aphakia during infancy: a randomized clinical trial of HOTV optotype acuity at age 4.5 years and clinical findings at age 5 years. JAMA Ophthalmol. 2014;132(6):676–82.

van Rijn GA, Mourik JE, Teeuwisse WM, Luyten GP, Webb AG. Magnetic resonance compatibility of intraocular lenses measured at 7 Tesla. Invest Ophthalmol Vis Sci. 2012;53(7):3449–53.

Werner L, Apple DJ, Escobar-Gomez M, Ohrstrom A, Crayford BB, Bianchi R, et al. Postoperative deposition of calcium on the surfaces of a hydrogel intraocular lens. Ophthalmology. 2000;107(12):2179–85.

Yong JL, Lertsumitkul S, Killingsworth MC, Filipic M. Calcification of intraocular hydrogel lens: evidence of dystrophic calcification. Clin Experiment Ophthalmol. 2004;32(5):492–500.

Ophthalmic Imaging and Neuroimaging of the Effects of Glaucoma Treatment

4

Daniel Thomas Ginat, Lili Farrokh-Siar, Fatoumata Yanoga, and Louis Pasquale

4.1 Overview

Glaucoma is a group of conditions that can lead to irreversible vision loss. There are many different types of glaucoma that can be broadly categorized into open-angle and closed-angle subtypes; these subtypes can be further stratified into primary and secondary types. Primary open-angle glaucoma is the most common type of glaucoma in the United States and is a diagnosis considered in the context of unremarkable gonioscopic findings, no apparent slit lamp biomicroscopic abnormalities, and glaucomatous optic disk cupping, accompanied by visual field loss localizing to the nerve fiber layer. On the other hand, primary closed-angle glaucoma results from obstruction of aqueous humor flow through the pupil into the anterior

D.T. Ginat, MD, MS (✉)
Director of Head and Neck Imaging,
Department of Radiology, University of Chicago,
5841 S Maryland Avenue, Chicago, IL 60637, USA
e-mail: ginatd01@gmail.com

L. Farrokh-Siar, MD
Department of Ophthalmology,
Illinois Glaucoma Center, Chicago, IL USA

F. Yanoga, MD
Department of Ophthalmology,
University of Chicago, Chicago, IL USA

L. Pasquale, MD
Department of Ophthalmology, Massachusetts Eye
and Ear Infirmary, Boston, MA, USA

Division of Network Medicine, Brigham
and Women's Hospital, Boston, MA, USA

chamber (pupillary block), which increases the pressure behind the iris and forces the iris anteriorly to occlude the anterior chamber angle. Secondary forms of glaucoma are caused by various ocular or systemic diseases, such as uveitis, corticosteroid use, lens dislocation or swelling, pigment dispersion syndrome, and intraocular hemorrhage. Chronic glaucoma affects the anterior visual pathway up to the optic chiasm and radiations and beyond, which manifests as volume loss and T2 hyperintensity on MRI (Fig. 4.1). These changes correlate with optic nerve damage, and MRI of the visual pathway may be useful for evaluating glaucomatous damage.

Numerous medical, laser, and surgical options are available for treating the various forms of glaucoma. Occasionally, B-scan ultrasound and ultrasound biomicroscopy can play a role in the diagnosis and follow-up of angle closure glaucoma, particularly when the mechanism of angle closure is called into question or gonioscopic findings are equivocal. Diagnostic imaging also serves a role in the post-therapeutic setting. B-mode ultrasound, CT, and MRI can depict certain glaucoma drainage implants, which may be encountered incidentally and should be appropriately recognized. In addition, these modalities can provide insight into the function of implants and are useful for the evaluation of certain complications, such as infection, hemorrhage, and device malposition, and to assess for the presence of underlying lesions that may be responsible for postoperative proptosis and ocular dysmotility.

D.T. Ginat, S.K. Freitag (eds.), *Post-treatment Imaging of the Orbit*,
DOI 10.1007/978-3-662-44023-0_4, © Springer-Verlag Berlin Heidelberg 2015

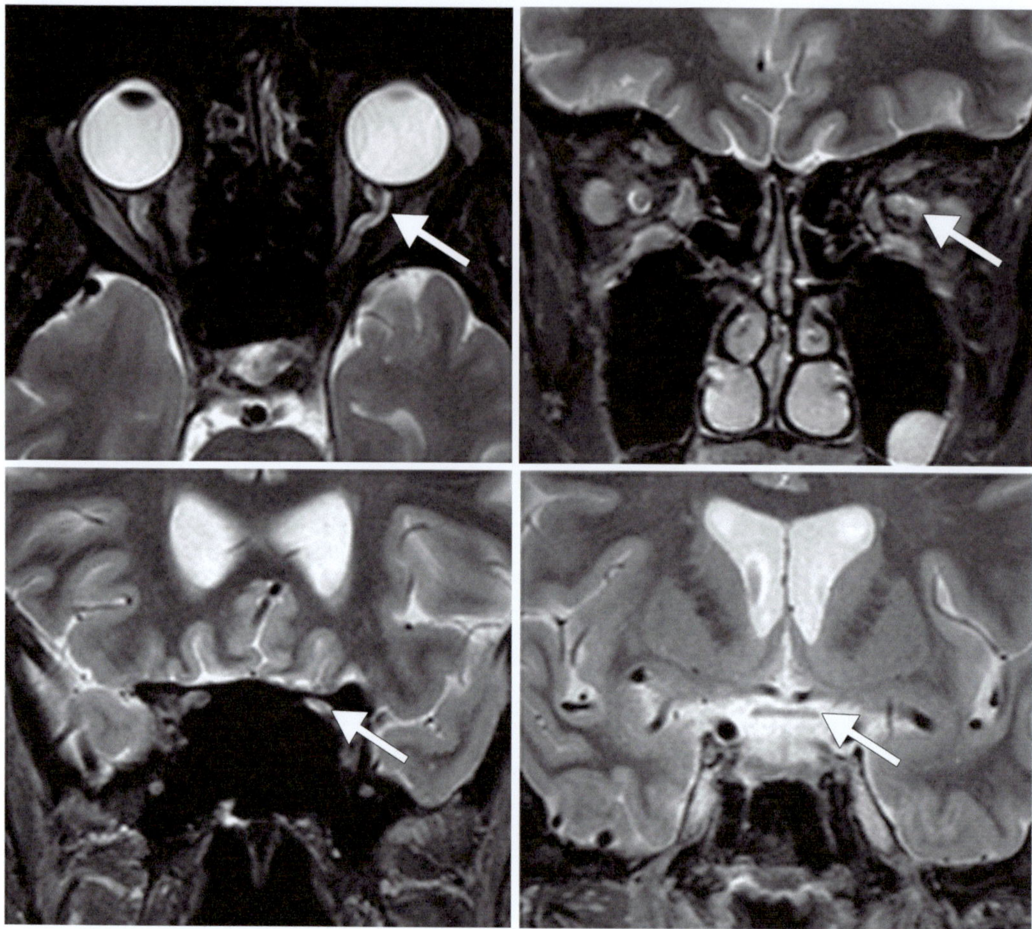

Fig. 4.1 Optic nerve and chiasm changes in chronic glaucoma. The patient has a history of long-standing normal tension glaucoma, left greater than right, treated with multiple topical medications. Axial (**a**) and coronal (**b–d**) T2-weighted MR images show diffuse optic nerve atrophy and hyperintensity as well as also atrophy of the optic chiasm, particularly on the left (*arrows*)

However, B-mode ultrasound, CT, and MRI have limited capacity for delineating the minute alterations of the fine anterior segment structures. When these structures must be assessed with adjunctive imaging, for which OCT and UBM are recommended. The particular indications for imaging and corresponding findings are described in further detail in the subsequent sections.

4.2 Pharmacological Management

Medical or pharmacological treatment is directed toward lowering intraocular pressure, which has been demonstrated to protect against further damage to the optic nerve head. Pharmaceuticals can decrease intraocular pressure by decreasing the production of aqueous humor by the ciliary body or by increasing the outflow through the trabecular meshwork or through the uveoscleral pathway. There are five major classes of drugs used for the long-term management of glaucoma: β-adrenergic antagonists, prostaglandin analogs, α-adrenergic agonists, carbonic anhydrase inhibitors, and cholinergic agonists. Conventional first-line treatment of glaucoma usually consists of a topical selective or non-selective β-blocker or a topical prostaglandin analog. Second-line drugs include α-agonists

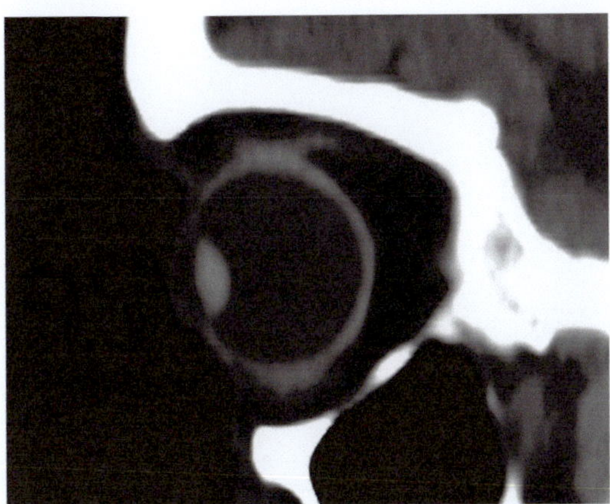

Fig. 4.2 Prostaglandin-associated periorbitopathy. The patient has a long history of topical prostaglandin use and displays upper lid ptosis and enophthalmos on exam. Sagittal CT image shows deepening of the upper eyelid sulcus, loss of the inferior orbital fat pads, and enophthalmos

and topical carbonic anhydrase inhibitors. Parasympathomimetic agents, most commonly pilocarpine, are considered third-line treatment options. Hyperosmotic agents such as glycerol, isosorbide, and mannitol can be administered to lower intraocular pressure from very high levels in emergency situations, but not for long-term management. The effects of cholinergic inhibitors can be discerned on UBM or OCT, whereby successful therapy results in an observable increase in size of the aqueous outflow pathway, due to pupillary constriction. Topical prostaglandin analogs can also result in changes that are visible on diagnostic imaging, in the form of prostaglandin-associated periorbitopathy. This condition consists of atrophy of orbital and periorbital fat associated with enophthalmos due to inhibition of adipogenesis through FP receptor stimulation. Prostaglandin–associated perioribitopathy is fairly common with an incidence of 70 to over 90 %, depending upon the particular analog that is used. Orbit/maxillofacial CT or MRI can be used to depict the decreased orbital and periorbital fat volume without inflammatory changes (Fig. 4.2), which is particularly evident if the process is unilateral, and to exclude other conditions that may result in enophthalmos, such as silent sinus syndrome.

4.3 Iridectomy and Laser Peripheral Iridotomy (LPI)

Surgical iridectomy and laser peripheral iridotomy (LPI) are procedures designed to minimize pupillary block, reduce peripheral iris-trabecular meshwork contact, and promote aqueous humor egress from the eye. Thus, these procedures are indicated for patients with acute-angle-closure glaucoma with pupillary block, although the LPI has largely supplanted surgical iridectomy but may be used in cases in which laser iridotomy fails. Alternatively, laser peripheral iridoplasty can be performed, which results in thinning of the peripheral iris, allowing for more aqueous humor exposure to contact the trabecular meshwork. Laser peripheral iridoplasty can be used for a crisis of acute angle closure and also in non-acute situations where there is residual angle closure despite a patent LPI. LPI can be performed using either Nd:YAG, argon laser, or both lasers in combination to create an opening that is usually 150–200 μm wide, which can be discerned by retroilluminating the iris using slit lamp biomicroscopy. In addition, the anterior chamber depth typically increases and the filtration angle widens following iridotomy, which can be measured on UBM or OCT (Fig. 4.3). UBM or OCT may also be obtained following LPI in order to evaluate residual angle closure. Several conditions can result in residual angle closure, such as plateau iris syndrome, pseudo-plateau iris syndrome, lens swelling, and failure to attain patency of an iridotomy. Plateau iris syndrome consists of angle closure due to anterior displacement of the peripheral iris despite an otherwise patent iridotomy. The ciliary body is rotated forward producing obliteration of the ciliary sulcus, resulting in an S-like morphology of the iris (Fig. 4.4). Pseudo-plateau iris syndrome is related to the presence of ciliary body or iris cysts which may not be readily apparent on slit lamp exam but can also produce angle closure. The formation of cystic and sheet-like epithelial invasion after surgical penetration of the anterior segment is rare. These lesions are best delineated on OCT or UBM (Fig. 4.5).

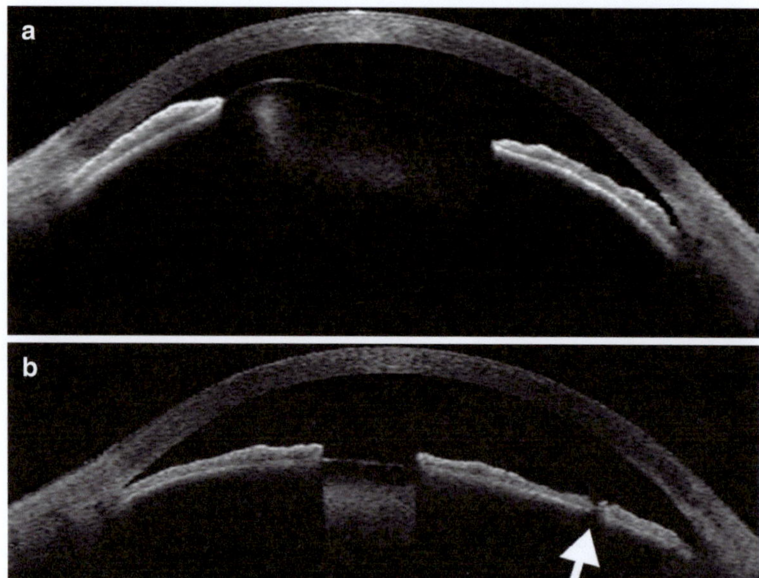

Fig. 4.3 Peripheral laser iridotomy. The patient incurred blunt trauma to the eye. Anterior segment OCT (**a**) shows anterior dislocation of the crystalline lens, which resulted in pupillary block angle-closure glaucoma. Following peripheral laser iridotomy, OCT (**b**) shows a patent peripheral iridotomy (*arrow*) and the deeper anterior chamber

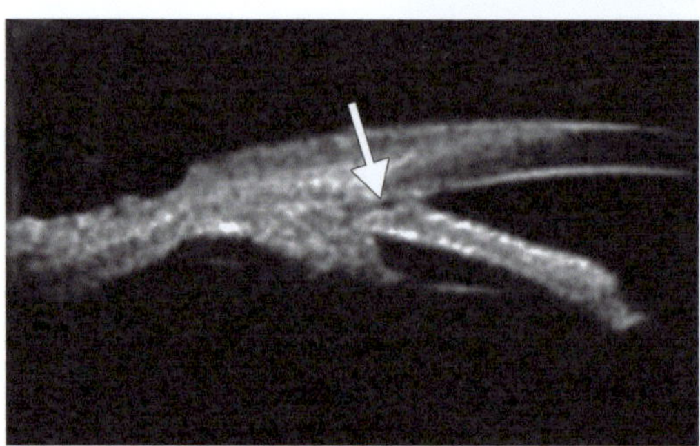

Fig. 4.4 Plateau iris syndrome. UBM shows anterior displacement of the lateral aspect of the iris at the site of iridotomy (*arrow*), where it blocks the canal of Schlemm

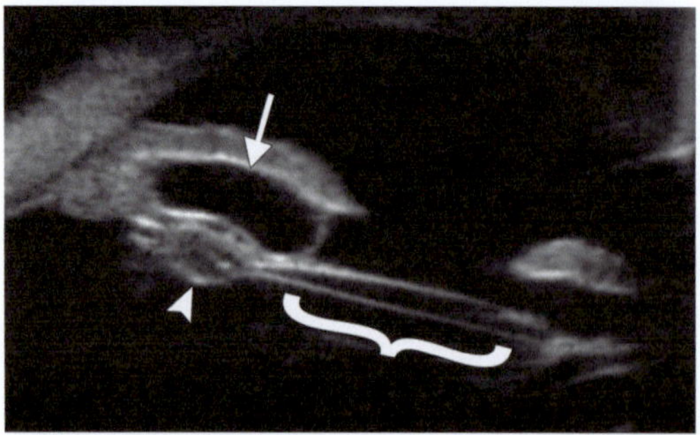

Fig. 4.5 Iris cyst. UBM shows an anechoic ovoid structure in the anterior chamber (*arrow*), obstructing the canal of Schlemm. An intraocular lens implant (*bracket*) is present and there is also retained intraocular lens cortical material (*arrowhead*) (Courtesy of Karen Capaccioli and Lois Hart)

4.4 Filtering Microsurgery (Trabeculectomy)

Trabeculectomy is often considered for patients who have failed laser surgery or pharmacotherapy. The procedure consists of creating a partial thickness scleral flap and removing an inner block of underlying corneal-scleral tissue, which typically includes trabecular tissue. In order to retain an opening (sclerostomy) from the anterior chamber to the subconjunctival space, a surgical iridectomy is typically performed to prevent peripheral iris prolapse into the sclerostomy. Subsequently, the scleral flap is sutured down over the sclerostomy at a desired tension to control the rate of outflow. Finally, the scleral wound is covered by conjunctiva and sutured tightly such that aqueous humor egress across the partial thickness sclerostomy is retained in the subconjunctival space creating a filtration bleb, which appears anechoic or hyporeflective on UBM and OCT, respectively. While tonometry provides an assessment of whether trabeculectomy is functioning, anterior segment imaging via OCT and UBM can provide a detailed assessment of the altered anterior ocular anatomy after trabeculectomy. In particular, the

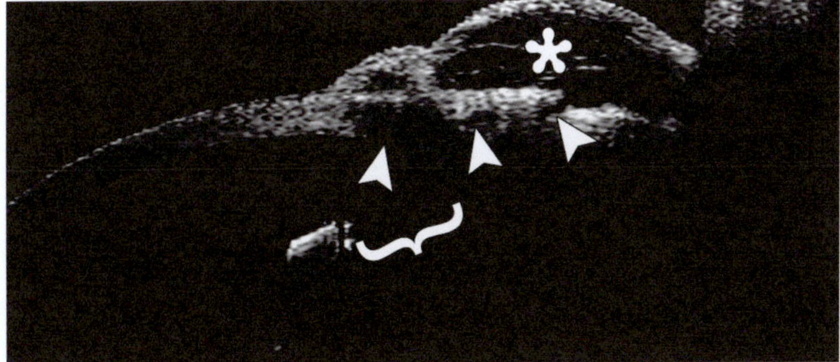

Fig. 4.6 Trabeculectomy. Anterior segment OCT shows the peripheral iridectomy (*bracket*), the sclerostomy site with fluid under the scleral flap (*arrowheads*), and the elevated conjunctival filtering bleb (*)

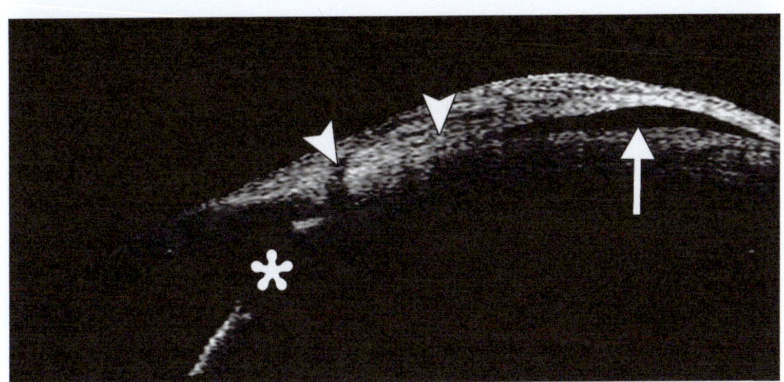

Fig. 4.7 Failed bleb after trabeculectomy. OCT image shows that the iridectomy site is patent (*), but there is scarring of the conjunctiva and Tenon's down to the sclera (*arrowheads*), and the bleb is flattened (*arrow*)

peripheral iridectomy and the sclerostomy site with fluid under the scleral flap can be delineated on UBM and OCT (Fig. 4.6). Bleb wall anatomy is better assessed by OCT, while in evaluating deeper structures, UBM is more effective. Due to its noncontact nature, OCT is particularly useful in the early postoperative stage. Furthermore, OCT can demonstrate features of bleb morphology that are not visible with the slit lamp examination. In particular, with respect to the appearance of blebs on imaging, two phenomena occur during the early post-trabeculectomy period in successful filtering operations: shading and stripping. With the shading phenomenon, there is poor visibility of sclera beneath the bleb. This decrease in visibility represents an increased diffuse water content commonly associated with successful filters. On the other hand, with the stripping phenomenon, there are multiple parallel hyporeflective layers or strips inside the Tenon's capsule surrounded by hyperreflective areas representing fluid-filled channels with fine connective tissue septa. "Stripping" may indicate the presence of multiple drainage channels in successful filters.

A major complication of trabeculectomy is scarring at the level of the conjunctiva–Tenon's–episcleral interface, the scleral flap, the overlying episclera, or the internal ostium. This is often associated with reduction in size or absence of the bleb and effacement of the aqueous drainage pathway on imaging (Fig. 4.7). There are several options for minimizing the risk of scarring after trabeculectomy, including the use of mitomycin C (MMC) and collagen matrix implants. MMC is an antimetabolite used intraoperatively during trabeculectomy in order to prevent excessive postoperative scarring and thus reduce the risk of failure. Porous biodegradable collagen matrix implants, such as Ologen, may serve as an alternative to traditional antimetabolites such as mitomycin C and 5-fluorouracil in glaucoma filtration procedures. New blebs tend to contain microcysts that indicate the presence of aqueous flow channels, while older blebs tend to contain macrocysts with thin septations. In addition, older blebs associated with the use of antimetabolic agents tend to form avascular areas with thinning of the overlying conjunctiva (Fig. 4.8). The use of Ologen implants may result in fewer side effects.

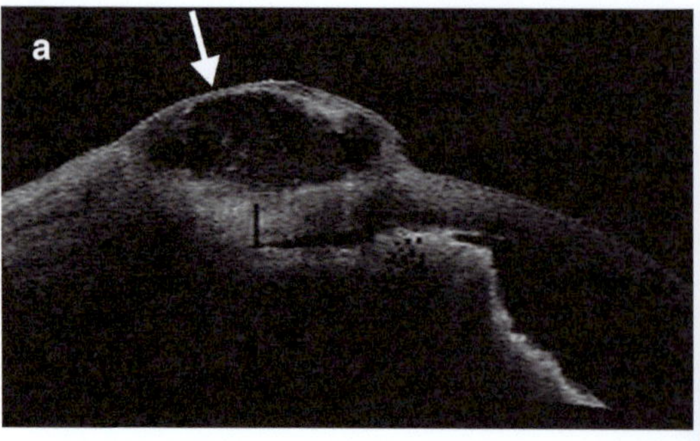

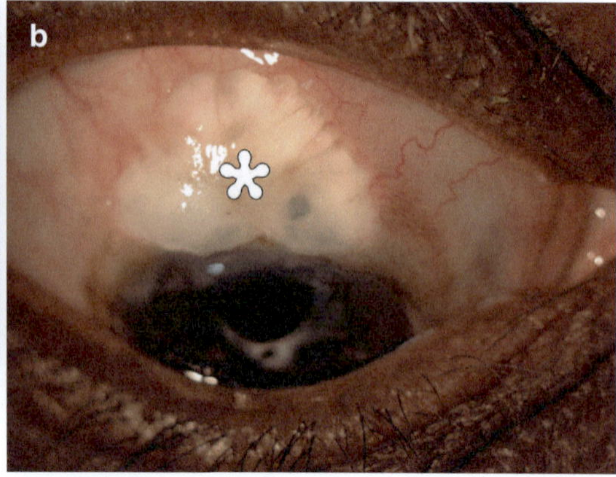

Fig. 4.8 Trabeculectomy with MMC and avascular macrocystic bleb. Anterior segment OCT (**a**) shows thinning of the conjunctiva overlying the bleb (*arrow*), which contains scattered thin hyperreflective septations. The corresponding clinical photograph (**b**) shows decreased vascularity in the conjunctiva overlying the bleb (*) (Courtesy of Rebecca Tudor)

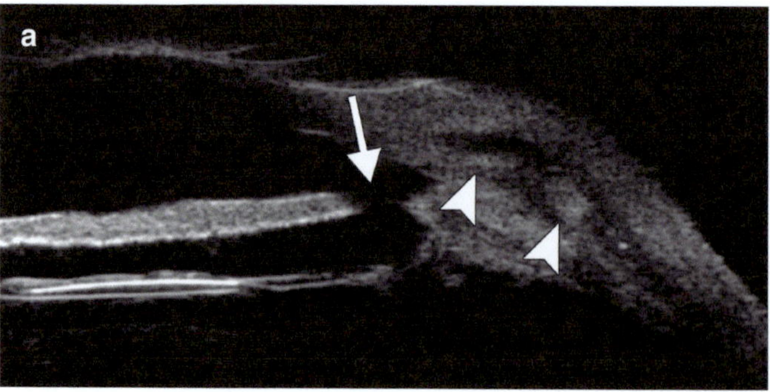

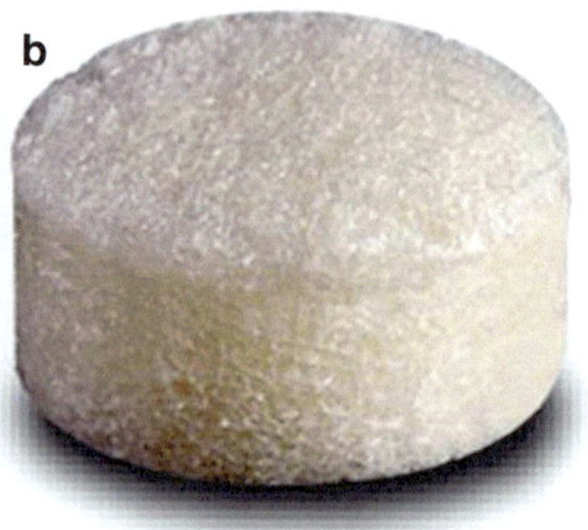

Fig. 4.9 Bleb revision with collagen matrix implant (Ologen). Anterior segment UBM (**a**) shows a patent surgical iridectomy (*arrow*) and an elevated filtrating bleb containing the collagen matrix (*arrowheads*). An intraocular lens implant is also present. Photograph of the Ologen Collagen Matrix (**b**) (Courtesy of Kestrel Ophthalmics)

Ologen is designed to minimize scar formation by dissipating the fibroblasts, which randomly proliferate throughout the matrix pores. During the early postoperative period, the bleb is relatively prominent due to the space occupied by the collagen matrix implant, which can be discerned as a spongy appearing echogenic structure on UBM (Fig. 4.9).

A flat anterior chamber can result from overfiltration in the early postoperative period after trabeculectomy. This complication is usually attributable to decreased resistance to aqueous outflow through the sclera with resultant hypotony. It may be associated with the development of a choroidal effusion that may further decrease aqueous fluid formation. Left untreated, a flat anterior chamber may lead to secondary complications, including synechiae, cataract progression, and corneal endothelial decompensation. Detailed delineation of a shallow anterior chamber via OCT enables accurate measurements of the anterior chamber depth to be obtained, without applying pressure to the globe (Fig. 4.10). The normal depth of the anterior chamber is 3.13 ± 0.34 mm in women and 3.27 ± 0.28 mm in men.

Another rare complication of trabeculectomy is the formation of an overhanging cystic bleb, which lies on the surface of Bowman's layer of the cornea and is covered by conjunctival epithelium. UBM or OCT often reveals multiple loculations with

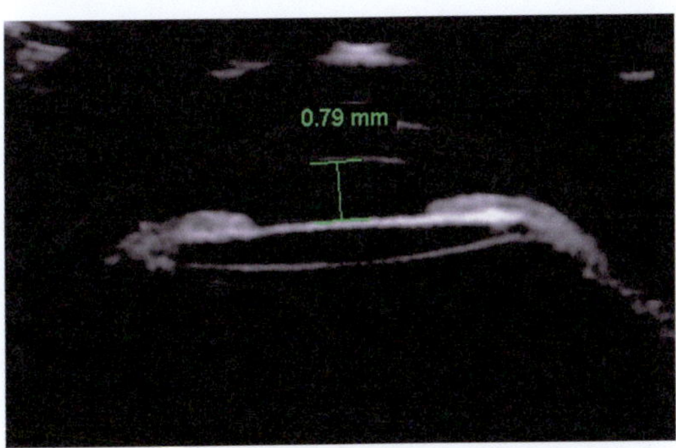

Fig. 4.10 Shallow anterior chamber. UBM shows an anterior chamber with central depth of 0.79 mm. An intraocular lens implant is also present (Courtesy of Karen Capaccioli and Lois Hart)

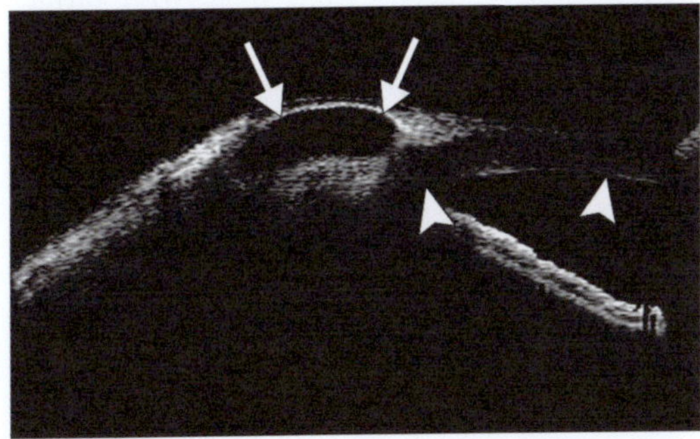

Fig. 4.11 Overhanging cystic bleb. The anterior segment OCT image shows a hypoechoic cystic bleb (*arrows*) that extends over the surface of the cornea (*arrowheads*)

thin septa inside the bleb (Fig. 4.11). Indications for intervention include overfiltration leading to hypotony, foreign body sensation, lid retraction, lagophthalmos, and compromised visual acuity.

4.5 Nonpenetrating Deep Sclerectomy

Nonpenetrating deep sclerectomy is a filtering surgery that is indicated to reduce the incidence of the postoperative complications encountered with the penetrating surgeries and is indicated for most of glaucoma (primary open-angle glaucoma, pseudoexfoliative glaucoma, pigmentary glaucoma, glaucoma associated with myopia, aphakic glaucoma, pseudophakic glaucoma, open-angle uveitic glaucoma, normal-tension

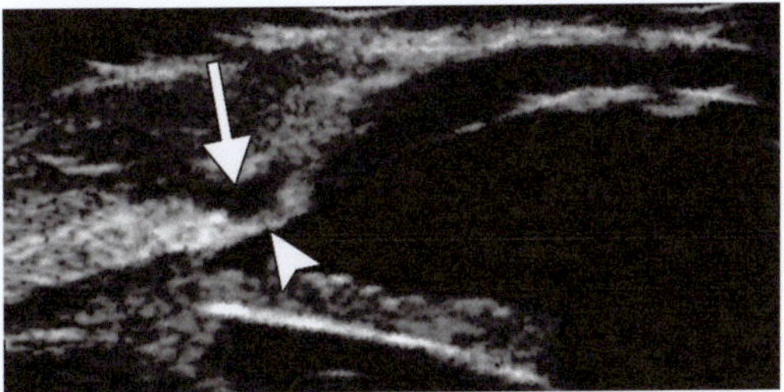

Fig. 4.12 Nonpenetrating deep sclerectomy. UBM shows the trabeculocorneal membrane (*arrowhead*) and the intrascleral lake of fluid (*arrow*) (Courtesy of Paul Harasymowycz MD)

glaucoma, and steroid-induced glaucoma), except angle closure and neovascular cases. The procedure consists of dissecting the conjunctiva and Tenon's capsule and creating a limbus-based superficial scleral flap. A deeper scleral flap is dissected and the roof of Schlemm's canal is removed. A space maintainer, such as a cylindrical collagen implant measuring 4 mm in length for a 0.5 mm diameter, is inserted, and the flap and conjunctiva are closed. Other space maintainer materials may include viscoelastics, HEMA (hydroxyethylmethacrylate), high reticulated hyaluronic acid, and polymethyl methacrylate (PMMA). Ultimately, the deep sclerectomy procedure creates a new outflow pathway for the drainage of the aqueous humor through the thin remaining trabeculo-Descemet's membrane into the intrascleral reservoir without even entering the anterior chamber. The trabeculo-Descemet's membrane prevents overfiltration and ensures a reproducible postoperative intraocular pressure. In addition, the presence of an intrascleral filtering space decreases the reliance on a subconjunctival filtering bleb. UBM and OCT are useful imaging modalities for evaluating the outflow mechanisms after nonpenetrating deep sclerectomy, since the bleb morphology correlates with intraocular pressure. In particular, successful surgery is indicated by the presence of high filtering blebs, a thin trabeculocorneal membrane, a hyporeflective suprachoroidal space, and blebs with low echogenicity based on UBM (Fig. 4.12) and thin bleb walls, large subconjunctival fluid spaces, and low bleb tissue reflectivity based on OCT. Furthermore, enhanced depth imaging spectral domain OCT can depict cupping reversal after nonpenetrating deep sclerectomy, which is mainly due to changes in prelaminar tissue thickness.

## 4.6	Tube Shunt Surgery

Glaucoma drainage devices consist of an end plate, without or with a valve mechanism, and a tube (Fig. 4.13). The glaucoma (aqueous) drainage devices channel aqueous humor from the anterior chamber through a tube to an equatorial end plate in the posterior subconjunctival space, promoting bleb formation and tutoplast can be used to reinforce the tube and prevent erosion. Occasionally, the tube may be inserted into the posterior chamber sulcus in patients with pseudophakia, so as to reduce the likelihood of corneal endothelial loss and avoid the need for pars plana vitrectomy. Glaucoma drainage devices may be considered for glaucoma treatment that does not respond to pharmaceutical therapy or trabeculectomy. In addition, glaucoma drainage device insertion is commonly considered as the primary intervention for neovascular glaucoma, iridio-corneal syndrome, penetrating keratoplasty with glaucoma, and glaucoma following retinal detachment surgery. The drainage devices are most frequently positioned in the superotemporal quadrant of the orbit (Fig. 4.14). The

inferotemporal quadrant (and occasionally the inferonasal quadrant) can also be used when the superior quadrant is not available for surgery (Fig. 4.15). However, the superonasal quadrant is generally avoided, due to the proximity to the trochlea.

Several glaucoma drainage devices are commercially available, each with a unique design, biomaterials composition, and end-plate configuration. The Molteno and Baerveldt devices do not include valves. The single-plate Molteno has a surface area of 130 mm^2, the double-plate Molteno implant has a surface area of 270 mm^2, and the Baerveldt glaucoma implant (Advanced Medical Optics, Inc., Santa Ana, CA) has a large barium-impregnated silicone plate with surface areas of 250, 350, or 425 mm^2; the Ahmed glaucoma valve has a surface area of 185 mm^2 and the Krupin disk implant has a surface area of 184 mm^2. These devices are made of different biomaterials: the Molteno and Ahmed devices are made of polypropylene whereas the Krupin and the Baerveldt are made of silicone. The end-plate biomaterial of the Ahmed valve was recently changed to silicone.

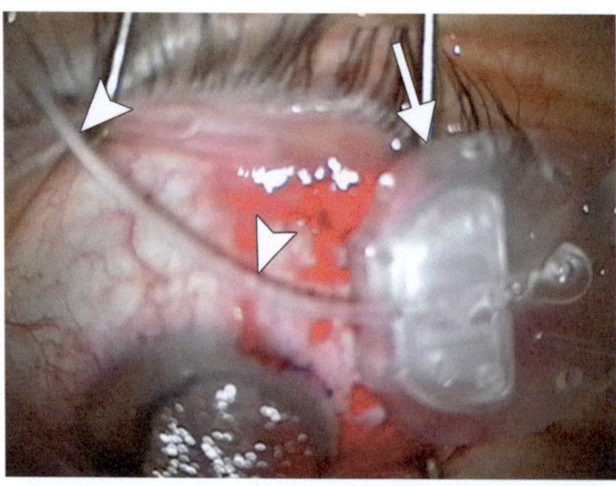

Fig. 4.13 Intraoperative photograph of an Ahmed valve shows the end plate (*arrow*) and tube (*arrowheads*) components prior to implantation in the posterior subconjunctival space

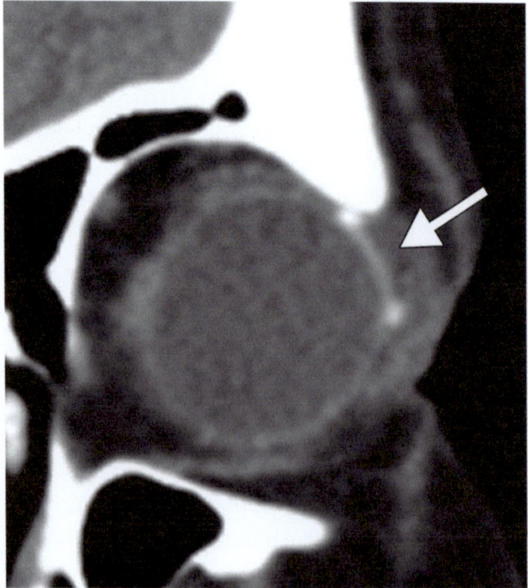

Fig. 4.14 Superotemporal glaucoma drainage device. Coronal CT image shows the end plate with associated small bleb positioned along the superotemporal surface of the left globe (*arrow*)

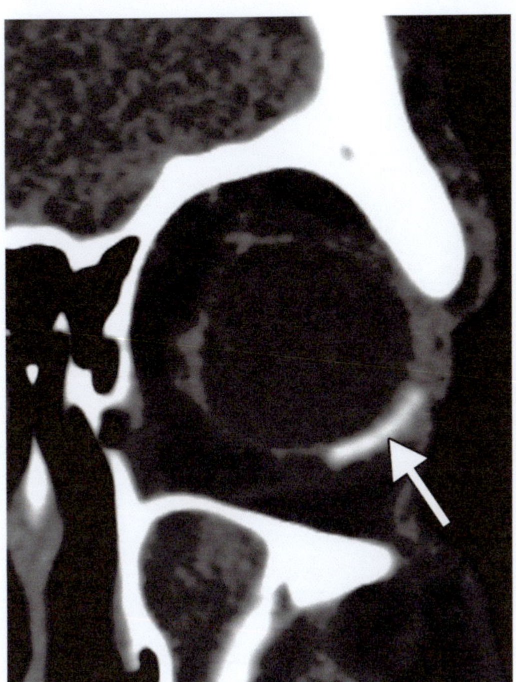

Fig. 4.15 Inferotemporal glaucoma drainage device depicted on CT. The coronal CT image shows the hyperattenuating end plate of a silicone Ahmed valve along the inferolateral aspect of the left globe (*arrow*)

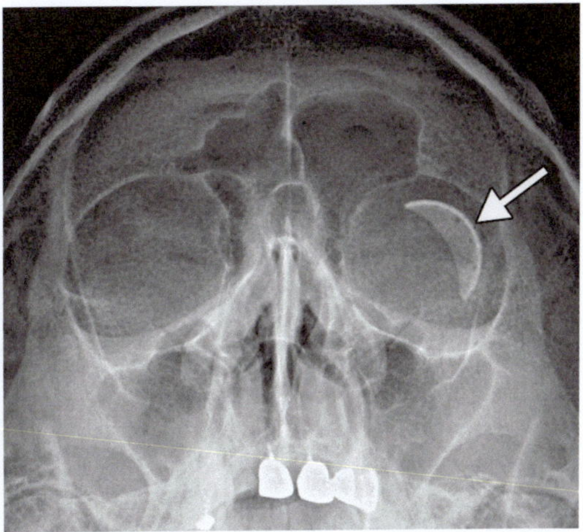

Fig. 4.16 Barium-impregnated glaucoma drainage device (Baerveldt shunt) depicted on radiography. The radiograph shows the radio-opaque implant in the superotemporal quadrant of the left orbit (*arrow*). The radiograph was obtained to screen for metallic foreign bodies prior to MRI

The barium-impregnated devices appear very radio-opaque, but should not be misconstrued as metallic foreign bodies on radiographs or CT (Figs. 4.16 and 4.17). On the other hand, the polypropylene devices are radiolucent, with similar attenuation as the orbital fat (Fig. 4.18). On MRI, the devices appear as low signal intensity on all sequences and are typically surrounded by a variable amount of fluid in the bleb (Figs. 4.19 and 4.20). However, the bleb should not exert significant mass effect upon the surrounding tissues. A mild degree of enhancement surrounding the bleb is typical. The blebs can be difficult to portray on B-mode ultrasound but appear as anechoic collections adjacent to the hyperechoic plate (Fig. 4.21). The tube portion of the glaucoma drainage device is best depicted on OCT or UBM (Figs. 4.22 and 4.23). The tube is typically implanted through the scleral limbus into the anterior chamber.

The anterior chamber may not be the optimal site for tube implantation when there is underlying posterior segment disease, such as in cases of neovascular glaucoma in proliferative diabetic retinopathy. Rather, glaucoma drainage device tube insertion through the pars plana during vitrectomy is an effective option for managing complex cases of glaucoma. As with standard glaucoma device tube implantations, UBM and OCT can effectively delineate the pars plana tube insertions (Fig. 4.24).

A variety of complications can occur in association with the glaucoma drainage devices. These include hypotony, choroidal hemorrhage, infection, diplopia, strabismus, proptosis, tube obstruction, tube malposition, corneal decompensation, and dystrophic calcification.

Hypotony is generally defined as an intraocular pressure of less than 5 mmHg, although it is recognized that some eyes maintain normal anatomic structure and physiologic function at lower intraocular pressure. Hypotony can lead to serous choroidal detachment and vision loss. If absolutely necessary, ultrasound should be performed with caution in patients with known or suspected hypotony. There can be associated choroidal hemorrhage, which can be identified on CT, MRI, OCT, and ultrasound. However,

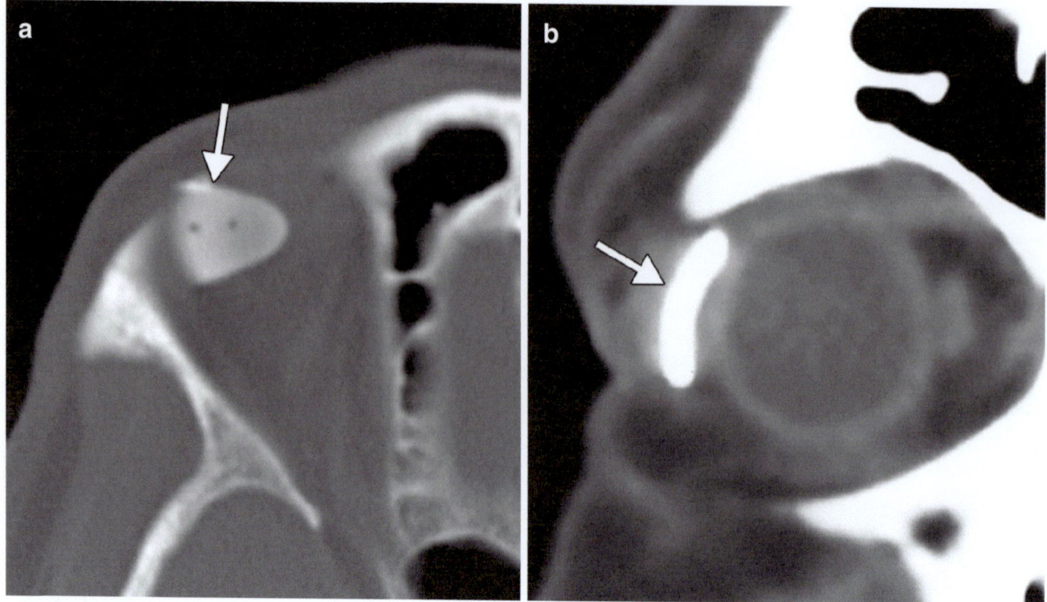

Fig. 4.17 Baerveldt shunt depicted on CT. Axial (**a**) and coronal (**b**) CT images show a thick, hyperattenuating superotemporal device (*arrows*)

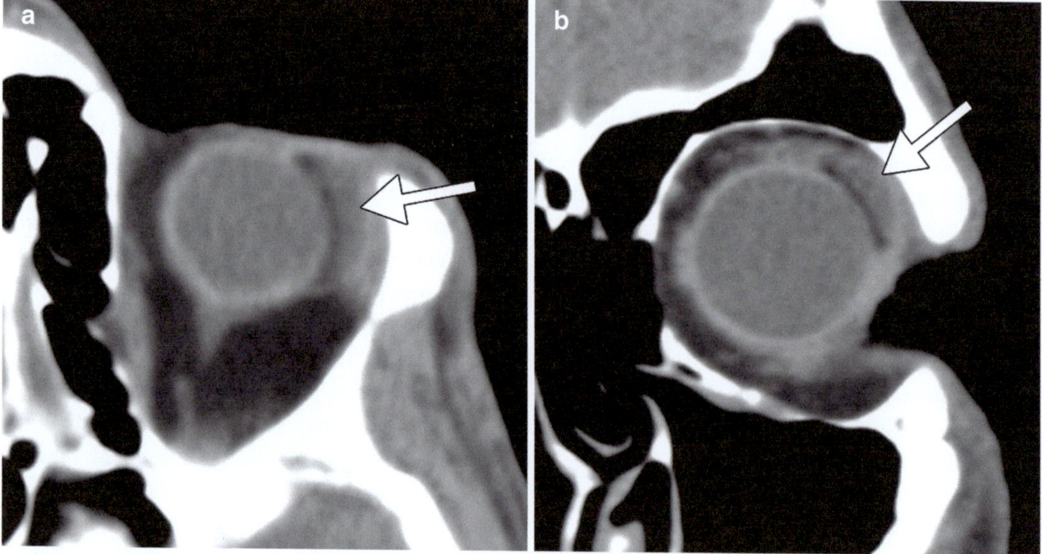

Fig. 4.18 Radiolucent Ahmed valve with bleb depicted on CT. Axial (**a**) and coronal (**b**) CT images show a fluid-filled bleb (*arrows*) adjacent to a superotemporal radiolucent drainage device

serial ultrasound is recommended to evaluate the size of the hemorrhage and also the liquefaction of the clot. Initially, the hemorrhage appears as echogenic (Fig. 4.25) and eventually becomes hypoechoic. Small hemorrhages can resolve spontaneously with conservative treatment, while larger ones may require drainage. Drainage is usually performed once liquefaction occurs.

Orbital cellulitis is an uncommon complication of aqueous drainage device implantation. Early recognition and intervention is important to achieve resolution of the infection. CT and MRI

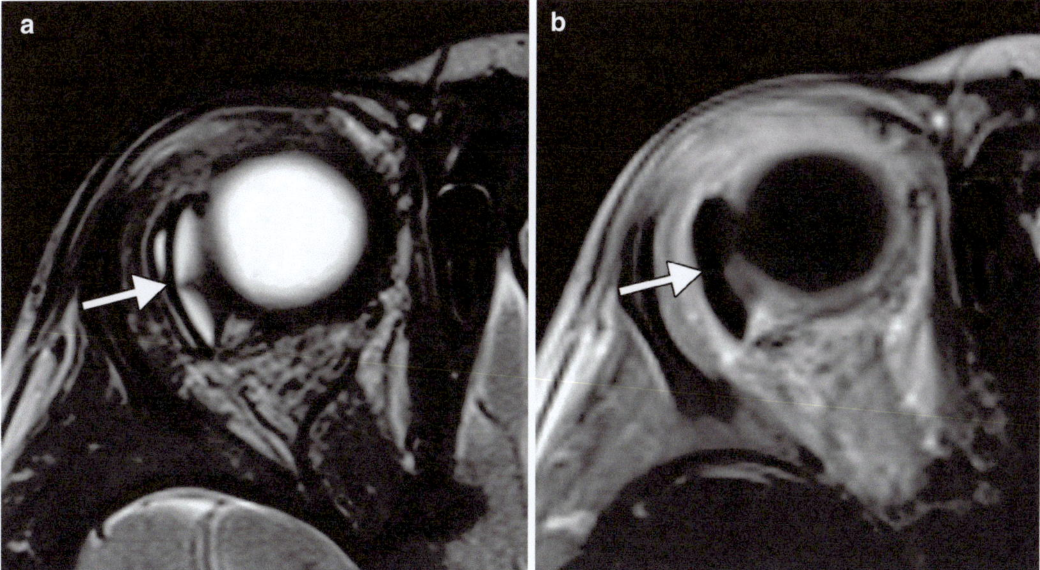

Fig. 4.19 Baerveldt shunt depicted on MRI. Axial T2 (**a**) and post-contrast T1 (**b**) MR images show a small amount of fluid surrounding the hypointense plate (*arrows*) in the superotemporal quadrant of the orbit. There is expected enhancement of the bleb walls

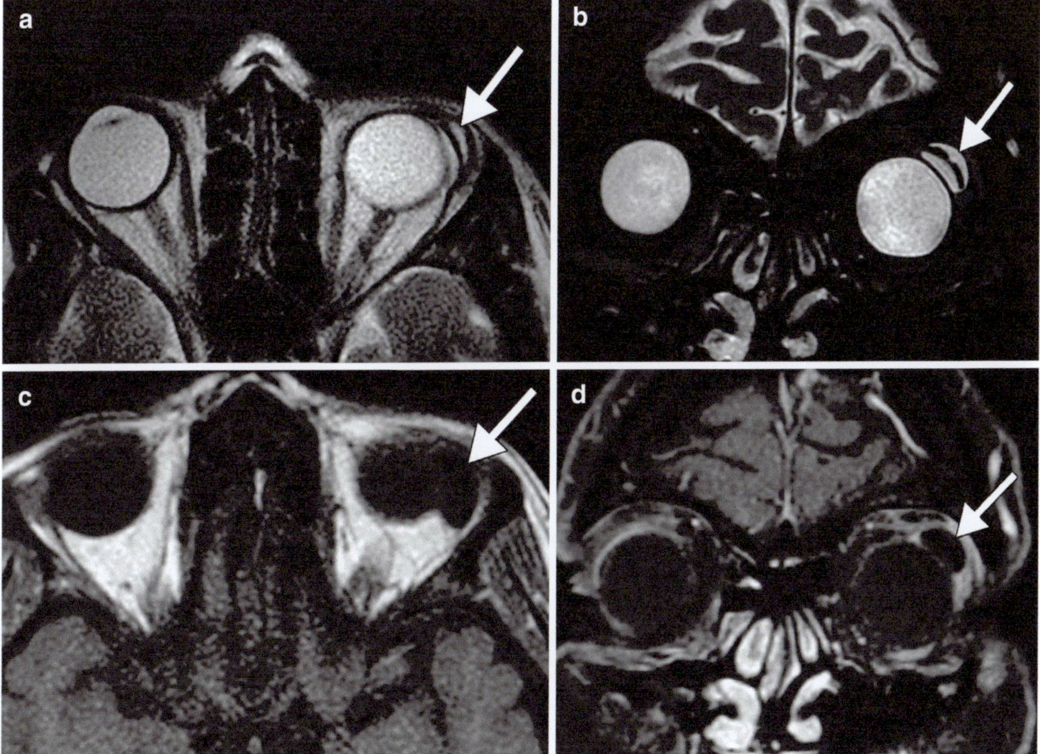

Fig. 4.20 Ahmed valve with bleb depicted on MRI. Axial T2-weighted (**a**), coronal fat-suppressed T2-weighted (**b**), axial T1-weighted (**c**), and post-contrast fat-suppressed coronal T1-weighted (**d**) MR images show the low-signal curvilinear drainage device, surrounded by a contained fluid collection (*arrows*). There is mild enhancement of the bleb wall. The bleb indents the wall of the globe in (**c**) and (**d**)

are both appropriate modalities for the evaluation of postoperative infection (Fig. 4.26). Contrast administration is not crucial for the depiction of cellulitis, which manifests as stranding of the fat on CT and low T1-weighted and high T2-weighted signal on MRI. However, contrast administration can be useful for the delineation of abscess formation and intracranial extension of the infectious process. Infected fluid collections can cause displacement of the aqueous drainage devices deep in the orbit, which can be observed on cross-sectional imaging. Endophthalmitis can also be apparent on CT and MRI and appears as thickening and enhancement of the sclera, as well as hyperattenuation or signal abnormality within the vitreous chamber on occasion. Alternatively, ultrasound is a useful modality for the diagnosis and assessment of endophthalmitis, whereby findings may include organization of opacities in the vitreous, membrane formation, thickening of the choroid, posterior vitreous membrane detachment, detachment of the choroid, retinal detachment, choroidal abscess or granuloma, edema of the optic nerve head and thickening of the sclera (Fig. 4.27).

The introduction of a biomaterial such as the end plate of any glaucoma drainage device appears to be associated with a fibrovascular response in the subconjunctival space. The introduction of glaucomatous aqueous humor from patients with elevated intraocular pressure into the subconjunctival space in itself can stimulate fibrovascular proliferation in the episcleral tissue. Excessive proliferative changes appear to be associated with bleb failure and elevated intraocular pressure. UBM may be useful for identifying and localizing the source of any obstruction, such as fibrosis at the tip of the tube, which can appear as amorphous hyperechoic material (Fig. 4.28).

Although small encapsulated blebs are expected postoperative findings, the formation

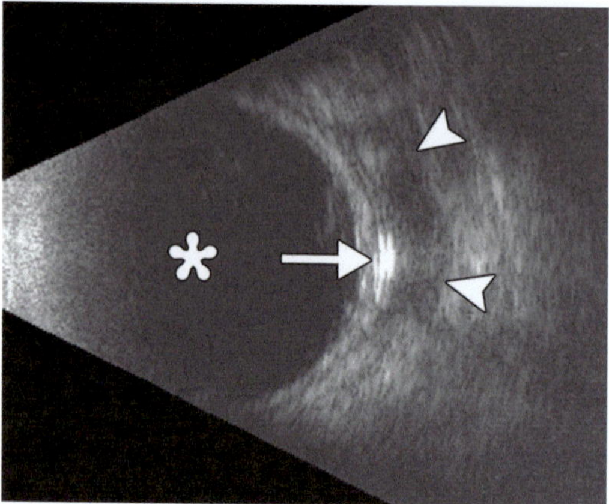

Fig. 4.21 Glaucoma drainage implant and bleb depicted on B-mode ultrasound. The B-mode ultrasound shows the echogenic plate (*arrow*) along the contour of the globe (*) and the surrounding anechoic bleb (*arrowheads*) (Courtesy of Karen Capaccioli and Lois Hart)

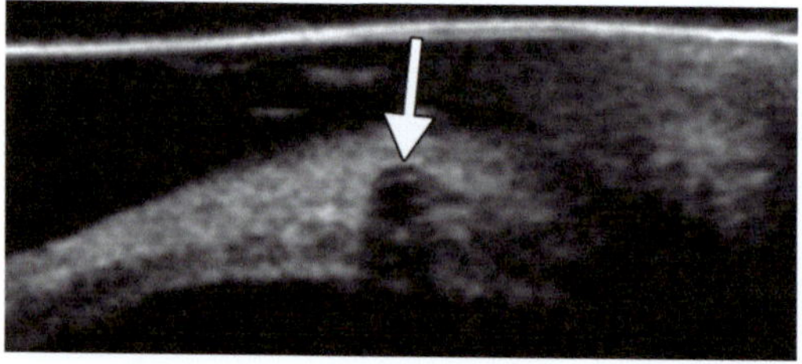

Fig. 4.22 Glaucoma drainage implant depicted on UBM. The cross section of the tube is depicted as it courses through the sclera (*arrow*) (Courtesy of Karen Capaccioli and Lois Hart)

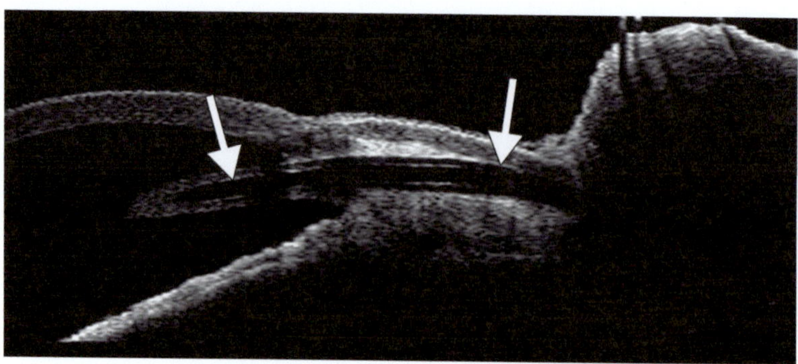

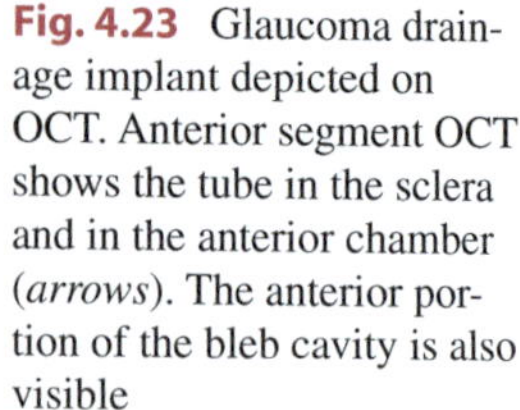

Fig. 4.23 Glaucoma drainage implant depicted on OCT. Anterior segment OCT shows the tube in the sclera and in the anterior chamber (*arrows*). The anterior portion of the bleb cavity is also visible

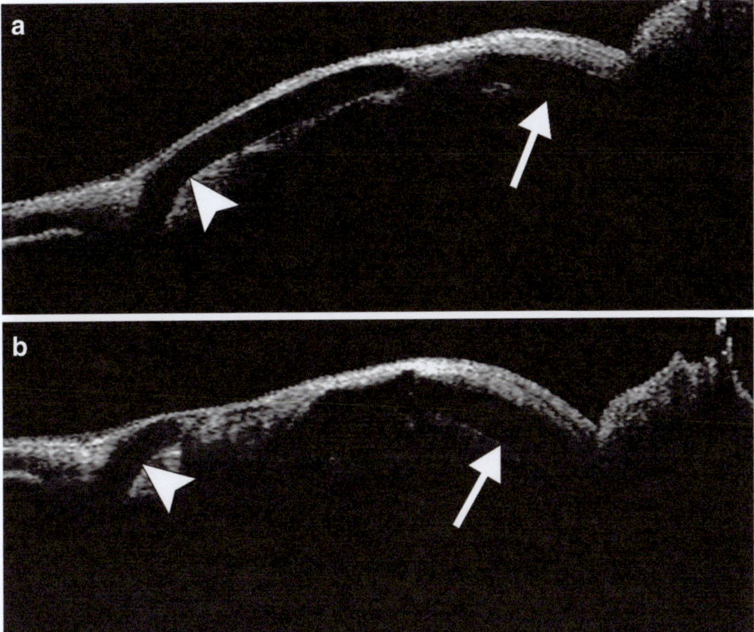

Fig. 4.24 Glaucoma drainage device inserted in pars plana. Anterior segment OCT images (**a**, **b**) show the plate of the drainage device (*arrows*) and the tube within the pars plana (*arrowheads*)

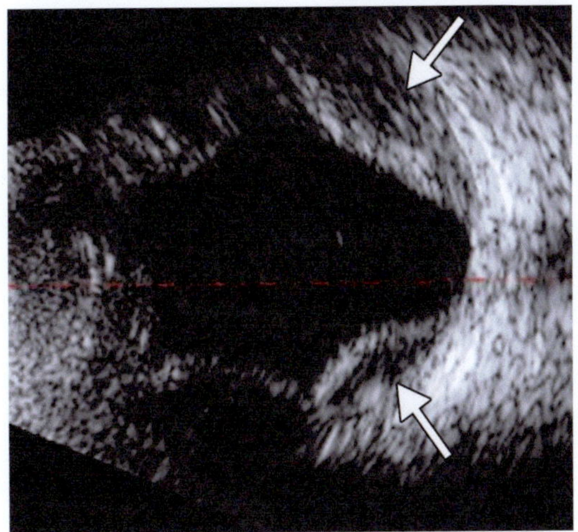

Fig. 4.25 Hemorrhagic choroidal detachment after glaucoma device tube repositioning. B-scan ultrasound image shows the echogenic hemorrhagic choroidal detachments (*arrows*). There was associated hypotony

of an unusually large fluid collection, a so-called giant reservoir, around glaucoma valve implants can cause progressive proptosis. Although other cystic lesions of the superotemporal orbit, such as a dermoid cyst, can present with similar imaging findings, the characteristic morphology and location and presence of the implant should lead to the correct identification of this cystic lesion. The incidence of diplopia in the setting of a tube shunt is in the range of 6 to 18 %, with the highest incidence of diplopia associated with the Baerveldt implant, likely related to its large size and positioning deep to the muscle belly. In addition to an enlarged bleb, compression of extraocular muscle and flattening of the adjacent globe contour can be depicted on imaging (Fig. 4.29), hinting at a possible restrictive strabismus etiology in correlation with clinical findings. In particular, high-resolution, multiplanar orbital MRI or CT can adequately delineate the affected anatomical structures and provide information for planning revision surgery. Bleb revision with needling of the bleb is an option for both non-valved and valved implants with encapsulated blebs producing diplopia. Surgical excision of the encapsulated bleb has been recommended in cases that do not respond to needling.

Malpositioned glaucoma drainage plates can be depicted on MRI and CT. Although end plates can be positioned posterior to the limbus while remaining away from the optic nerve, there is an increased risk that the plates may impinge upon the optic nerve if positioned too far posteriorly

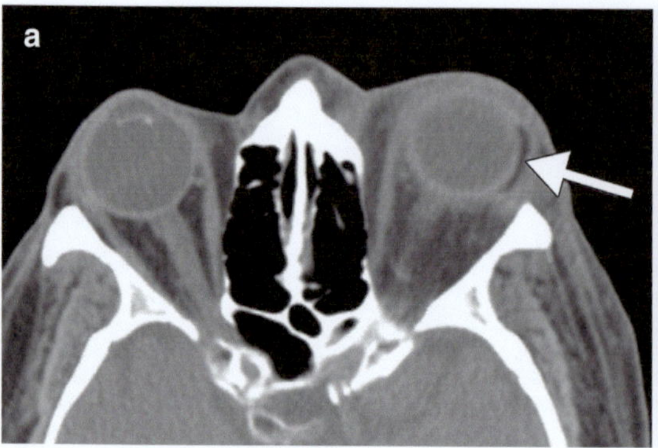

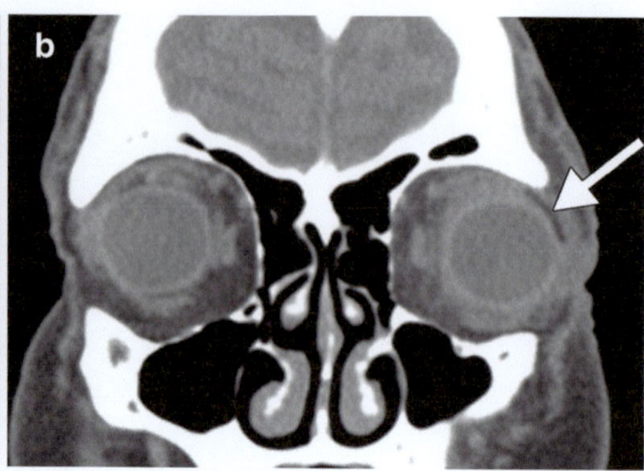

Fig. 4.26 Infected Ahmed valve depicted on CT. Axial (**a**) and coronal (**b**) non-contrast CT images demonstrate diffuse preseptal and postseptal swelling and stranding, as well as circumferential uveoscleral thickening OS, with an Ahmed valve present (*arrows*)

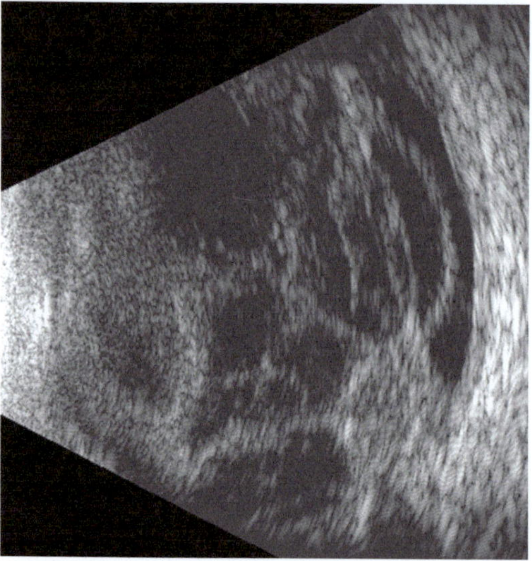

Fig. 4.27 Endophthalmitis after glaucoma device implantation. B-scan ultrasound shows extensive membrane formation within the globe (Courtesy of Arun Singh MD)

Calcium deposits are uncommonly associated glaucoma drainage devices. The development of dystrophic calcification associated with implanted biomaterials can be intrinsic (material dependent) or extrinsic (host dependent). Intrinsic calcification can be secondary to a defect in the biodevice, such as remnants of manufacturing material on the surface. Extrinsic calcification can result from breakdown of the blood–aqueous barrier from surgery, trauma, infection, or inflammation. If sufficiently large, the dystrophic calcifications can be discerned on CT (Fig. 4.32) and may warrant further investigation of associated complications. However, these calcifications may be encountered incidentally on imaging and may not carry any clinical significance.

(Fig. 4.30). Encroachment upon the optic nerve can damage the nerve and lead to visual loss. This has been demonstrated in rabbit models if then edge of the end plate is inserted within 1 mm of the optic nerve, at least in rabbit models. Alternatively, the glaucoma drainage tube may also be malpositioned and can be best delineated via UBM or OCT. For example, if inserted too far into the anterior chamber, the tube can contact the iris and result in pigment dispersion (Fig. 4.31). This complication can exacerbate the patient's glaucoma.

4.7 Novel Glaucoma Devices

Several devices and procedures that have US Food and Drug Administration clearance or are currently in phase III clinical trials in the United States include: the Fugo blade (Medisurg Ltd., Norristown, PA), Ex-PRESS mini glaucoma shunt (Alcon, Inc., Hunenberg, Switzerland), SOLX Gold Shunt (SOLX Ltd., Boston, MA), excimer laser trabeculotomy (AIDA, Glautec AG, Nurnberg, Germany), trabeculotomy by internal approach (Trabectome, NeoMedix, Inc., Tustin, CA), and trabecular micro-bypass stent (iStent, Glaukos Corporation, Laguna Hills,

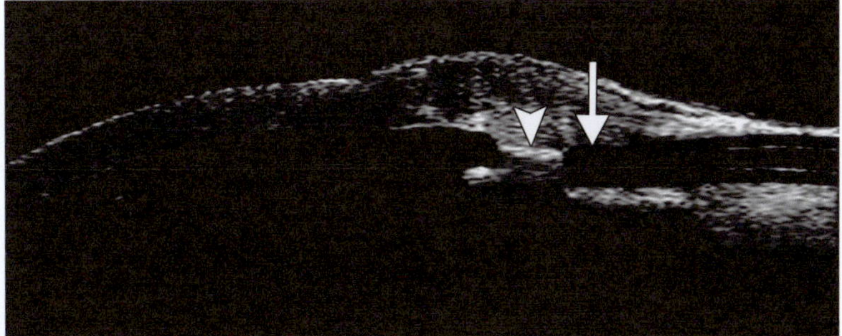

Fig. 4.28 Glaucoma drainage device tube occlusion by fibrosis. The anterior segment OCT image shows a glaucoma drainage implant retracted into the sclera and the tip of the tube (*arrow*) is effaced by fibrotic tissues (*arrowhead*)

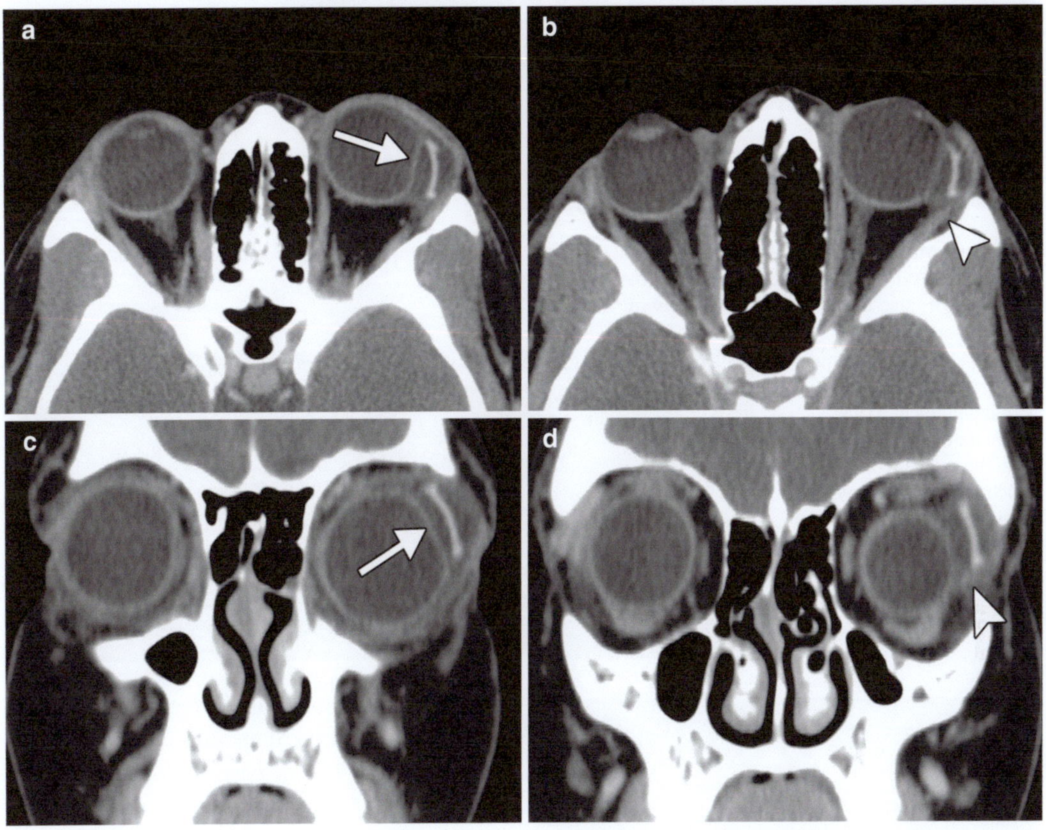

Fig. 4.29 Giant bleb with restricted ocular motility. The patient had a Krupin valve implanted for glaucoma associated with trauma and presented with proptosis and diplopia. Axial (**a**, **b**) and coronal (**c**, **d**) CT images show a large fluid collection surrounding the left superotempo- ral glaucoma valve device with resultant flattening of the adjacent globe (*arrows*) and inferolateral displacement of the lateral rectus muscle (*arrowheads*). As expected, the posterior aspect of the end plate that is not secured to the sclera can float freely within the bleb cavity

CA). All of these devices yield a statistically significant reduction in intraocular pressure and, in some cases, glaucoma medication use. Among these, the Ex-PRESS mini glaucoma shunt and Gold Shunt are described and depicted further.

The Ex-PRESS mini glaucoma shunt is a biocompatible stainless steel device less than 3 mm long with an external diameter of approximately 400 μm and a 50 μm diameter lumen. The device has an external disk at one end and a spur-like extension on the other to prevent extrusion and is typically inserted under a scleral flap (Fig. 4.33). The device shunts aqueous from the anterior chamber to a subconjunctival reservoir

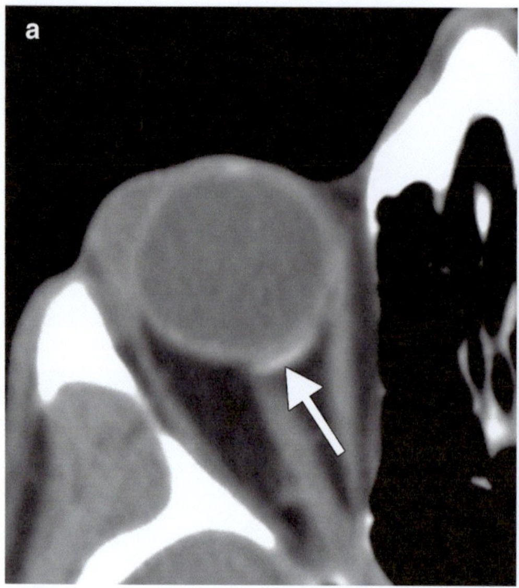

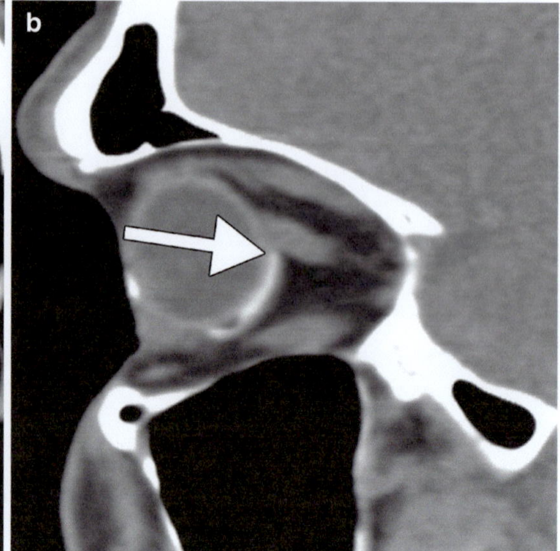

Fig. 4.30 Malpositioned Ahmed valve contacting the optic nerve. Axial (**a**) and sagittal (**b**) CT images show the posterior edge of the plate in contact with the optic nerve (*arrows*). The patient developed optic neuropathy as a result

Fig. 4.31 Glaucoma drainage device tube in contact with the pigment. UBM shows that the tube impinges upon the pigment (*arrow*), which resulted in pigment dispersion syndrome (Courtesy of Karen Capaccioli and Lois Hart)

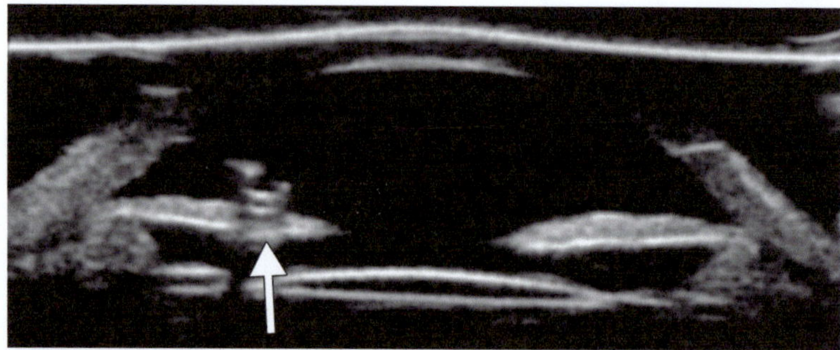

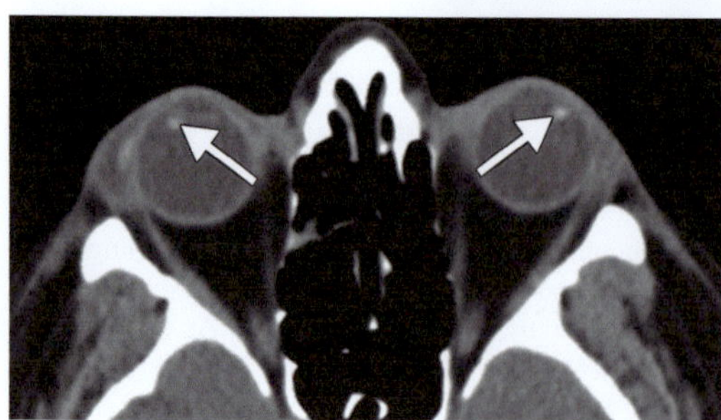

Fig. 4.32 Ahmed valve with dystrophic calcifications. Axial CT image shows coarse calcifications involving the tubes of the bilateral implants (*arrows*). The presence of calcification was an incidental finding in this patient

in a similar fashion as trabeculectomy, but without removal of sclera or iris tissue. The success rate at 3 years after surgery is approximately 95 %. The most common device-related complication is obstruction of the tube, which occurs in approximately 2 % of cases and can be treated with Nd:YAG laser. Hypotony occurs in approximately 4 % of cases, which is less common than with trabeculectomy. The Ex-PRESS glaucoma shunt is readily depicted on CT as a punctate focus of high attenuation in the anterior globe (Fig. 4.34) and should not be mistaken as an unintended foreign body. The Ex-PRESS shunt appears to be MRI compatible at 1.5 and 3.0 T, in which no significant torque has been reported. Although the implant can produce mild distortion due to metallic susceptibility artifact (Fig. 4.35), the interpretation of MRI scans of the orbit and brain is unaffected by the focal artifacts. The shunt and surrounding structures

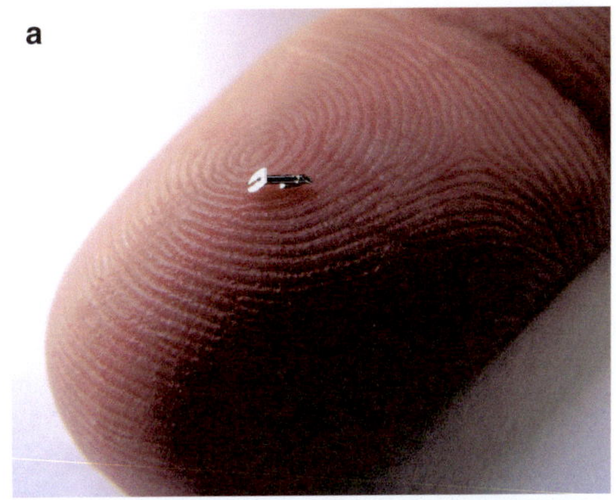

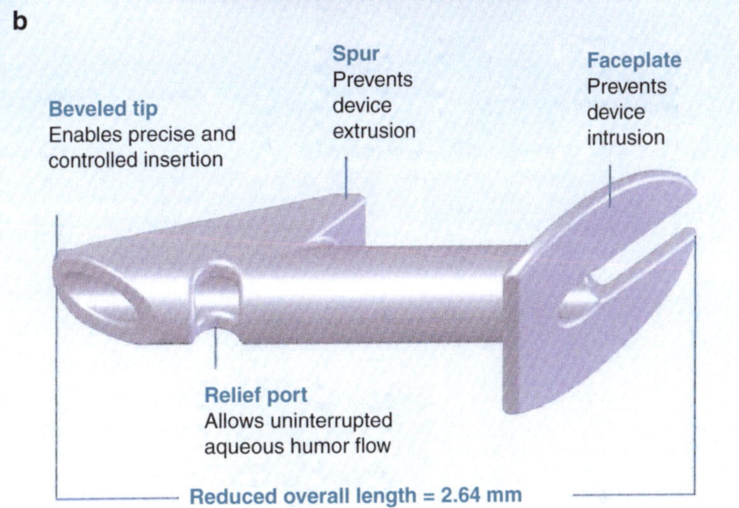

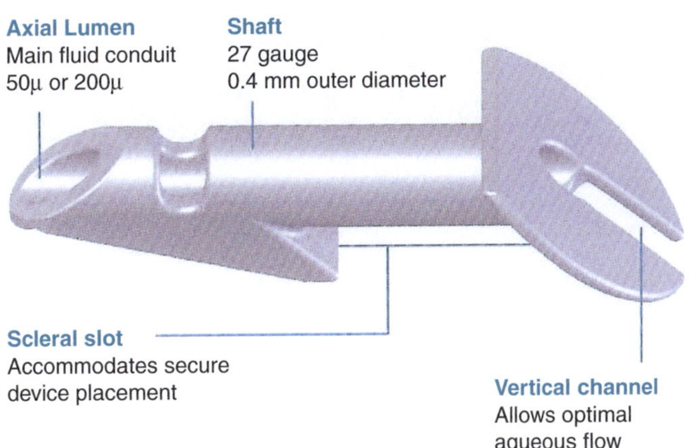

Fig. 4.33 Ex-PRESS shunt (Model P50/200). Photograph of the device (**a**). Schematic of the device dimensions and components (**b**) (Courtesy of the Alcon manufacturing company)

can be delineated in exquisite detail using OCT or UBM, in which the device appears as bright or echogenic with associated shadowing (Fig. 4.36). Often, fluid is observed beneath the scleral flap and small blebs can be expected to form.

The gold micro shunt (SOLX Ltd, Boston, Massachusetts) is also indicated for treatment of

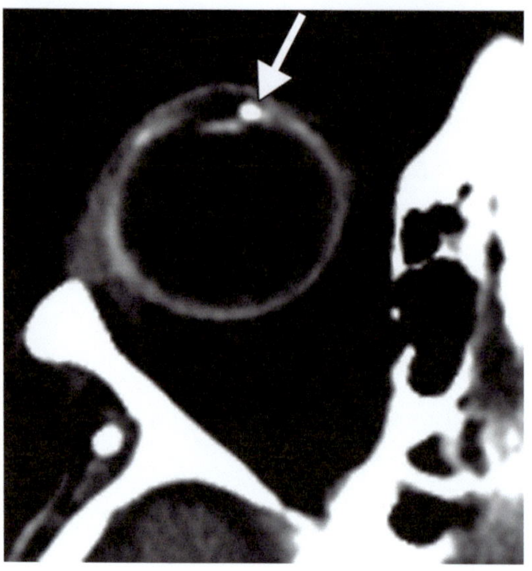

Fig. 4.34 Ex-PRESS mini glaucoma shunt depicted on CT. Axial CT image shows a punctate metallic structure within the nasal aspect of the anterior chamber of the right globe (*arrow*)

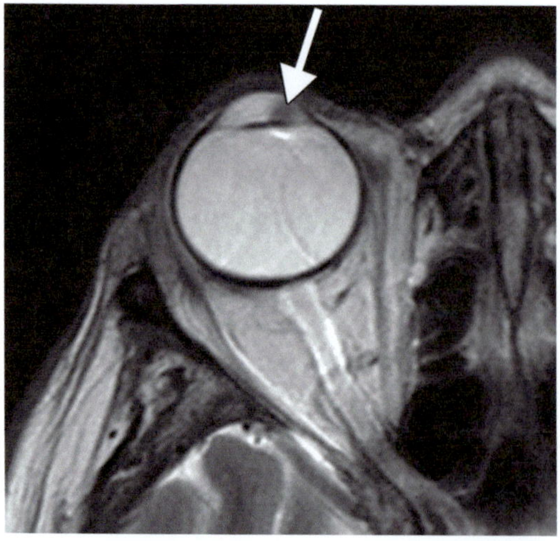

Fig. 4.35 Ex-PRESS mini glaucoma shunt depicted on MRI. Axial T2-weighted MRI shows susceptibility effect within the nasal aspect of the anterior chamber (*arrow*), which corresponds to the shunt. An intraocular lens implant is also present and the optic nerve is diffusely hyperintense and atrophic due to chronic glaucoma

open-angle glaucoma and consists of two parallel ultrathin 24-karat gold sheets (Fig. 4.37). The device contains multiple tubules to facilitate

aqueous flow between the anterior chamber and the supraciliary/suprachoroidal space without the creation of a bleb. Gold is used for its biocompatibility and it is also MRI compatible. The implant is inserted via what is essentially a deep nonpenetrating sclerectomy. A surgical success rate of nearly 80 % has been reported in patients receiving the gold micro shunt for uncontrolled severe glaucoma. The position of the device can be readily confirmed using UBM or OCT (Fig. 4.38). A spongy appearance of the sclera adjacent to the plate may observed, which is suggestive of fluid absorption.

4.8 Canaloplasty

Canaloplasty is a procedure that involves circumferential viscodilation and tensioning of Schlemm's canal using an ophthalmic microcannula (iScience Interventional Corp., Menlo Park, CA). Canaloplasty refines the older viscocanalostomy by using a microcatheter to clear the entire canal rather than just a segment. In a canaloplasty, the 250-μm fiber-optic microcannula is introduced through a small incision to enlarge the main drainage channel. After 360° of canal cannulation, the microcannula is then used to insert a 10-0 prolene suture into the entire circumference of the canal. The suture ends are tied together to provide tension to the inner wall of the canal and the associated trabecular meshwork. Once the suture is tied, the tension stretches the trabecular meshwork to facilitate better outflow into the canal, keeping the canal open and preventing its collapse. The suture and patency of the canal of Schlemm can be discerned on high-resolution imaging, such as UBM or OCT (Figs. 4.39 and 4.40).

4.9 Summary

- Ultrasound, OCT, and diagnostic neuroimaging (CT and MRI) all have important roles in the posttreatment evaluation of glaucoma.

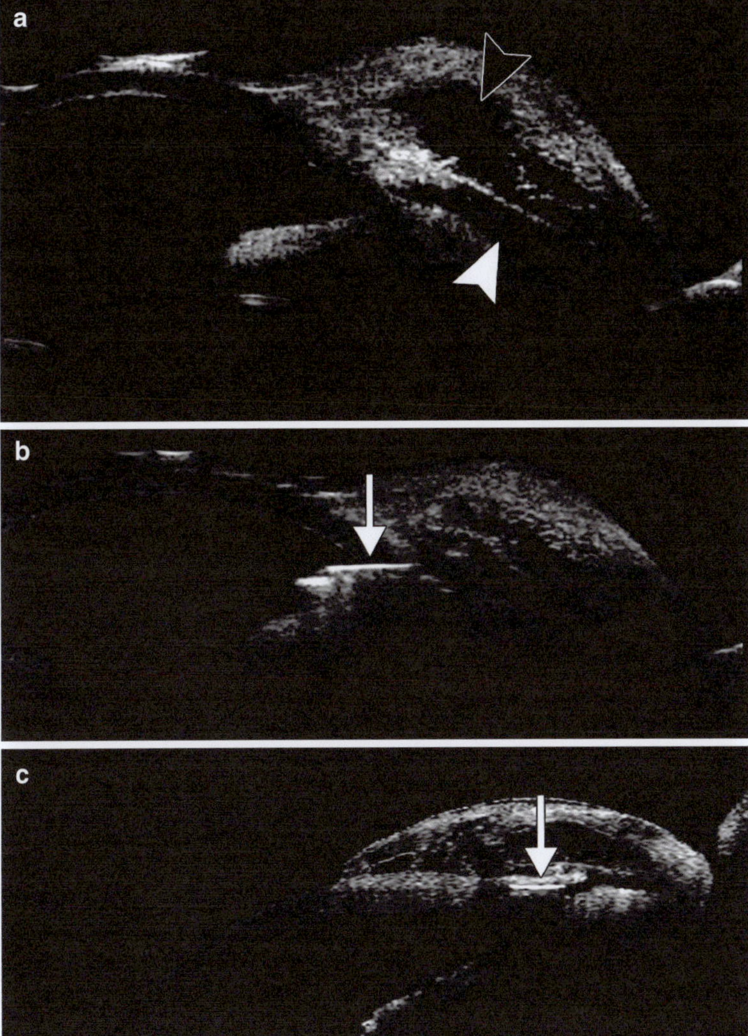

Fig. 4.36 Express shunt depicted on UBM. Anterior segment UBM (**a–c**) shows fluid under the scleral flap (*white arrowhead*) and an elevated conjunctival bleb (*black arrowhead*). The reflective metal plate of express shunt within the anterior chamber and within the sclera (*arrows*)

- Ophthalmologists and neuroradiologists should be aware that glaucoma causes atrophy of the entire visual pathway from the retrobulbar optic nerve to visual cortex and that these changes can be encountered on imaging even after treatment of glaucoma has been instituted.
- The high spatial resolution of OCT and UBM makes these excellent modalities for depicting the expected and complicated results of glaucoma surgery.
- CT and MRI are useful for depicting the end plates of glaucoma drainage devices, surrounding structures, and associated complications.
- It is important to be aware that there is increased usage of prosthetic devices for the surgical management of glaucoma and that these devices will be encountered as incidental findings in patients who undergo neuroimaging for non-ophthalmic indications and that these should not be misinterpreted as unintended foreign bodies or lesions.

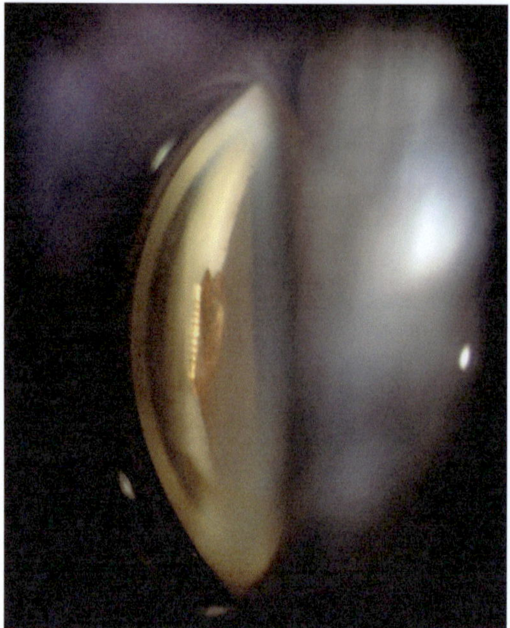

Fig. 4.37 Slit lamp photograph of the Gold Mini Shunt (Courtesy of Rebecca Tudor)

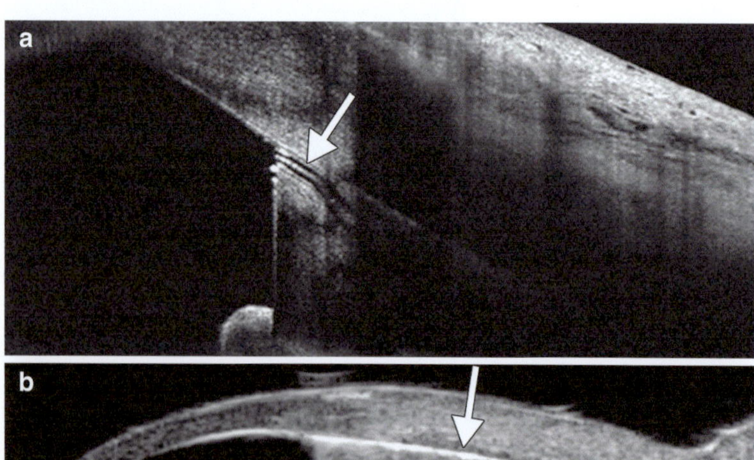

Fig. 4.38 Anterior segment OCT images (**a**, **b**) show the reflective gold plate (*arrows*) that extends from the margin of the anterior chamber into the suprachoroidal space

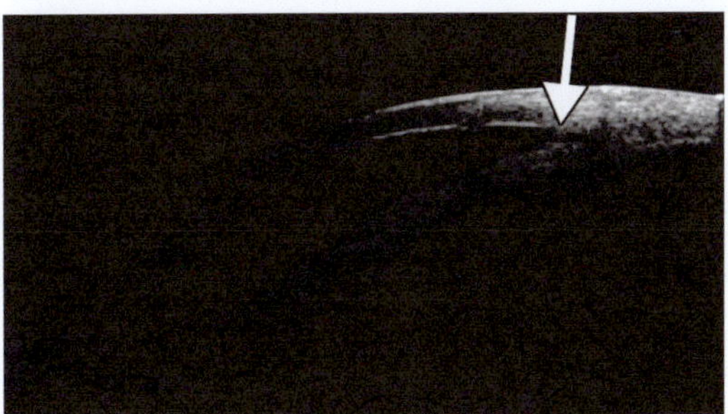

Fig. 4.39 Canaloplasty depicted on UBM. The anterior segment UBM image shows that the prolene suture (*arrow*) appears as a punctate echogenic focus in the canal of Schlemm, which is otherwise patent

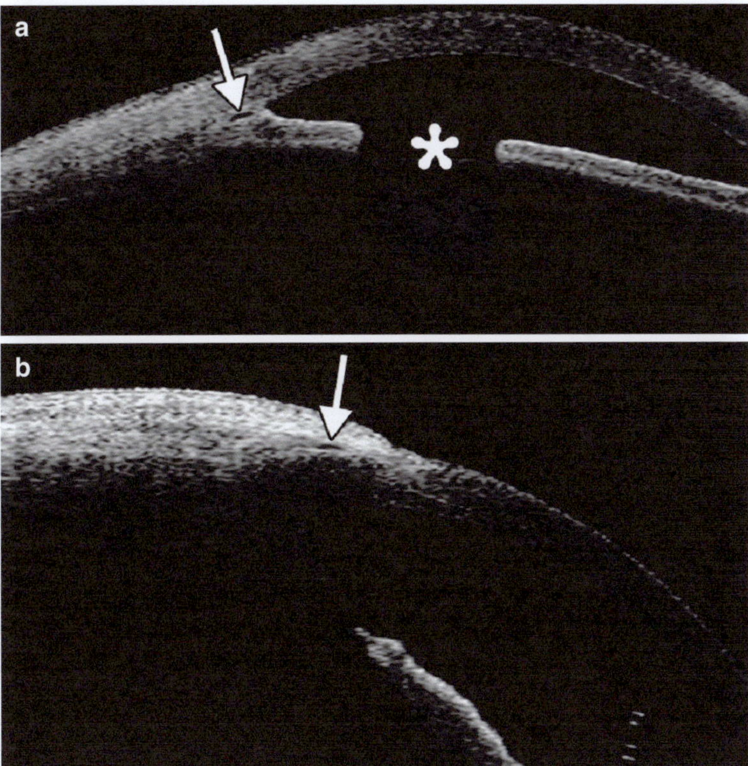

Fig. 4.40 Canaloplasty depicted on OCT. Anterior OCT demonstrates a patent Schlemm's canal (*arrow*). Iridectomy was also performed previously (*)

Further Reading

Aktas Z, Korkmaz S, Hasanreisoglu M, Onol M, Hasanreisoglu B. Trabeculectomy with large area mitomycin-C application as a first-line treatment in advanced glaucoma: retrospective review. Int J Ophthalmol. 2014;7(1):104–9.

Alward WL. Medical management of glaucoma. N Engl J Med. 1998;339(18):1298–307.

Aptel F, Dumas S, Denis P. Ultrasound biomicroscopy and optical coherence tomography imaging of filtering blebs after deep sclerectomy with new collagen implant. Eur J Ophthalmol. 2009;19(2):223–30.

Ates H, Andac K, Uretmen O. Non-penetrating deep sclerectomy and collagen implant surgery in glaucoma patients with advanced field loss. Int Ophthalmol. 1999;23(3):123–8.

Ayyala RS, Parma SE, Karcioglu ZA. Optic nerve changes following posterior insertion of glaucoma drainage device in rabbit model. J Glaucoma. 2004;13(2):145–8.

Barbosa DT, Levison AL, Lin SC. Clear lens extraction in angle-closure glaucoma patients. Int J Ophthalmol. 2013;6(3):406–8.

Barrancos C, Rebolleda G, Oblanca N, Cabarga C, Muñoz-Negrete FJ. Changes in lamina cribrosa and prelaminar tissue after deep sclerectomy. Eye (Lond). 2014;28(1):58–65.

Bissig A, Rivier D, Zaninetti M, Shaarawy T, Mermoud A, Roy S. Ten years follow-up after deep sclerectomy with collagen implant. J Glaucoma. 2008;17(8):680–6.

Buys YM. Trabeculectomy with ExPRESS: weighing the benefits and cost. Curr Opin Ophthalmol. 2013;24:111–8.

Cabrejas L, Rebolleda G, Muñoz-Negrete FJ, Losada D. An ultrasound biomicroscopy study of filtering blebs after deep sclerectomy with a new acrylic implant. Eur J Ophthalmol. 2011;21(4):391–9.

Chaudhry IA, Shamsi FA, Morales J. Orbital cellulitis following implantation of aqueous drainage devices. Eur J Ophthalmol. 2007;17(1):136–40.

Coats DK, Paysse EA, Orenga-Nania S. Acquired Pseudo-Brown's syndrome immediately following Ahmed valve glaucoma implant. Ophthalmic Surg Lasers. 1999;30(5):396–7.

de Barros DS, Navarro JB, Mantravadi AV, Siam GA, Gheith ME, Tittler EH, Baez KA, Martinez SM, Spaeth GL. The early flat anterior chamber after trabeculectomy: a randomized, prospective study of 3 methods of management. J Glaucoma. 2009;18(1):13–20.

Engelhorn T, Michelson G, Waerntges S, Struffert T, Haider S, Doerfler A. Diffusion tensor imaging detects rarefaction of optic radiation in glaucoma patients. Acad Radiol. 2011;18:764–9.

Faghihi H, Hajizadeh F, Mohammadi SF, Kadkhoda A, Peyman GA, Riazi-Esfahani M. Pars plana Ahmed valve implant and vitrectomy in the management of neovascular glaucoma. Ophthalmic Surg Lasers Imaging. 2007;38(4):292–300.

Francis BA, Singh K, Lin SC, Hodapp E, Jampel HD, Samples JR, Smith SD. Novel glaucoma procedures: a report by the American Academy of Ophthalmology. Ophthalmology. 2011;118(7):1466–80.

Geffen N, Trope GE, Alasbali T, Salonen D, Crowley AP, Buys YM. Is the Ex-PRESS glaucoma shunt magnetic resonance imaging safe? J Glaucoma. 2010;19(2):116–8.

Golez 3rd E, Latina M. The use of anterior segment imaging after trabeculectomy. Semin Ophthalmol. 2012;27(5–6):155–9.

Hendrick AM, Kahook MY. Ex-PRESS mini glaucoma shunt: surgical technique and review of clinical experience. Expert Rev Med Devices. 2008;5(6):673–7.

Hong CH, Arosemena A, Zurakowski D, Ayyala RS. Glaucoma drainage devices: a systematic literature review and current controversies. Surv Ophthalmol. 2005;50(1):48–60.

Hoyng PF, van Beek LM. Pharmacological therapy for glaucoma: a review. Drugs. 2000;59(3):411–34.

Jayaprakasam A, Ghazi-Nouri S. Periorbital fat atrophy – an unfamiliar side effect of prostaglandin analogues. Orbit. 2010;29(6):357–9.

Jeon TY, Kim HJ, Kim ST, Chung TY, Kee C. MR imaging features of giant reservoir formation in the orbit: an unusual complication of Ahmed glaucoma valve implantation. AJNR Am J Neuroradiol. 2007;28(8):1565–6.

Kahook MY, Noecker RJ, Pantcheva MB, Schuman JS. Location of glaucoma drainage devices relative to the optic nerve. Br J Ophthalmol. 2006;90(8):1010–3. Epub 2006 Apr 13.

Kashiwagi K, Okubo T, Tsukahara S. Association of magnetic resonance imaging of anterior optic pathway with glaucomatous visual field damage and optic disc cupping. J Glaucoma. 2004;13:189–95.

Kass MA, Heuer DK, Higginbotham EJ, Johnson CA, Keltner JL, Miller JP, Parrish 2nd RK, Wilson MR, Gordon MO. The Ocular Hypertension Treatment Study: a randomized trial determines that topical ocular hypotensive medication delays or prevents the onset of primary open-angle glaucoma. Arch Ophthalmol. 2002;120(6):701–13; discussion 829–30.

Kassam F, Lee BE, Damji KF. Concurrent endophthalmitis and orbital cellulitis in a child with congenital glaucoma and a glaucoma drainage device. Digit J Ophthalmol. 2011;17(4):58–61.

Khan AO, Al-Katan H, Edward DP. Nummular dystrophic calcification of an Ahmed glaucoma valve in a child. J AAPOS. 2012;16(4):401–2.

Kim WK, Seong GJ, Lee CS, Kim YG, Kim CY. Anterior segment optical coherence tomography imaging and histopathologic findings of an overhanging filtering bleb. Eye (Lond). 2008;22(12):1520–1.

Kojima S, Inoue T, Kawaji T, Tanihara H. Filtration bleb revision guided by 3-dimensional anterior segment optical coherence tomography. J Glaucoma. 2014;23:312–5 [Epub ahead of print].

Lachkar Y, Neverauskiene J, Jeanteur-Lunel MN, Gracies H, Berkani M, Ecoffet M, Kopel J, Kretz G, Lavat

P, Lehrer M, Valtot F, Demailly P. Nonpenetrating deep sclerectomy: a 6-year retrospective study. Eur J Ophthalmol. 2004;14(1):26–36.

Lee DA, Higginbotham EJ. Glaucoma and its treatment: a review. Am J Health Syst Pharm. 2005;62(7):691–9.

Leske MC, Heijl A, Hussein M, Bengtsson B, Hyman L, Komaroff E, Early Manifest Glaucoma Trial Group. Factors for glaucoma progression and the effect of treatment: the early manifest glaucoma trial. Arch Ophthalmol. 2003;121(1):48–56.

Liebmann JM, Ritch R. Laser surgery for angle closure glaucoma. Semin Ophthalmol. 2002;17(2):84–91.

Mansouri K, Burgener ND, Bagnoud M, Shaarawy T. A prospective ultrasound biomicroscopy evaluation of changes in anterior segment morphology following laser iridotomy in European eyes. Eye (Lond). 2009;23(11):2046–51.

Melamed S, Ben Simon GJ, Goldenfeld M, Simon G. Efficacy and safety of gold micro shunt implantation to the supraciliary space in patients with glaucoma: a pilot study. Arch Ophthalmol. 2009;127(3):264–9.

Ng DS, Ching RH, Yam JC, Chan CW. Safe excision of a large overhanging cystic bleb following autologous blood injection and compression suture. Korean J Ophthalmol. 2013;27(2):145–8.

Papaconstantinou D, Georgalas I, Karmiris E, Diagourtas A, Koutsandrea C, Ladas I, Apostolopoulos M, Georgopoulos G. Trabeculectomy with OloGen versus trabeculectomy for the treatment of glaucoma: a pilot study. Acta Ophthalmol. 2010;88(1):80–5.

Pirouzian A, Scher C, O'Halloran H, Jockin Y. Ahmed glaucoma valve implants in the pediatric population: the use of magnetic resonance imaging findings for surgical approach to reoperation. J AAPOS. 2006;10(4):340–4.

Reiter M, Schwope R, Walker K, Suhr A. Imaging of glaucoma drainage devices. J Comput Assist Tomogr. 2012;36((2):277–9.

Rosentreter A, Schild AM, Jordan JF, Krieglstein GK, Dietlein TS. A prospective randomised trial of trabeculectomy using mitomycin C vs an ologen implant in open angle glaucoma. Eye (Lond). 2010;24(9):1449–57.

Roy S, Mermoud A. Deep sclerectomy. Dev Ophthalmol. 2012;50:29–36.

Saffra N, Smith SN, Seidman CJ. Topiramate-induced refractive change and angle closure glaucoma and its ultrasound bimicroscopy findings. BMJ Case Rep. 2012;2012.

Sarkisian Jr SR. Tube shunt complications and their prevention. Curr Opin Ophthalmol. 2009;20(2):126–30.

Schwartz KS, Lee RK, Gedde SJ. Glaucoma drainage implants: a critical comparison of types. Curr Opin Ophthalmol. 2006;17(2):181–9.

Scott IU, Alexandrakis G, Flynn Jr HW, Smiddy WE, Murray TG, Schiffman J, Gedde SJ, Budenz DL, Fantes F, Parrish RK. Combined pars plana vitrectomy and glaucoma drainage implant placement for refractory glaucoma. Am J Ophthalmol. 2000;129(3):334–41.

Seibold LK, Rorrer RA, Kahook MY. MRI of the Ex-PRESS stainless steel glaucoma drainage device. Br J Ophthalmol. 2011;95(2):251–4.

Singh M, Chew PT, Friedman DS, Nolan WP, See JL, Smith SD, Zheng C, Foster PJ, Aung T. Imaging of trabeculectomy blebs using anterior segment optical coherence tomography. Ophthalmology. 2007;114(1):47–53.

Stein JD, Herndon LW, Brent Bond J, Challa P. Exposure of Ex-PRESS Miniature Glaucoma Devices: case series and technique for tube shunt removal. J Glaucoma. 2007;16(8):704–6.

Suominen S, Harju M, Ihanamäki T, Vesti E. The effect of deep sclerectomy on intraocular pressure of normal-tension glaucoma patients: 1-year results. Acta Ophthalmol. 2010;88(1):27–32.

Taketani Y, Yamagishi R, Fujishiro T, Igarashi M, Sakata R, Aihara M. Activation of the prostanoid FP receptor inhibits adipogenesis leading to deepening of the upper eyelid sulcus in prostaglandin-associated periorbitopathy. Invest Ophthalmol Vis Sci. 2014;55(3):1269–76.

Tan J, Berke S. Latanoprost-induced prostaglandin-associated periorbitopathy. Optom Vis Sci. 2013;90(9):e245–7; discussion 1029.

Tello C, Espana EM, Mora R, Dorairaj S, Liebmann JM, Ritch R. Baerveldt glaucoma implant insertion in the posterior chamber sulcus. Br J Ophthalmol. 2007;91(6):739–42.

Ventura MP, Vianna RN, Souza Filho JP, Solari HP, Curi RL. Acquired Brown's syndrome secondary to Ahmed valve implant for neovascular glaucoma. Eye (Lond). 2005;19(2):230–2.

Wallsh JO, Gallemore RP, Taban M, Hu C, Sharareh B. Pars plana Ahmed valve and vitrectomy in patients with glaucoma associated with posterior segment disease. Retina. 2013;33(10):2059–68.

Whitson JT. Glaucoma: a review of adjunctive therapy and new management strategies. Expert Opin Pharmacother. 2007;8(18):3237–49.

Wilkins M, Indar A, Wormald R. Intra-operative mitomycin C for glaucoma surgery. Cochrane Database Syst Rev. 2005;(4):CD002897.

Imaging After Oculoplastic Surgery

5

Daniel Thomas Ginat, Gul Moonis, and Suzanne K. Freitag

5.1 Overview

Oculoplastic surgery encompasses a wide variety of procedures involving the ocular adnexa, including the eyelids and periorbital soft tissues, the orbital space and its contents, the bony orbital walls, and the nasolacrimal drainage system. Goals of surgery are not only to correct the problem but to maintain the cosmesis and functionality of this important facial region. Many of these procedures involve the use of grafts and implants, which are often apparent on CT and MRI. While the postoperative findings may be encountered incidentally on radiological imaging, diagnostic radiology serves an important role in excluding or evaluating potential postoperative complications. The spectrum of non-oncological oculoplastic surgeries and corresponding expected and complicated results on imaging are reviewed in the subsequent sections. Oncological cases are discussed in a dedicated chapter.

D.T. Ginat, MD, MS (⊠)
Director of Head and Neck Imaging,
Department of Radiology, University of Chicago,
5841 S Maryland Avenue, Chicago, IL 60637, USA
e-mail: ginatd01@gmail.com

G. Moonis, MD
Department of Radiology, Beth Israel Deaconess
Medical Center, Boston, MA, USA

S.K. Freitag, MD
Director, Ophthalmic Plastic Surgery Service,
Department of Ophthalmology, Massachusetts Eye
and Ear Infirmary, Harvard Medical School,
Boston, MA, USA

5.2 Periorbital Cosmetic Fillers

Injectable fillers are a minimally invasive option for periorbital augmentation and facial rejuvenation. Among the more commonly used filler agents in the periorbital region are hyaluronic acid gels. Since these fillers are comprised mostly of water, they appear as high signal intensity on STIR and T2-weighted MRI sequences (Fig. 5.1). The fillers usually do not display enhancement centrally, although they may elicit an inflammatory response that can result in enhancement and hypermetabolism on 18FDG-PET. Occasionally, the fillers may appear clumped and can mimic tumors on imaging. These fillers are temporary and gradually resorb over the course of months.

5.3 Punctal Plugs

Punctal and canalicular plugs are small devices used to occlude the lacrimal outflow system for treatment of dry eye syndrome and after surgical procedures such as penetrating keratoplasty or refractive surgery. A variety of plugs are available, including those composed of collagen, hydrogel, and silicone (Fig. 5.2). The silicone punctual plugs are radio-opaque (Fig. 5.3) and visible on radiographs, which can be used to localize the plugs if there is clinical uncertainty. The plugs should be appropriately recognized on radiographs so as to not mistake them for metal foreign bodies when screening patients prior to MRI.

D.T. Ginat, S.K. Freitag (eds.), *Post-treatment Imaging of the Orbit*,
DOI 10.1007/978-3-662-44023-0_5, © Springer-Verlag Berlin Heidelberg 2015

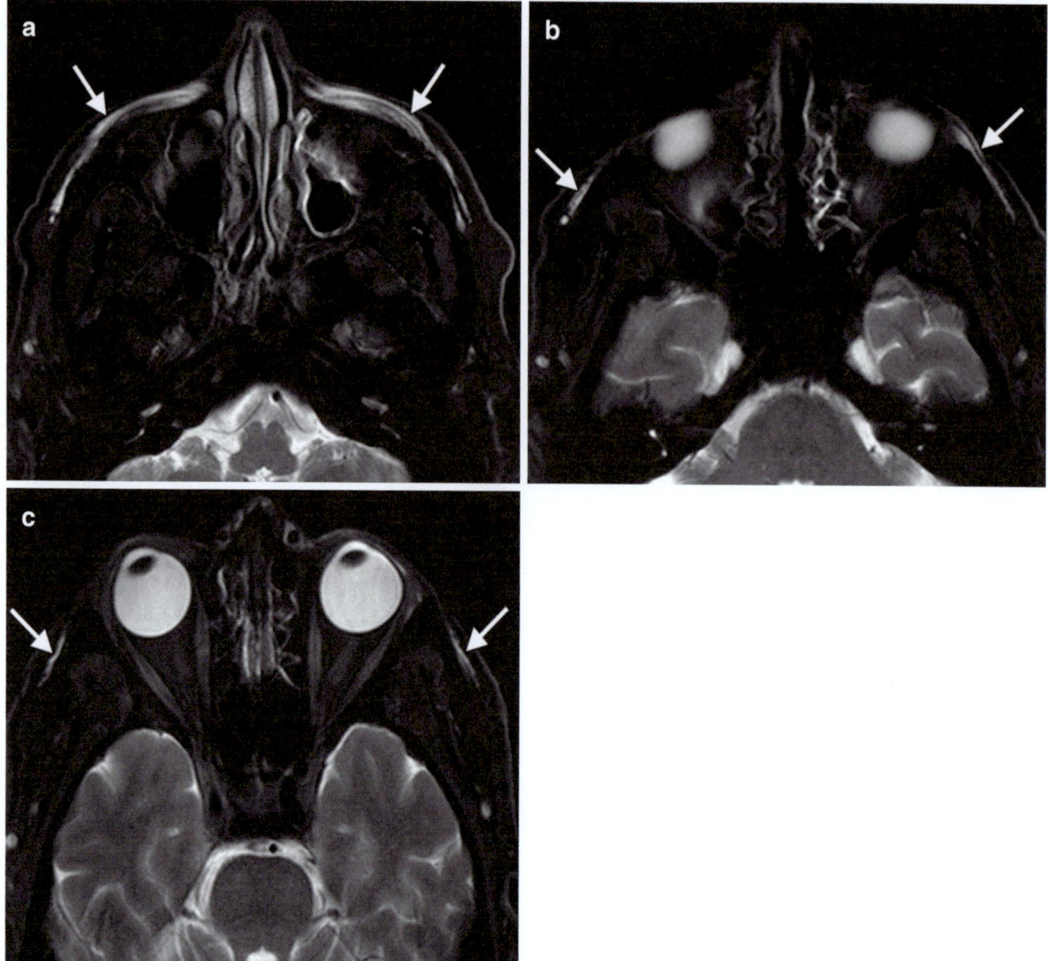

Fig. 5.1 Periorbital injectable fillers used for malar and temporalis augmentation. Axial fat-suppressed T2-weighted MR images (**a**–**c**) show streaky areas of high signal within the periorbital soft tissues, which correspond to the filler material (*arrows*). These were incidental findings on the MRI, which was performed for other reasons

5.4 Eyelid Weights

Facial nerve deficits can lead to keratitis secondary to lagophthalmos, eyelid retraction, and incomplete blink. Implantation of eyelid weights in the upper eyelid as a procedure for addressing this condition was introduced in 1958 by Illig. Platinum or gold weights are available in different sizes and shapes, including thin profile (Fig. 5.4). Standard sizes range from 0.6 to 1.8 g. The implants are contoured to fit the curvature of the globe and contain holes for fixation to the tarsus with sutures, which can be identified on plain radiographs (Fig. 5.5). Ingrowth of fibrous tissue through the holes also helps secure the weight in position. Flexible chains have also been designed to optimally match the curvature of the tarsal plate of the upper eyelid. Eyelid weights are typically implanted between the orbicularis oculi muscle and the tarsal plate and secured to the tarsus in the upper eyelid, enhancing upper eyelid excursion. The eyelid weights generally produce considerable streak artifact on CT, which can obscure surrounding anatomy (Fig. 5.6). Platinum and gold eyelid weights are considered MRI compatible but may also cause susceptibility effects

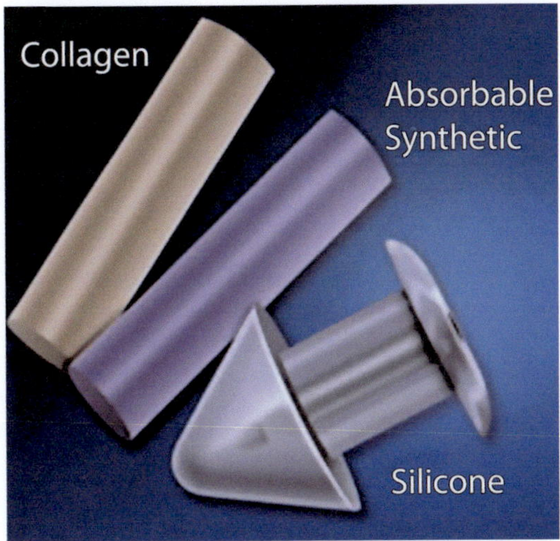

Fig. 5.2 Illustration of different types of commercially available punctual plugs (Courtesy of I-med Pharma, Inc)

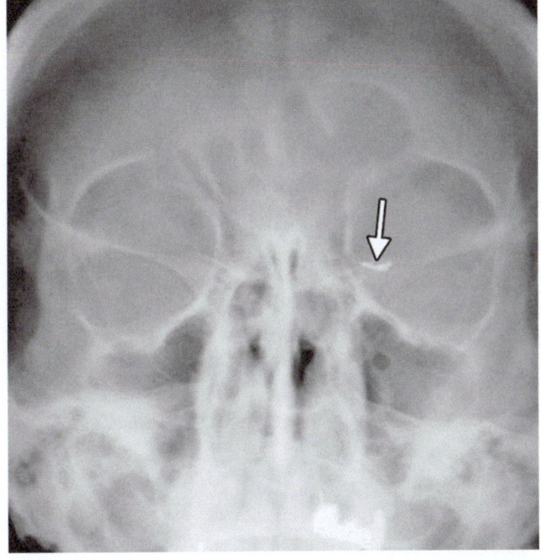

Fig. 5.3 Punctal plug. Frontal radiograph shows a radio-opaque linear structure projecting at the expected location of the left inferior lacrimal punctum and canaliculus (*arrow*)

that limit the visualization of surrounding structures (Fig. 5.7). Complications related to eyelid implantation include prominent implants visible through the skin, infection, allergic reaction, migration, and extrusion. Ultimately, the eyelid weight may be removed if sufficient facial nerve function is recovered.

5.5 Eyelid Springs

Eyelid (palpebral) springs are infrequently used to augment lid closure in patients with eyelid paralysis. The device is implanted via orbitotomy and consists of a palpebral branch and an orbital branch connected by a spring mechanism at the fulcrum (Fig. 5.8). The spring mechanism is sutured to the periosteum of the lateral orbital rim. The positioning and function of the device can be assessed on radiographs obtained in the open and closed lid positions, whereby the palpebral branch is expected to descend with lid closure (Fig. 5.9). This does not occur, however, if the device has been deactivated. The eyelid spring in relation to the soft tissues of the orbit can be better depicted on CT, however (Fig. 5.10). Potential complications include dislocation, metal fatigue resulting in failure, and exposure.

5.6 Lateral Canthotomy, Cantholysis, and Canthopexy

Lateral canthotomy and cantholysis is a procedure used to treat orbital compartment syndrome in the setting of acute orbital hemorrhage or other conditions causing high orbital pressure such as carotid cavernous fistula. It is also used

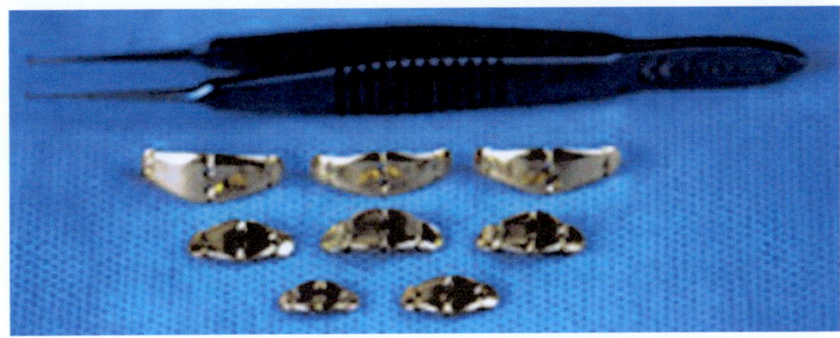

Fig. 5.4 Photograph of various sizes of gold eyelid weight implants (Courtesy of Osmed)

as a surgical approach to the lateral orbit. The procedure involves incising the lateral canthus of the eyelids and releasing one or both lateral canthal tendons. On imaging, disruption of one or both lateral canthal tendons can be discerned, and increased proptosis and herniation of orbital contents may be observed after the procedure (Fig. 5.11). Canthopexy, on the other hand, consists of repairing or reattaching the canthal ten-

dons. Occasionally metallic anchors, such as wire or screws, may be used to affix the ligament to the underlying bone, which should not be mistaken as an unintended foreign body on imaging (Fig. 5.12).

5.7 Orbital Tissue Expanders for Congenital Anophthalmia

Congenital or acquired anophthalmia in pediatric patients has significant cosmetic ramifications. In particular, growth of the orbit during early childhood is dependent on the presence and growth of the orbital contents. If untreated, an anophthalmic socket in a young child will result in a disproportionately small orbit and sometimes entire hemifacial bone structure compared to the contralateral side. Traditional methods for orbital expansion include using progressively enlarging static acrylic conformers, insertion of conventional static spherical orbital implants, dermis-fat grafts, or inflatable balloon expanders for orbital enlargement. However, these techniques may still result in suboptimal cosmetic outcomes, with delayed growth of the bony orbit and overlying soft tissues. Another option for stimulating bone growth in an anophthalmic socket is an integrated

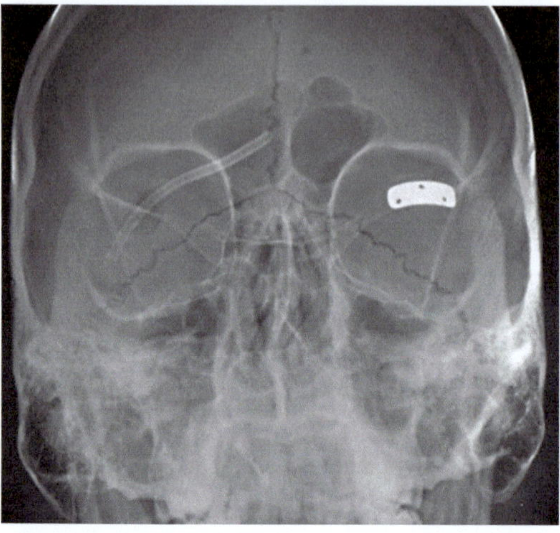

Fig. 5.5 Eyelid weight depicted on radiography. Frontal radiograph shows a rectangular, curved metal implant containing *three holes* for suture fixation at the level of the left upper eyelid

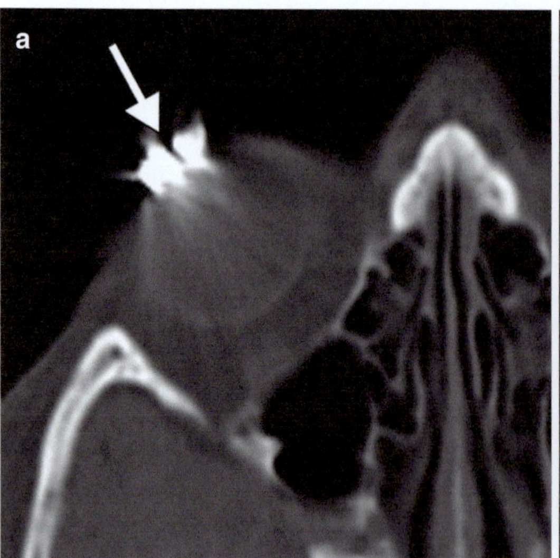
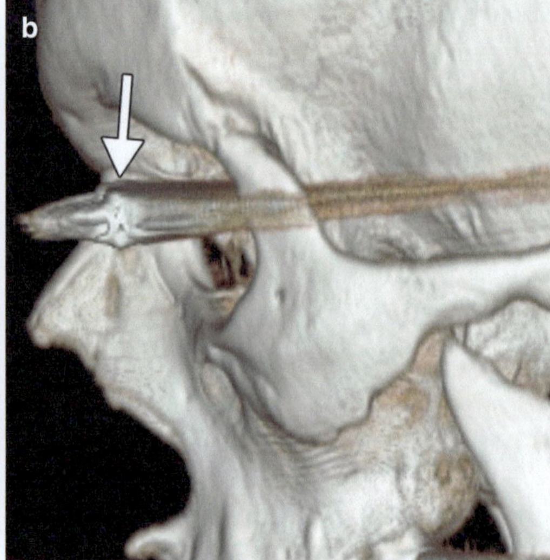

Fig. 5.6 Eyelid weight depicted on CT. The axial (**a**) and 3D CT (**b**) images show extensive streak artifact associated with the device (*arrows*)

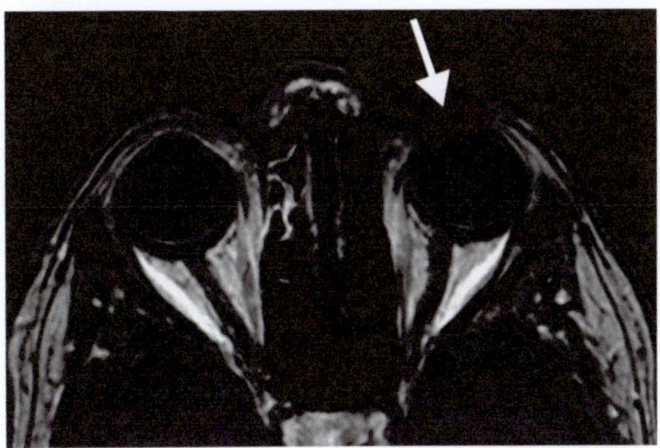

Fig. 5.7 The fat-suppressed post-contrast T1-weighted MRI shows that the presence of the eyelid weight (*arrow*) results in mild field inhomogeneity from metal artifact that obscures surrounding structures

orbital tissue expander comprised of an inflatable silicone globe on a sliding titanium T-plate secured to the lateral orbital rim with screws (Fig. 5.13). The sphere can be inflated via transconjunctival injection of saline. Saline expanders appear as spherical sacs containing fluid attenuation on CT adjacent to the metal density T-plate (Fig. 5.14). Hydrogel tissue expanders are an alternative therapy for the anophthalmic socket. The expanders are inserted in a dry, contracted state and expand gradually to full size via osmosis of fluid from surrounding tissues, with up to a tenfold increase in volume. Hydrogel orbital expanders are available in the form of spheres and hemispheres (Fig. 5.15). Hydrogel expanders appear as nearly fluid attenuation on CT due to the high water content. On MRI, these devices tend to display low T1 signal and high T2 signal, and do not enhance (Fig. 5.16). The increased orbital volume provided by the use of these devices can be delineated on imaging.

5.8 Evisceration, Enucleation, and Exenteration

When there is otherwise untreatable disease, it may become necessary to remove the eye or the entire orbital contents. The surgical options include evisceration, enucleation, and exenteration.

Evisceration consists of removing the globe contents while preserving the sclera and attached

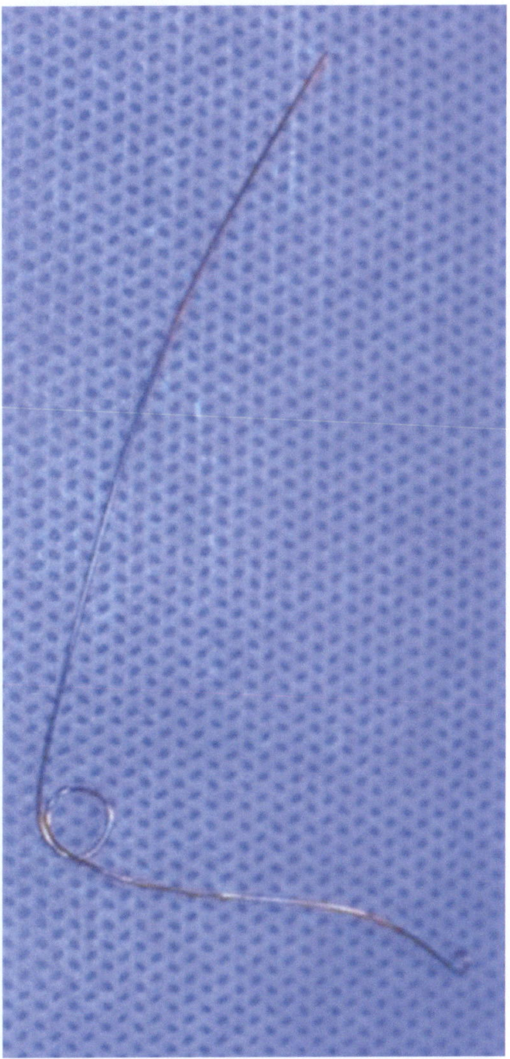

Fig. 5.8 Photograph of an eyelid spring (Courtesy of Dawn DeCastro MD)

extraocular muscles (Fig. 5.17). Occasionally, the cornea may be retained. Indications include endophthalmitis or a blind, painful eye due to a known etiology that would not be exacerbated by incomplete excision. The residual sclera can be discerned on CT and MRI. A spherical implant is often inserted within the residual sclera (Fig. 5.18). Alternatively, the scleral cavity may be filled with a dermis-fat graft (Fig. 5.19). Dermis fat graft placement is sometimes performed after complications related to initial placement of a synthetic implant. After proper healing, a prosthetic shell may be made

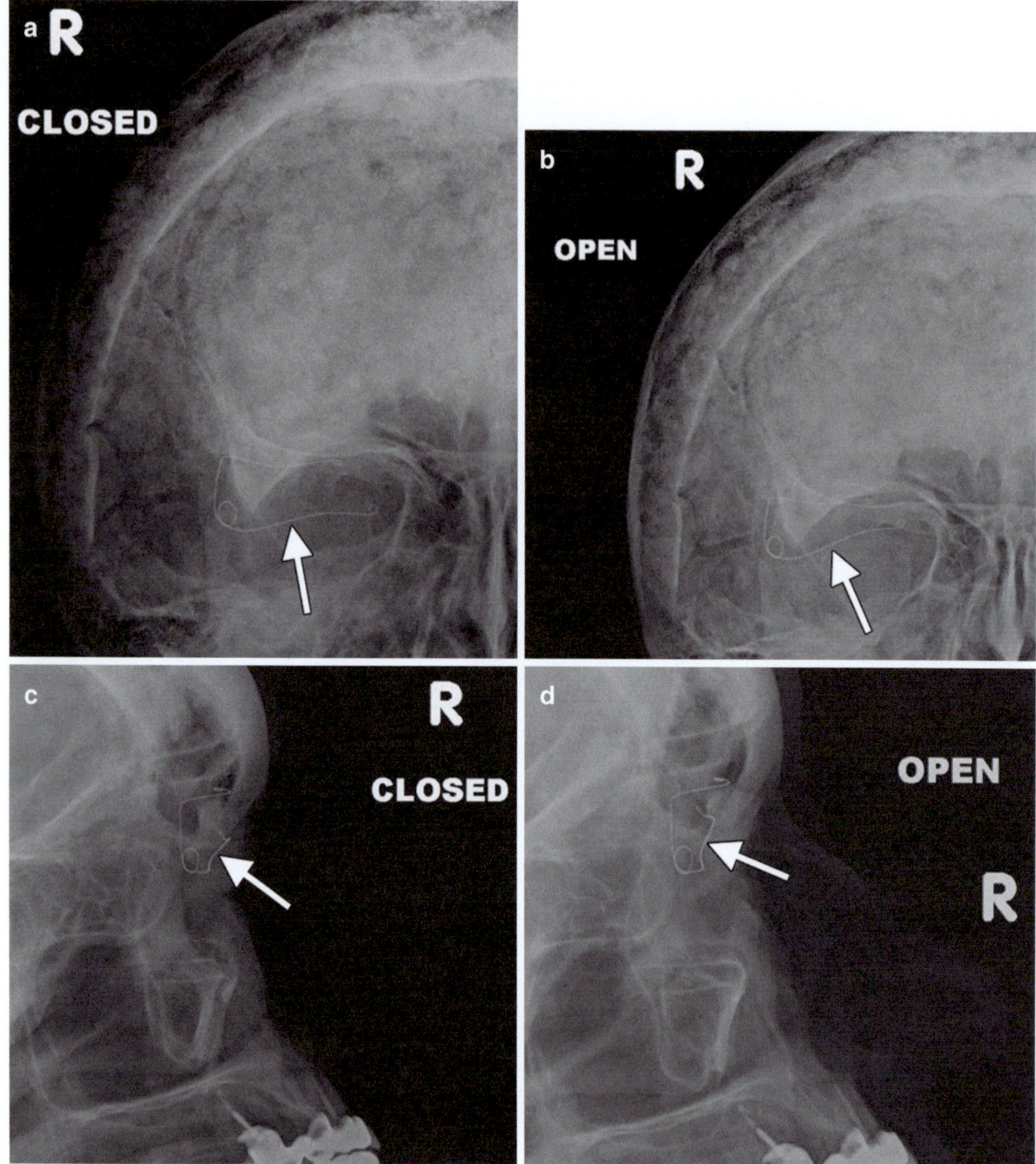

Fig. 5.9 Eyelid spring on dynamic radiographic imaging. Open and closed frontal and lateral radiographs (**a–d**) show the lower arm of the device (*arrows*) moves with the eyelid

to cover the socket and cosmetically match the contralateral eye.

Enucleation consists of removing the entire globe (Fig. 5.20). Indications for enucleation include a blind painful eye, intraocular tumor, trauma with risk of sympathetic ophthalmia, phthisis bulbi, microphthalmia, and panophthalmitis. The extraocular muscles may be imbricated in front of an orbital implant, sutured directly to the orbital implant or to the wrapping surrounding the implant, or, less commonly, allowed to fall back into the orbit. The orbital implant and wrapper may be made from a variety of materials, which are described below. As with evisceration, a prosthetic shell is usually made to cover the socket. Rarely, a shell may be used alone without an orbital implant filling the socket, particularly if a complication necessitated removal of the implant (Fig. 5.21).

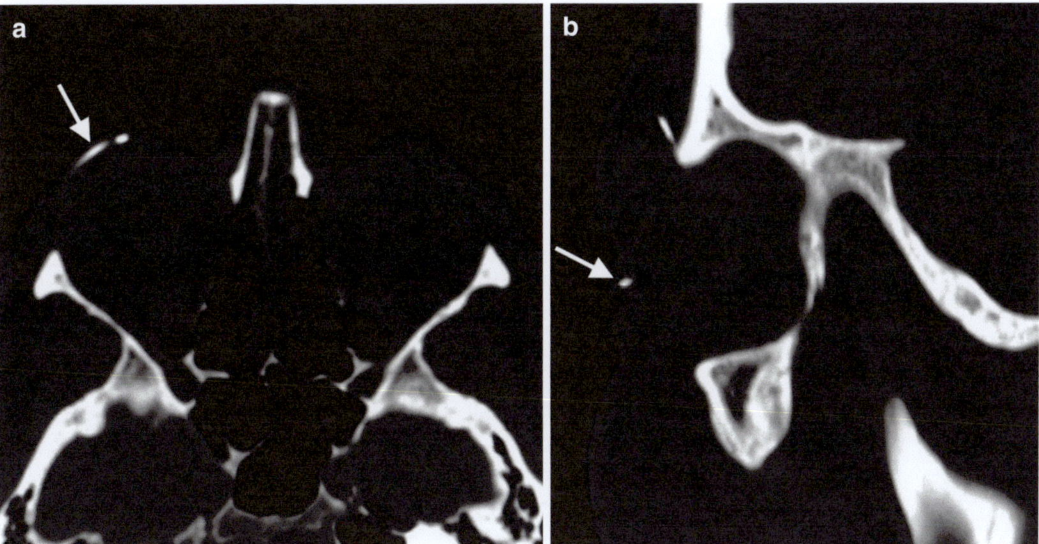

Fig. 5.10 Eyelid spring depicted on CT. Axial (**a**) and sagittal (**b**) CT images show the inferior limb of the spring positioned within the upper lid (*arrows*)

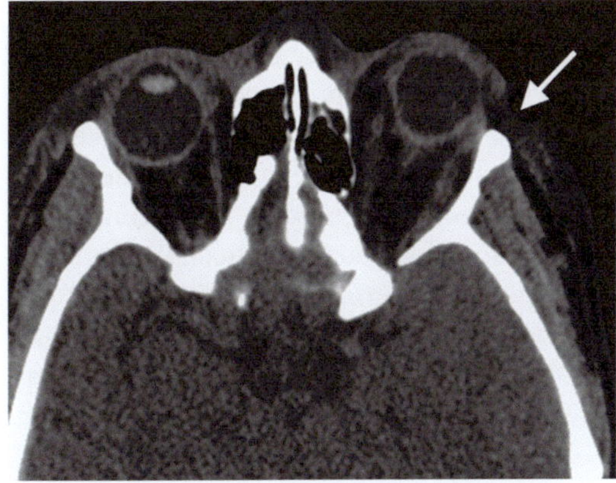

Fig. 5.11 Lateral canthotomy and cantholysis. Axial CT image shows a surgical defect in the left lateral canthal region (*arrow*) with mild anterior herniation of orbital fat and proptosis

Several types of orbital implants may be used after evisceration and enucleation. These can be composed of a variety of materials (Table 5.1) and are available in different shapes and sizes (Figs. 5.22, 5.23, 5.24, 5.25, 5.26, and 5.27). For example, implants may feature grooves for the extraocular muscles or have ovoid configurations that were designed to conform better to the enucleation cavity than standard spherical implants. Furthermore, the implants may be fitted with motility pegs that couple the ocular prosthesis with the ocular implant in order to optimally synchronize and transmit motion to the prosthesis when the extraocular muscles move the implant. These motility pegs have fallen out of favor in recent years because of frequent complications. MRI has a specific role in the evaluation of ocular implants for motility pegs; it serves to confirm sufficient fibrovascular ingrowth of the implant in order to accommodate the peg. Although modern implants are generally composed of hydroxyapatite, porous polyethylene (Medpor), and silicone, older implants composed of plastic, acrylic, glass, and metal may still be encountered on imaging (Fig. 5.28). Regardless of the implant type, signal changes within the optic nerve remnant on T2-weighted images and atrophy of the nerve remnant and the chiasm are to be expected following enucleation and should not be interpreted as necessarily indicating active pathology (Fig. 5.29).

Orbital exenteration is a radical procedure that involves removal of the globe and orbital contents (Fig. 5.30). The eyelids may be spared, depending on the pathology. Indications include cutaneous or conjunctival malignancies with orbital invasion, orbital or lacrimal gland malignancies, or orbital mucormycosis.

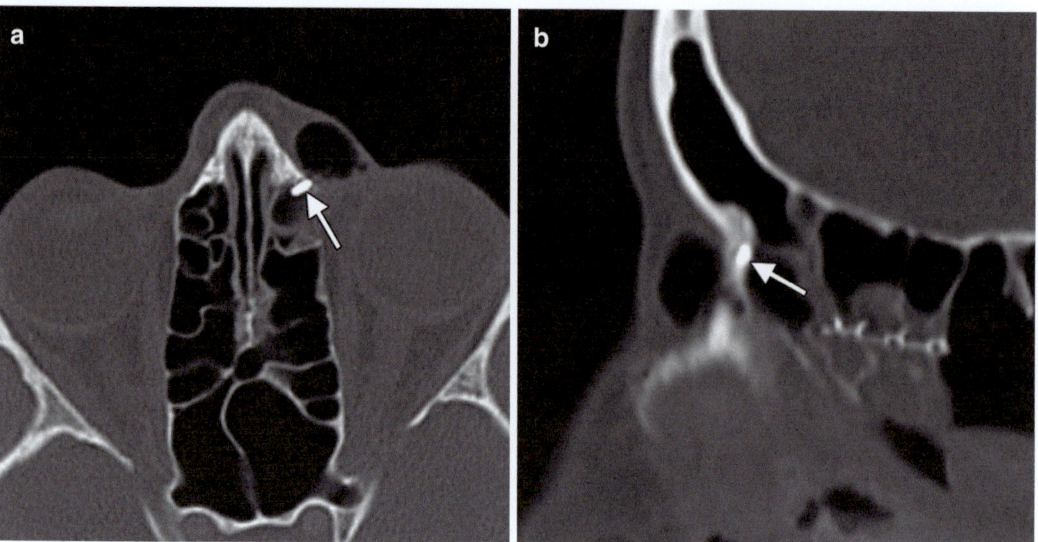

Fig. 5.12 Canthopexy with Mitek anchor. Axial (**a**) and sagittal (**b**) CT images show a metallic density structure embedded within the left frontal process of the maxilla (*arrows*)

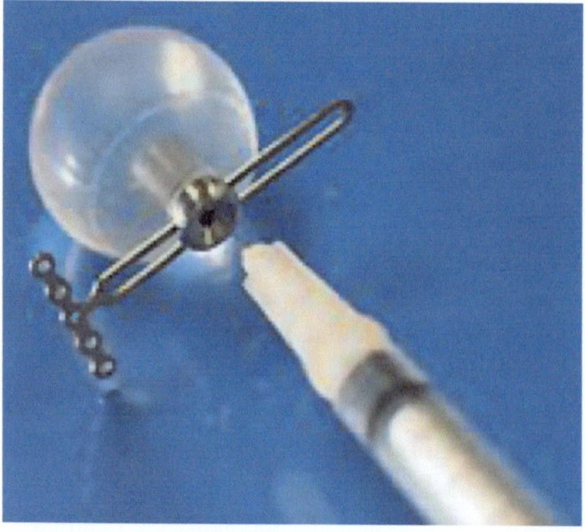

Fig. 5.13 Photograph of a saline orbital sphere, which consists of an inflatable silicone sphere held in place by a titanium bone plate anchored to the lateral orbital wall by screws with a slotted arm attached to the bone plate, providing multiple fixation areas. This allows for repeated fixation adjustments as the orbit enlarges (Courtesy of Innovia LLC)

Reconstructive techniques include ipsilateral temporalis muscle flaps, cutaneous or myocutaneous free flaps, and osseointegrated implants. Often the socket is left to granulate or is lined with a split-thickness skin graft, which allows for direct surveillance for recurrent disease.

Diagnostic imaging can be helpful for evaluating certain complications that may occur following evisceration, enucleation, and exenteration. Postoperative hemorrhage into the enucleation cavity may appear as hyperattenuating fluid outlined by the residual sclera (Fig. 5.31). Postoperative infection is particularly a concern when surgery is performed in the setting of preexisting endophthalmitis or panophthalmitis. On imaging, abnormal fluid collections, gas, fat stranding, and enhancement may be encountered within the enucleation cavity (Fig. 5.32). Likewise, infected fluid collections can form around the implants and prostheses (Fig. 5.33). In the setting of exenteration for rhino-orbitocerebral zygomycosis, serial imaging may show the need for repeated radical debridement. Nevertheless, this condition carries a poor prognosis due to complications such as arteritis and cerebral infarction (Fig. 5.34). Postoperative conjunctival dehiscence resulting in exposure of the orbital implant may result from inflammation or infection or improper selection of the orbital implant size. Although implant extrusion may be clinically apparent, imaging is useful for evaluating associated problems (Fig. 5.35). Finally, the stigmata of postenucleation/evisceration socket

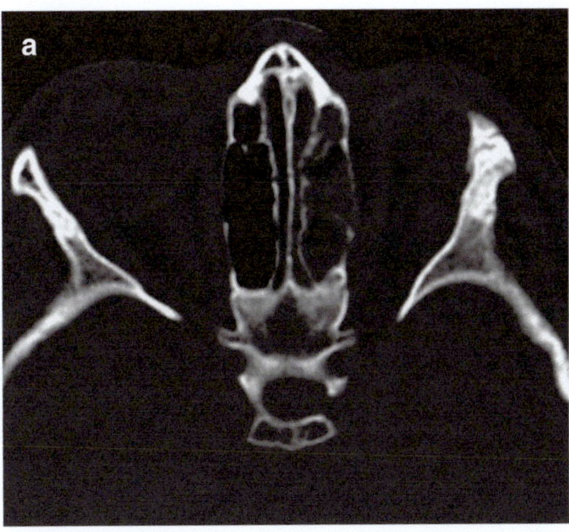

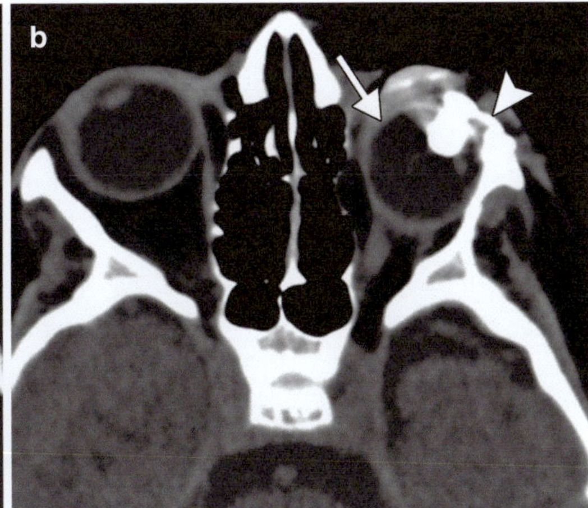

Fig. 5.14 Saline orbital expander. Preoperative axial CT image (**a**) shows a small left orbit. Postoperative axial CT image (**b**) shows a saline-filled left orbital expander (*arrow*) attached to the lateral orbital rim via the metal plate (*arrowhead*) (Courtesy of David Tse MD)

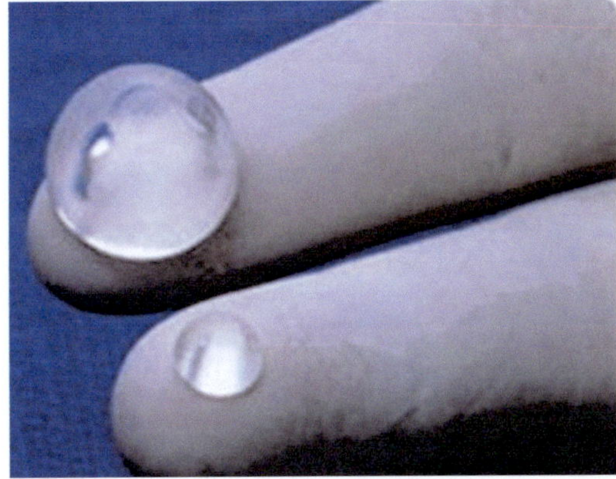

Fig. 5.15 Photograph of hydrogel hemispheric implants shows the degree to which the implants can expand. The material can be used to increase the orbital volume prior to permanent orbital implant insertion (Courtesy of Osmed)

5.9 Orbital Foreign Body Removal

Prompt detection and accurate localization of intraorbital foreign bodies are crucial for the optimal management of patients. Computed tomography (CT) is very useful in determining the size of foreign bodies and localizing them as intraocular, extraocular, or retro-ocular before, during, and after surgery if necessary. Metallic foreign bodies are readily recognizable on CT, although streak artifact can obscure surrounding structures. Plastic and wood foreign bodies may be less conspicuous on CT. In particular, wood can mimic air on CT. CT is generally considered the gold standard in the evaluation of foreign bodies because it is safe to use with metallic foreign bodies and it excludes orbitocranial extension and is also able to diagnose orbital wall fractures with high accuracy. CT is sometimes obtained after foreign body removal for verification (Fig. 5.37) and to assess potential complications such as orbital infection. However, many orbital foreign bodies, particularly those made of metal and those in posterior orbital locations, are not surgically removed. MRI is generally not recommended for the evaluation of the foreign bodies due to the risks associated with ferromagnetic metal.

volume loss can be encountered on diagnostic imaging. This syndrome is fairly common and consists of enophthalmos, deepening of the superior sulcus, tilting of the prosthesis, and sinking of the implant (Fig. 5.36). Correction of anophthalmic enophthalmos can be achieved using injectable filler agents, such as calcium hydroxyapatite and hyaluronic- or collagen-based gels.

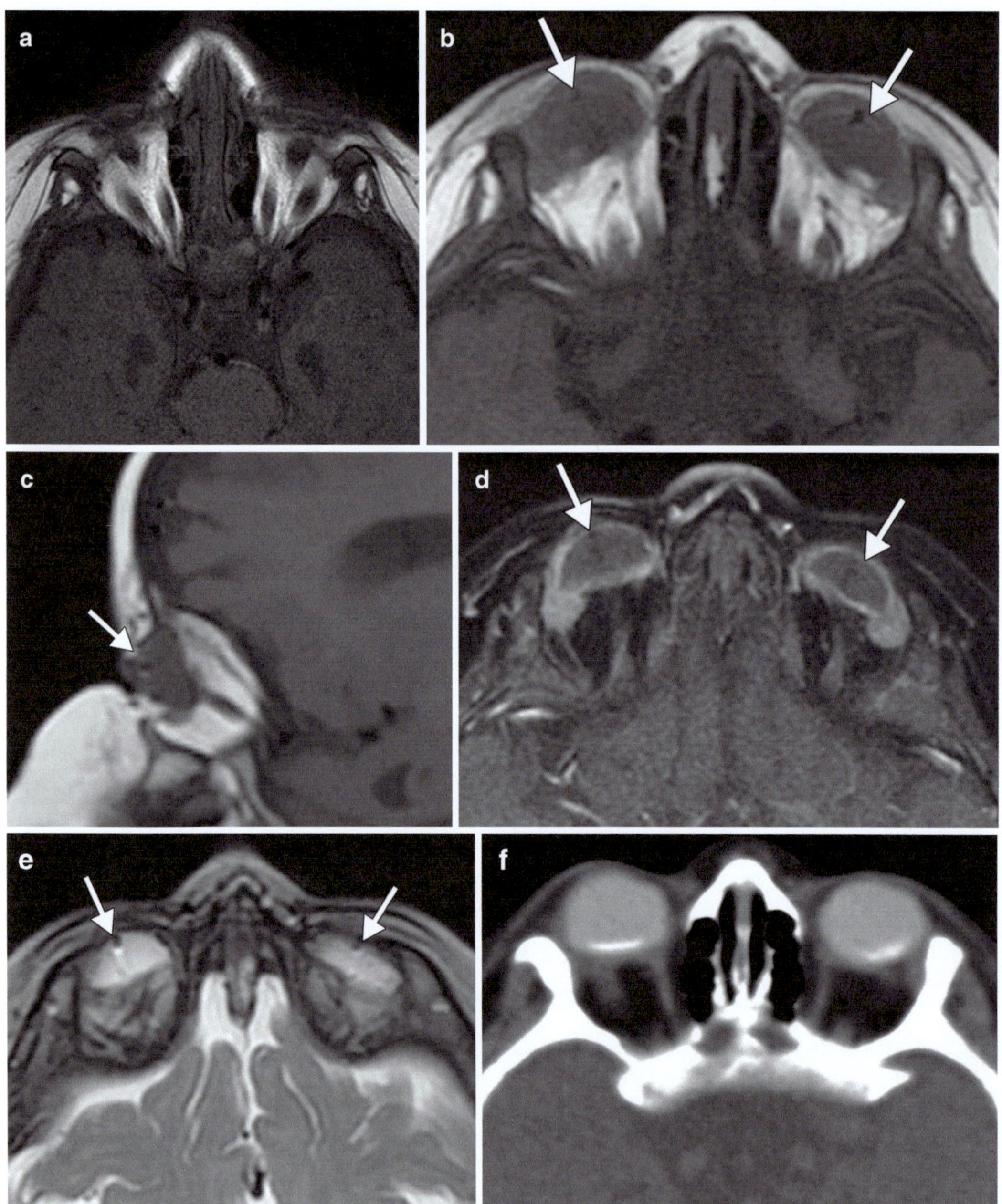

Fig. 5.16 Hydrogel orbital expander. Preoperative axial T1-weighted MRI (**a**) shows bilateral anophthalmos. Axial (**b**) and sagittal (**c**) T1-weighted, axial post-contrast T1-weighted (**d**), and axial T2-weighted (**e**), and MR images show bilateral hemispherical hydrogel expanders in position (*arrows*). The expanders have signal characteristics similar to fluid. Subsequent axial CT image (**f**) shows interval placement of bilateral orbital implants

5.10 Orbital Fracture Repair

A wide variety of materials can be used for orbital fracture repair (Table 5.2 and Figs. 5.38, 5.39, 5.40, and 5.41).

5.10.1 Orbital Wall and Rim Fracture Repair

The goal of managing orbital wall blow-in or blow-out fractures is to restore extraocular

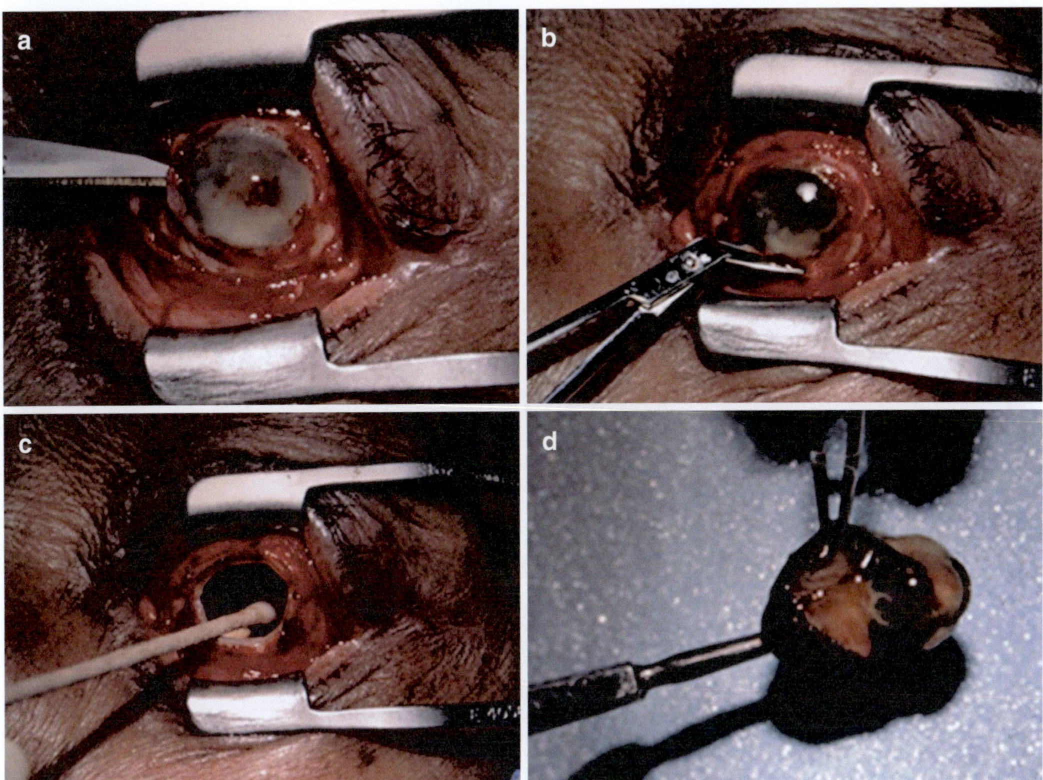

Fig. 5.17 Evisceration surgery. The patient has a history of endophthalmitis. Intraoperative photograph after circumferential conjunctival peritomy shows the anterior chamber is entered with a blade (**a**); the cornea is removed (**b**); the sclera is emptied of its contents and cleaned with absolute alcohol (**c**); the infected intra-ocular contents have been removed (**d**)

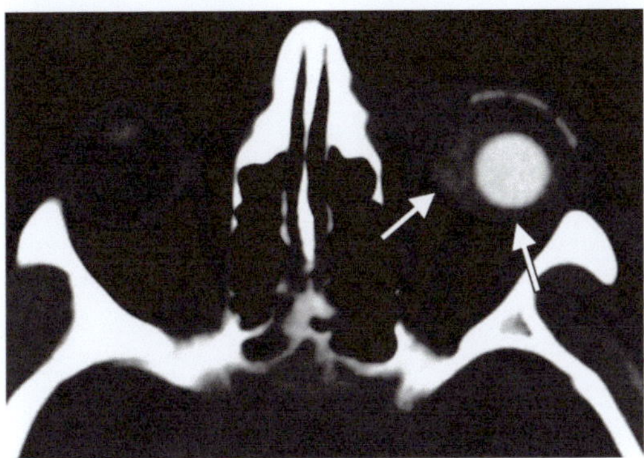

Fig. 5.18 Evisceration with intrascleral implant. Axial CT image shows a left evisceration socket containing a small spherical implant and hyperattenuating fluid that outlines the surrounding sclera (*arrows*)

motility and orbital volume, which can be impacted by herniation of orbital contents, displaced bone fragments, and expansion of the bony orbit. Although postoperative imaging after orbital fracture repair is mainly performed to assess complications, some practitioners request CT to verify correct positioning of orbital sheet implants and reduction of fracture fragments in the early postoperative period. Medial orbital wall fractures may be associated with diplopia due to herniation or entrapment of the medial rectus muscle. In large medial orbital wall fractures, complete coverage of the posterior aspect of the fracture with the implant can be difficult, and CT may be useful to define the extent to which there is remaining deficiency of the lamina papyracea (Fig. 5.42). Orbital floor fractures in children often do not require reduction, since the flexible bone assumes a near-anatomic alignment. However, pediatric trapdoor fractures may require urgent treatment in order to prevent ischemia and permanent damage to the affected extra-ocular muscle. Orbital roof fractures that are associated with dural tears may require an

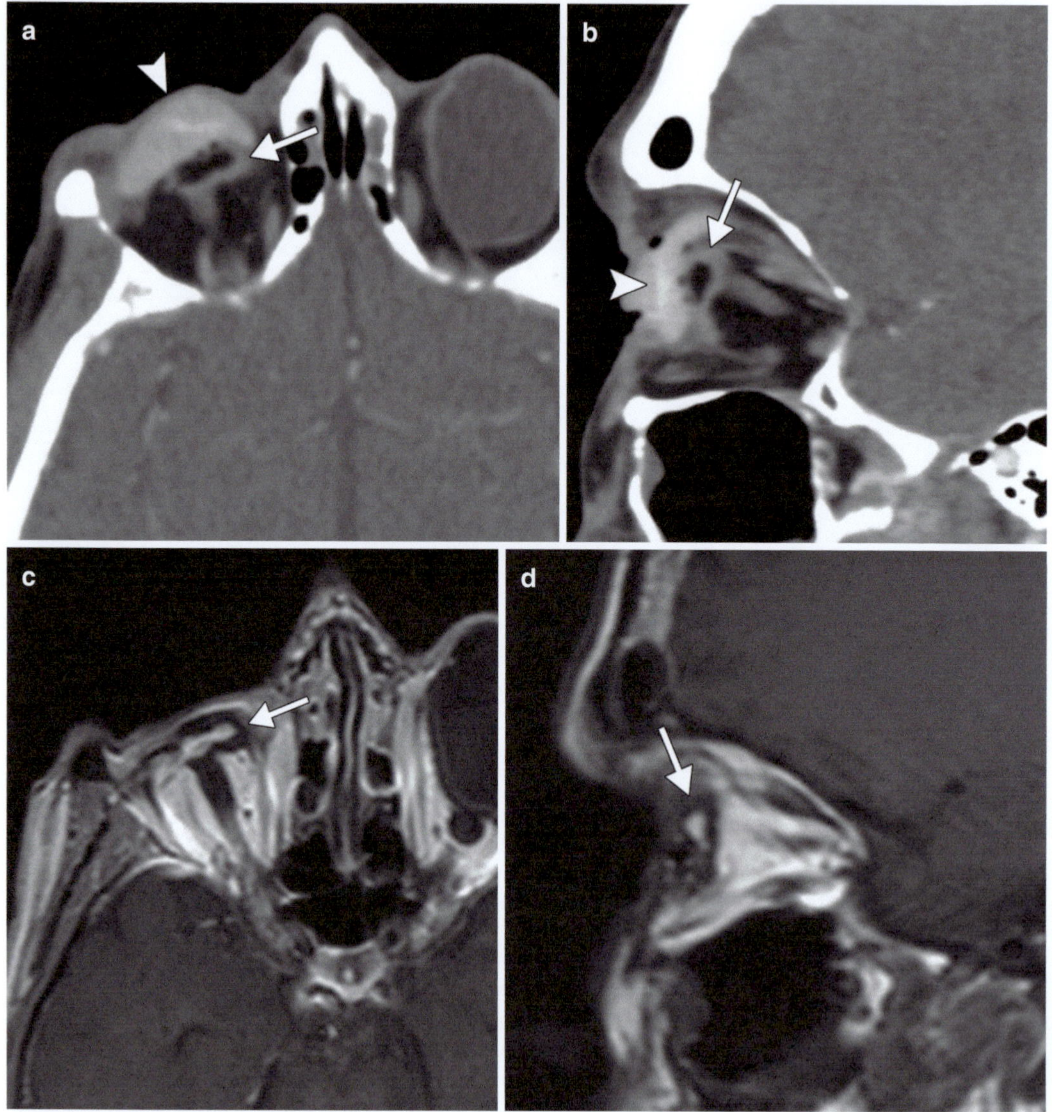

Fig. 5.19 Eviscerated sclera without orbital implant. Axial (**a**) and sagittal (**b**) CT images and axial (**c**) and sagittal (**d**) post-contrast T1 MRI images show the partially collapsed residual sclera within the right orbit (*arrows*). A scleral shell prosthesis is present on the CT (*arrowheads*) but absent on the MRI

intracranial approach, whereby fat, mesh, and/or fascial grafts are positioned over the orbital roof in order to reconstruct the defect and seal dural leaks (Fig. 5.43). Reconstructed orbital roof fractures sometimes have a flattened configuration, which can be associated with exophthalmos (Fig. 5.44). Superior orbital rim fractures associated with pneumatized frontal sinuses pose particular cosmetic and functional considerations.

Along with restoring the proper orbital contour, it is also important to maintain the integrity of the frontal sinus to minimize the risk of infection and obstruction of secretions. Comminuted fractures of this region can be secured via absorbable or low-profile titanium mesh for optimal cosmetic results (Fig. 5.45). Finally, small residual displaced bone fragments in the orbits or paranasal sinuses associated with comminuted orbital

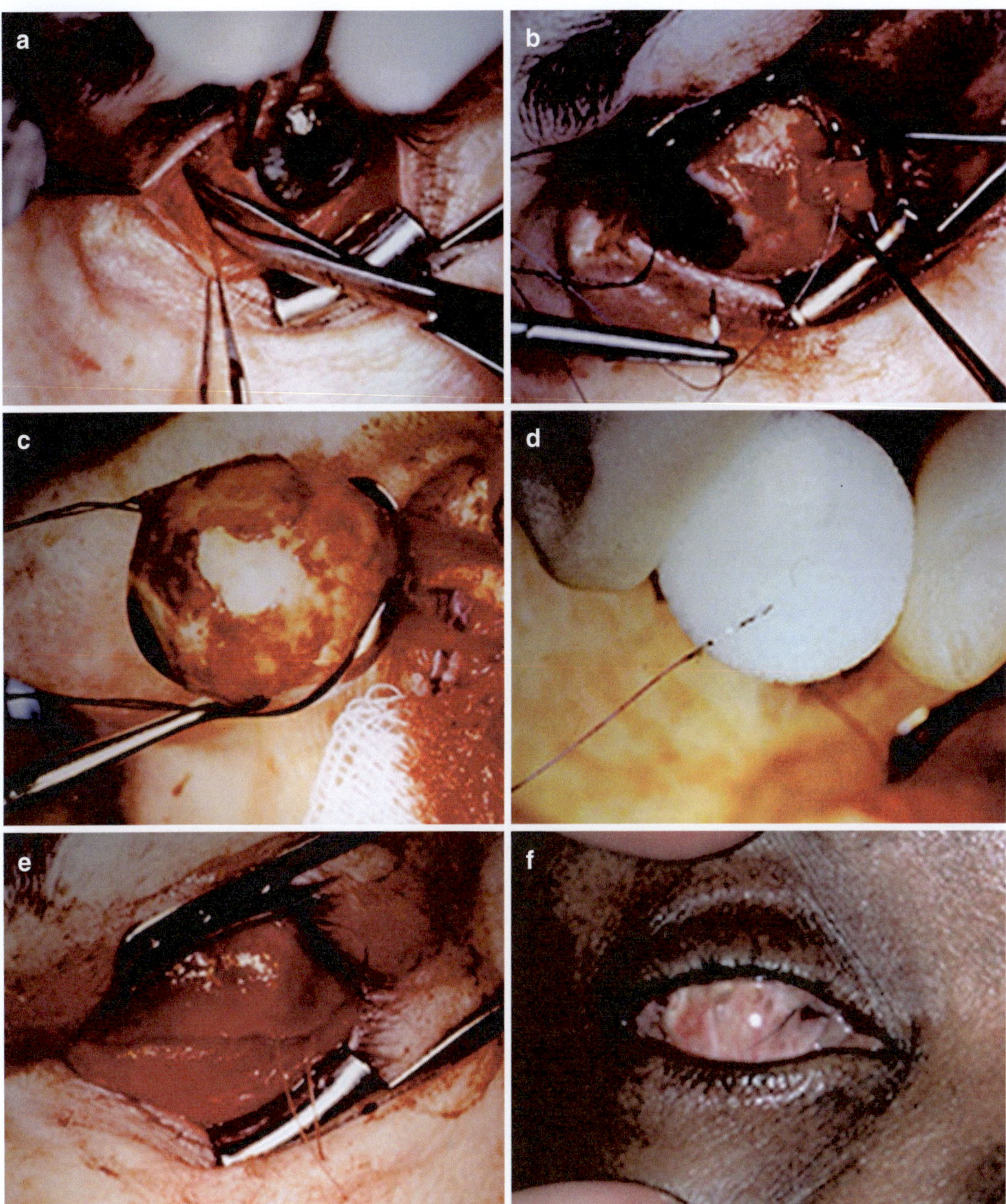

Fig. 5.20 Enucleation procedure. Photograph shows conjunctiva is being opened 360° to expose globe and extraocular muscles (**a**). Each extraocular muscle is isolated, sutured, and detached from the globe (**b**). The globe is removed from the orbit after the optic nerve has been transected (**c**). Extraocular muscles are sutured to implant (**d**). Tenon's capsule and conjunctiva are closed anterior to the implant (**e**). A well-healed anophthalmic socket with clear plastic conformer is shown in a different patient (**f**)

fractures are not uncommonly encountered and are typically left in position after repair, since these are generally innocuous and resorb over time (Fig. 5.46). Likewise, paranasal sinus opacification from hemorrhage and inflammation during the early postoperative period generally resolves spontaneously, unless there is outflow obstruction.

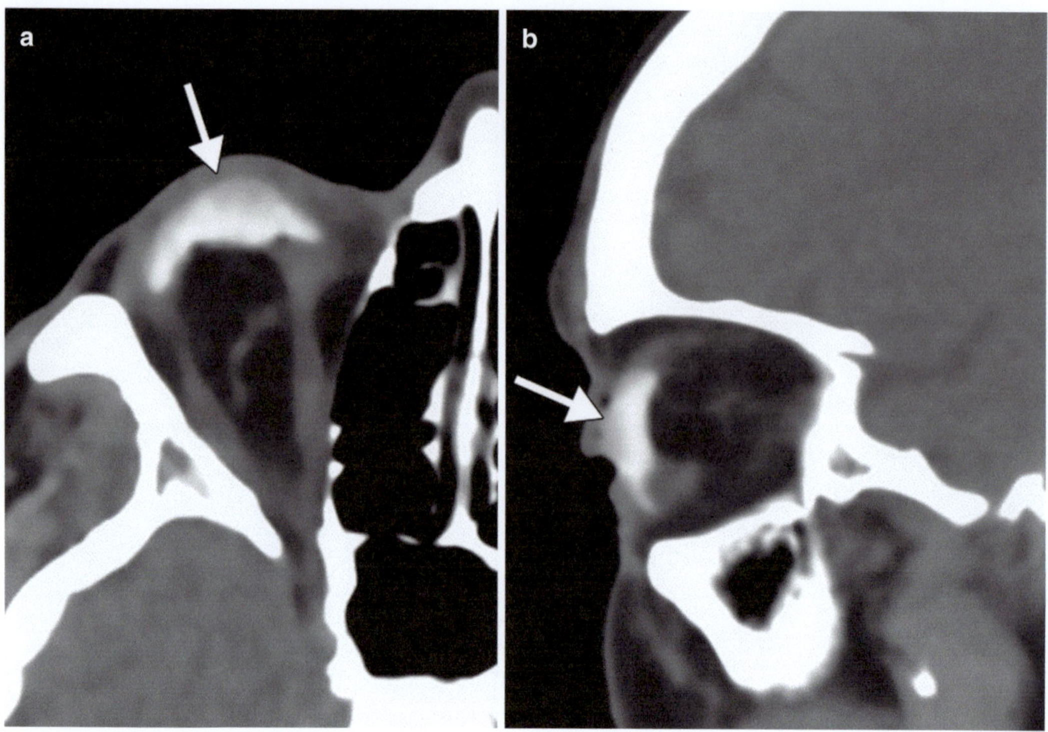

Fig. 5.21 Orbital prosthesis without orbital implant after enucleation. Axial (**a**) and sagittal (**b**) CT images show a hyperattenuating ocular prosthesis (*arrows*) supported by orbital fat after enucleation

Table 5.1 Imaging features of commonly used orbital implant materials

Material	CT	MRI
Hydroxyapatite and aluminum hydroxide ceramic	Hyperattenuating, similar to cortical bone	Low to intermediate signal on T1 and T2. Enhancement may occur with fibrovascular ingrowth
Silicone	Hyperattenuating but to a lesser degree than hydroxyapatite	Very low signal on T1 and T2
Porous polyethylene (Medpor)	Attenuation intermediate between fat and water	Low signal on T1 and high on T2. Enhancement after fibrovascular ingrowth

5.10.2 Nasoorbitoethmoid Fracture Repair

Nasoorbitoethmoid fractures involve the central upper midface, disrupting the confluence of the medial maxillary buttress with the upper transverse maxillary buttress, as well as their posterior extensions along the medial orbital wall and floor. The frontal sinus and frontoethmoid recesses are often obliterated using bone chips, fat graft, and other materials in order to prevent postoperative mucocele formation due to inad-

equate frontal sinus drainage. Fractures of the nasoorbitoethmoid complex can be difficult to accurately repair. Therefore, postoperative high-resolution maxillofacial CT is useful (Fig. 5.47). Even if the frontal process of the maxilla (superior portion of the medial maxillary buttress) is anatomically reduced, there can still be a residual rotational deformity or displaced bone fragment at the attachment of the medial canthus that disrupts the posterior extension of this buttress. This will increase the transverse distance between the medial orbital walls and the attachments

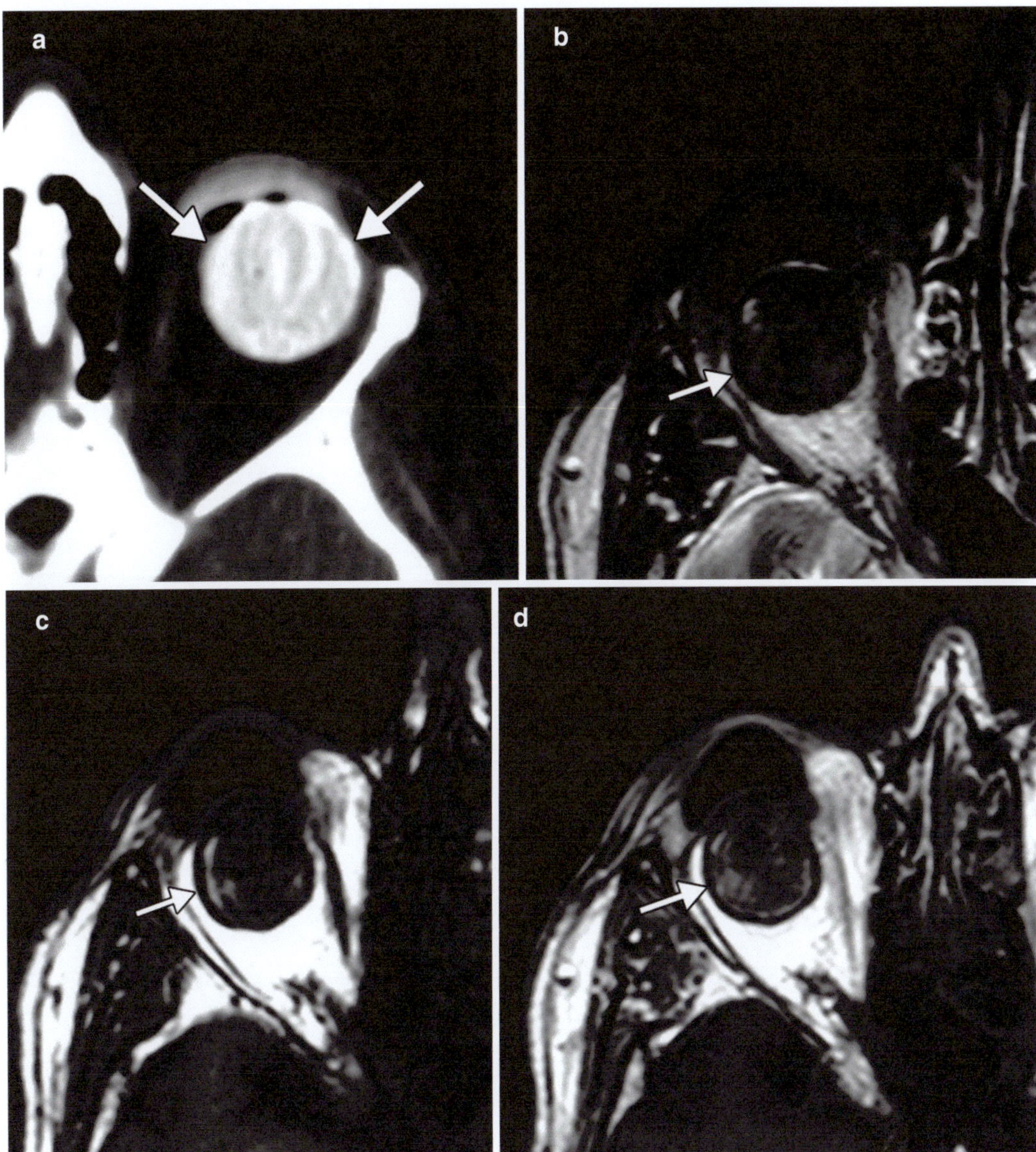

Fig. 5.22 Hydroxyapatite orbital implant after enucleation surgery. Axial CT image (**a**) shows a hyperattenuating spherical left implant (*arrows*). Axial T2-weighted (**b**), T1-weighted (**c**), and post-contrast T1-weighted (**d**) MR images in a different patient show that the hydroxyapatite implant (*arrows*) displays low to intermediate signal and mild enhancement

of the medial canthi, resulting in telecanthus (Fig. 5.48). Reduction and fixation of the frontal process of the maxilla to the frontal bone sometimes accompanied by a bone graft to the medial orbital wall may be used to treat the orbital relationship. However, a graft to the nasal dorsum may be required to restore nasal projection. Concomitant orbital floor reconstruction may be necessary in these patients given the proximity of the floor and involvement of the inferomedial wall of the orbit. Persistent nasolacrimal obstruction after open reduction and internal fixation of nasoorbitoethmoid fractures is uncommon but may be seen in 5–10 % of cases. This can lead to dacryocystocele (enlarged lacrimal sac) formation (Fig. 5.49).

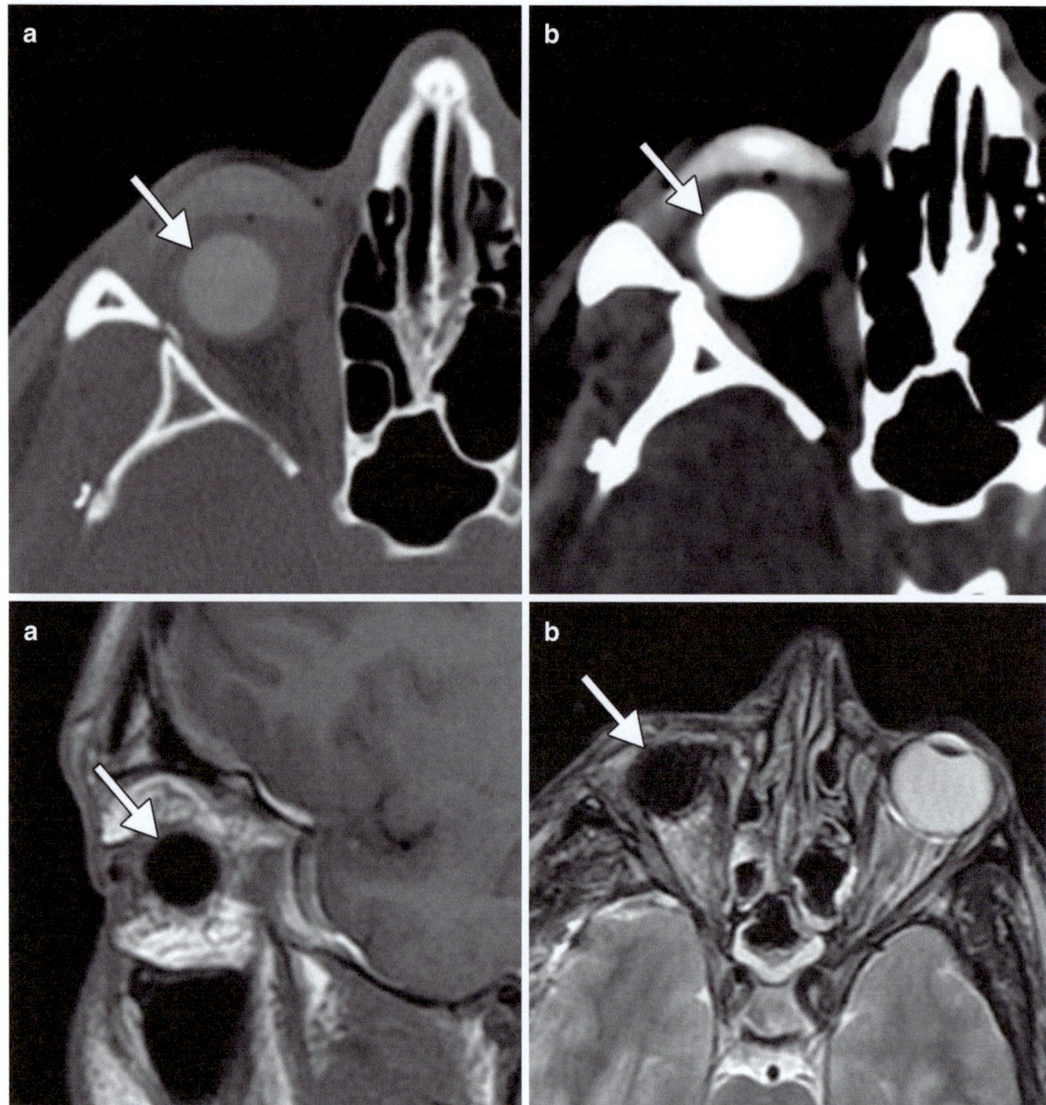

Fig. 5.23 Silicone orbital implant after enucleation surgery. Axial CT images in the bone (**a**) and soft tissue (**b**) windows show hyperattenuating right ocular implant (*arrows*) and prosthesis. The implant (*arrows*) displays low signal on both T1-weighted (**c**) and T2-weighted (**d**) MRI. The prosthesis is not present on the MRI

5.10.3 Zygomaticomaxillary Complex (ZMC) Fracture Repair

ZMC fractures involve the disruption of four buttresses, including the zygomaticomaxillary, frontozygomatic, zygomaticosphenoid, and zygomaticotemporal. Surgical indications for concomitant orbital fracture repair include significant fractures of the inferior orbital rim, orbital floor defects greater than 2 cm^2, and significant posterior displacement (>1 cm^2) of the ZMC body. Posterior displacement of the ZMC can cause the orbital floor to buckle as it is also displaced posteriorly. Subsequently, as the ZMC is anatomically reduced, it can unearth a significant orbital floor defect that requires reconstruction. Zygomaticomaxillary complex fractures

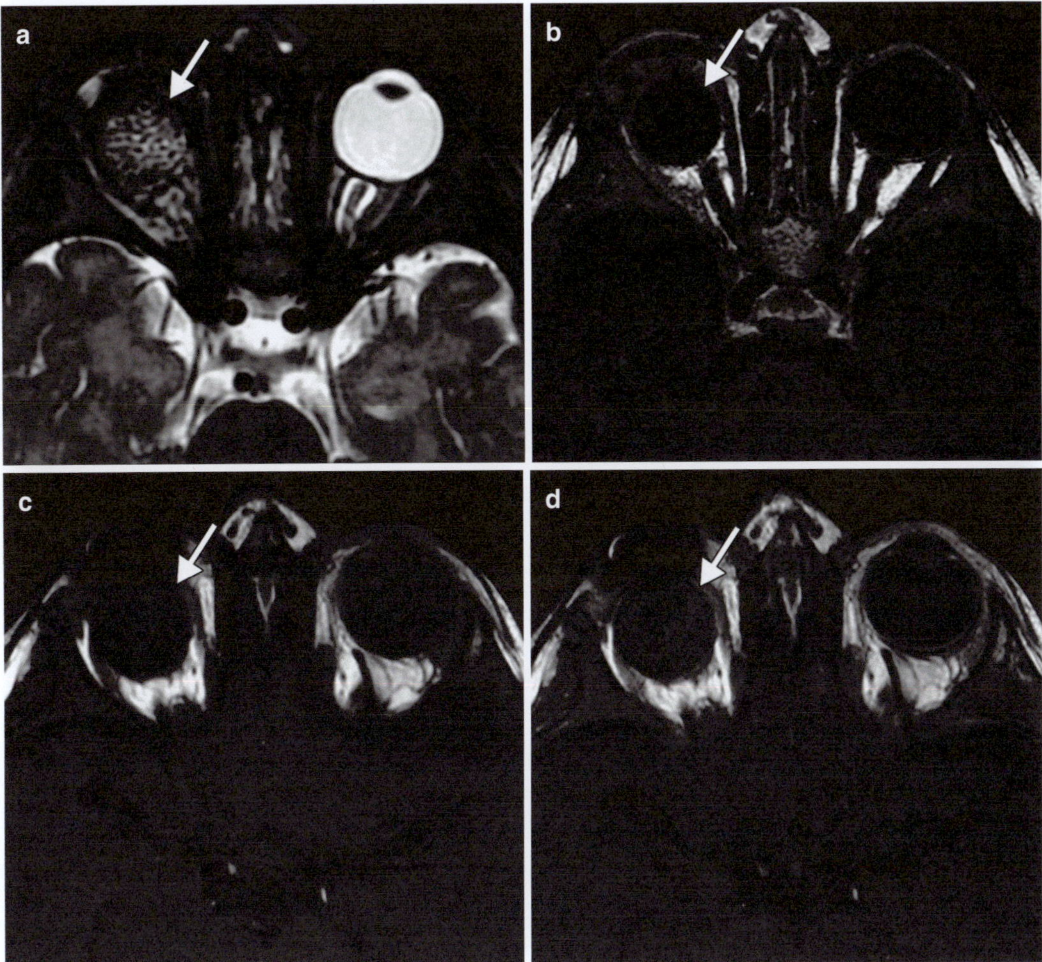

Fig. 5.24 Medpor ocular implant after evisceration. Initial axial T2-weighted (**a**) and post-contrast T1-weighted (**b**) MR images show a non-enhancing spherical right ocular prosthesis (*arrows*). Axial pre-contrast (**c**) and post-contrast (**d**) T1-weighted MR images obtained 6 months later show interval enhancement in the periphery of the prosthesis (*arrows*), indicating fibrovascular ingrowth

are most often reduced via open reduction and internal fixation. Often the lateral orbital wall and zygomatic arch fractures will be appropriately reduced by fixation of the maxillary buttress fracture (Fig. 5.50). Postoperative imaging can be helpful in assessing the adequacy of reduction and fixation of ZMC fractures, with particular attention to the alignment of the zygoma and lateral orbital wall, since angulation of these after fixation of the remaining buttresses may indicate a residual rotational deformity and an associated increased orbital volume (Fig. 5.51).

5.10.4 General Complications After Orbital Fracture Repair

It is important to detect the underlying cause of persistent symptoms following orbital wall reconstruction. Determining the etiology of postoperative complications may not be entirely possible by clinical examination, and imaging via CT and/or MRI is often required. A classic mistake when inserting the implant for an orbital floor fracture is to direct it straight back into the maxillary antrum rather than with a superior angulation towards a stable posterior ledge, which can result in persistent

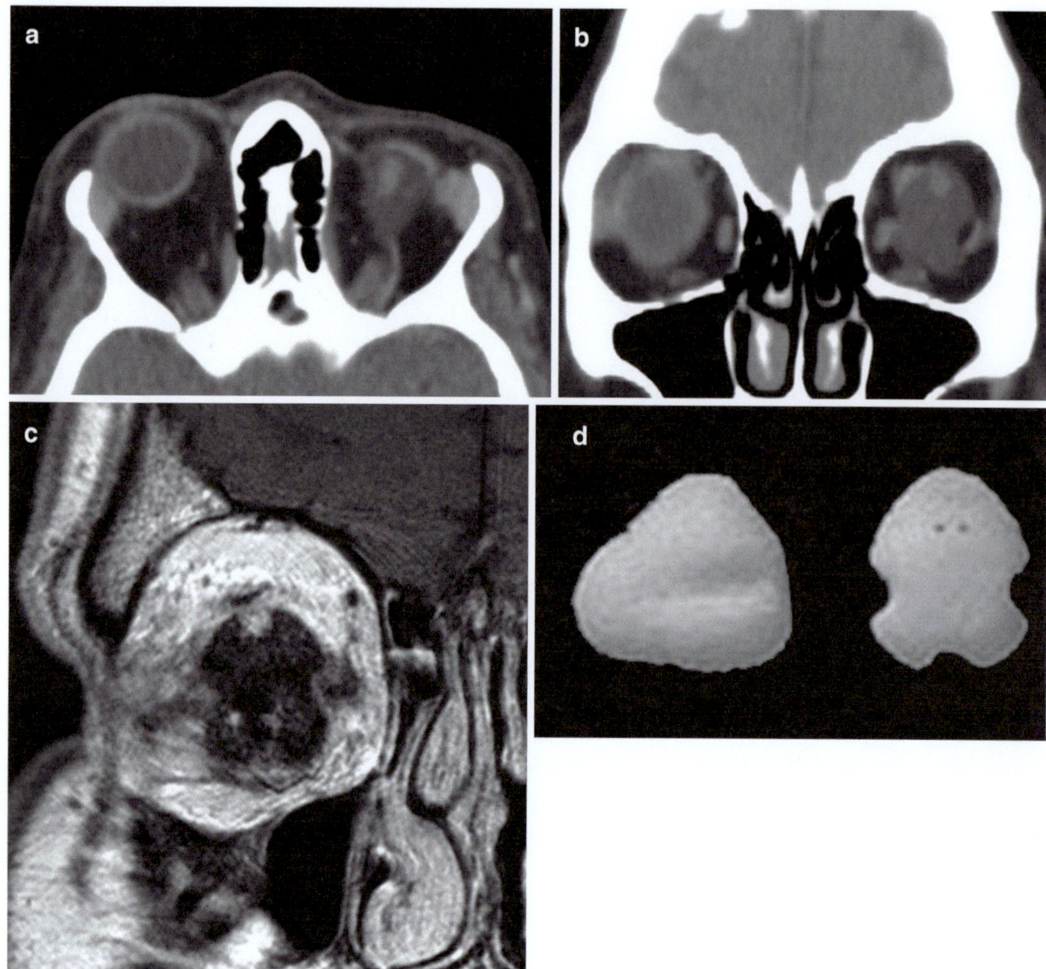

Fig. 5.25 Conical Medpor orbital implant. Axial (**a**) and coronal (**b**) CT images show longitudinal groves for the rectus muscles along the sides of the implant in the left orbit. Coronal T1-weighted MRI (**c**) shows multiple grooves in the right ocular implant. Front and side photographs of the conical Medpor implant (**d**)

orbital volume expansion and postoperative enophthalmos (Fig. 5.52). Postoperative enophthalmos can also result from herniation of orbital contents through a persistent orbital wall defect (Fig. 5.53). Exophthalmos following orbital wall fracture repair can result from hematic cysts, peri-implant infection, intraorbital sinus mucoceles, excessive orbital wall augmentation, and loss of the normal convex margins of the orbit, as shown earlier in the case of orbital roof fracture. Hematic cysts are collections of blood products contained by a fibrous capsule. This complication is more likely to occur with silicone implants than other materials and often occurs many years after surgery. The CT and MRI features of hematic cysts largely depend on the stage of the blood breakdown products but typically appear as a lenticular collection adjacent to the implant (Fig. 5.54). Alloplastic implants can serve as a nidus for infection. Peri-implant infections can manifest in the form of abscess, in which there is a rim-enhancing fluid collection, and/or cellulitis, in which there is stranding of the orbital fat (Fig. 5.55). MRI is particularly useful for evaluating intracranial extension of infection, which is especially a concern in the setting of superior orbital wall and rim fractures. Mucoceles can result from fractures or the related surgeries and represent trapped secretions that expand and become mass-like (Fig. 5.56). The appearance on imaging is variable depending upon the protein content and degree of hydration, but does not typically demonstrate internal enhancement. Occasionally multiple layers of reconstruction material are used to compensate for perceived orbital volume loss. Overcorrection can not only lead to proptosis but also impingement on critical intraorbital structures

and strabismus. These complications can be evaluated on CT, particularly if metal mesh was used in the reconstruction (Fig. 5.57). Alternatively, insertion of a plate with inadequate reduction or herniation of extraocular muscles can result in entrapment and strabismus (Fig. 5.58). Similarly, impingement upon intraorbital structures can result from excessively long fixation screws (Fig. 5.59). Late-onset postoperative strabismus can result from orbital adhesion due to scar formation. On CT or MRI, adhesions may appear as ill-defined soft tissue in the orbital fat in proximity to the surgical site. A distorted configuration of the rectus muscle may suggest the diagnosis (Fig. 5.60). Finally, migration of silastic sheet implants used during reconstruction of an orbital floor fracture can occur many years after insertion and present with sinusitis and nasolacrimal duct obstruction (Fig. 5.61). Such symptoms in patients with prior orbital wall fracture repair should be evaluated clinically and radiographically.

5.11 Orbital Wall Reconstruction for Sphenoid Wing Dysplasia

Sphenoid wing dysplasia is a characteristic manifestation of craniofacial neurofibromatosis type 1 in which the absence of the sphenoid greater

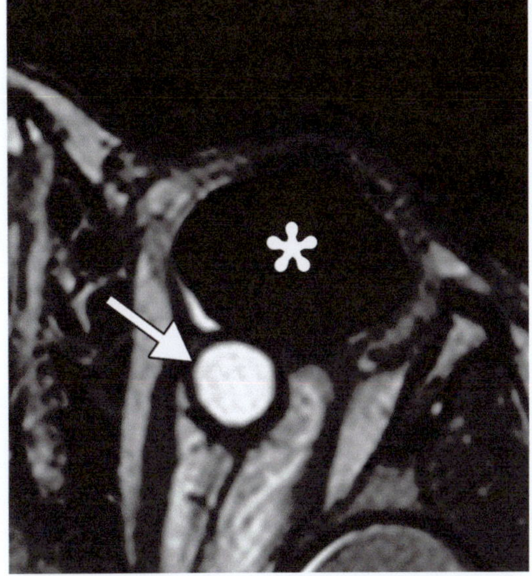

Fig. 5.26 Oval ocular implant. Axial T2-weighted MRI shows a left silicone implant (*) in a patient with anophthalmia. A cyst is present posterior to the implant (*arrow*)

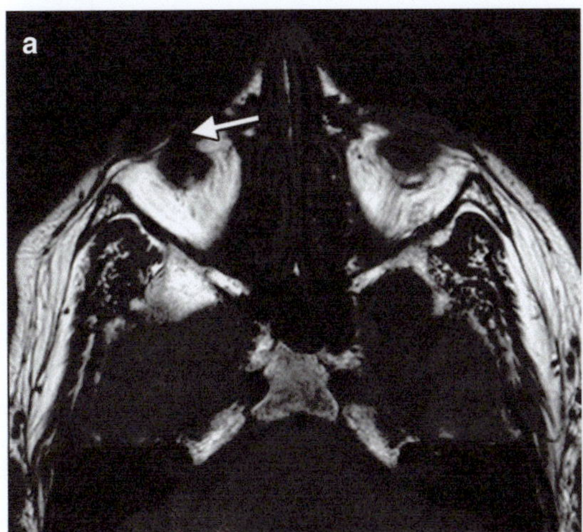

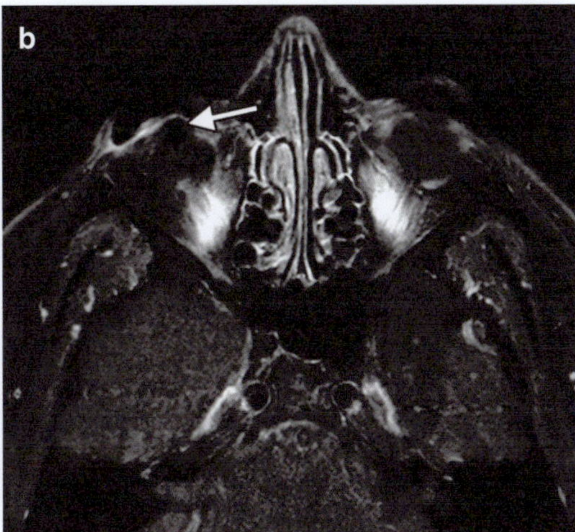

Fig. 5.27 Orbital implant with motility peg. Axial T-weighted (**a**) and post-contrast T1-weighted (**b**) MR images show the low signal peg extending from the enhancing implant (*arrows*). Peg placement allows the

implant to be directly coupled to the prosthesis. The peg is drilled into the implant after fibrovascular ingrowth is confirmed on MRI

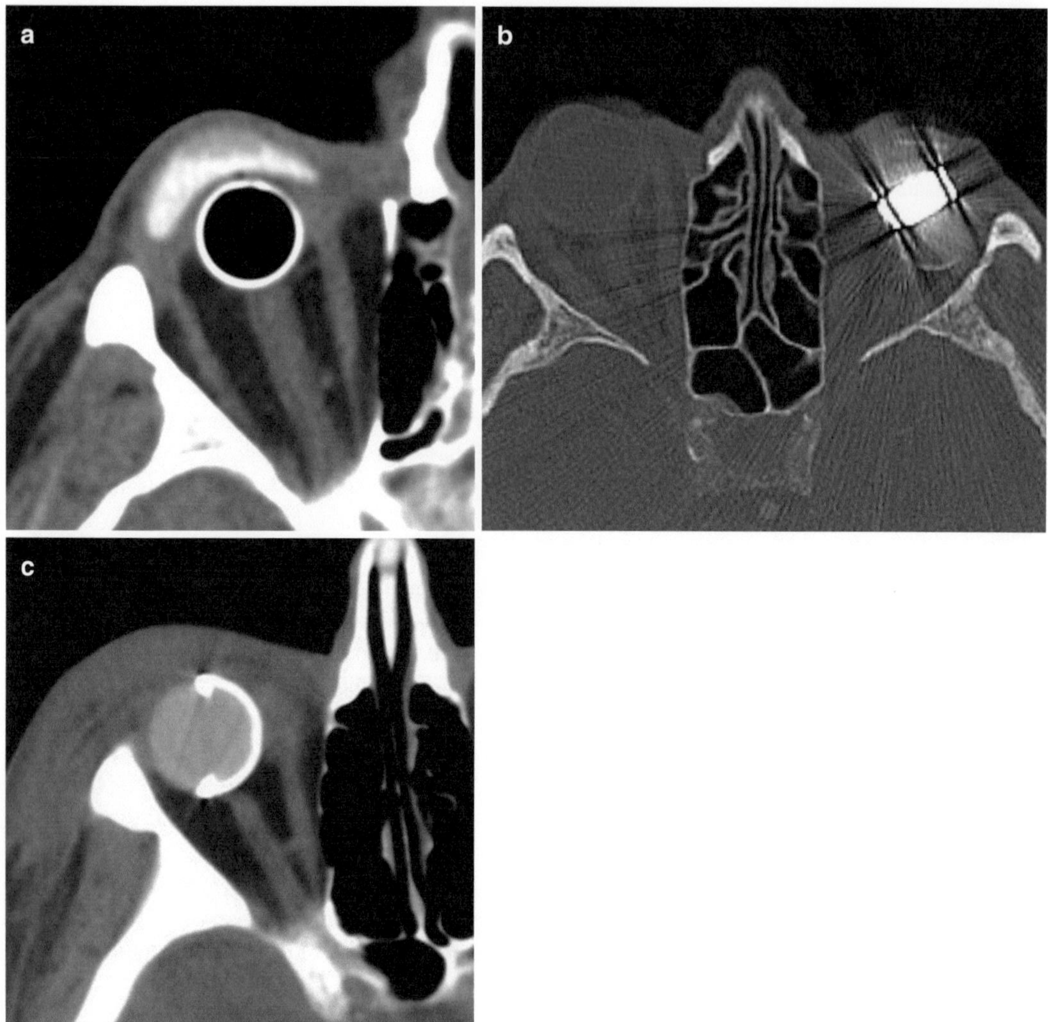

Fig. 5.28 Obsolete orbital implants. Axial CT image shows a hollow metal spherical implant and overlying hyperattenuating shell prosthesis in a patient who underwent enucleation in 1964 for trauma (**a**). Axial CT image shows a left orbital implant that consists of both plastic and metal components with considerable streak artifact (**b**). Axial CT image shows a hyperattenuating ocular implant with a hemispheric metal shell, which was placed after enucleation for trauma to the right globe during the Vietnam War (**c**)

wing allows the temporal lobe to prolapse into the orbit resulting in temporal base encephalocele and pulsatile exophthalmos. The goal of surgical intervention is to preserve vision, improve ocular motility, and cosmesis. This defect can be closed using bone grafts and/or titanium mesh (Fig. 5.62). Biomodelling and neuronavigation can be implemented in order to closely fit the reconstruction to the underlying anatomy. Nevertheless, the results of the procedure may be undermined due to bone graft resorption or displacement as well as mesh deformity, which is often related to elevated intracranial pressure and associated CSF pulsations. Thus, postoperative imaging may be useful to characterize the status of the reconstruction materials. In neurofibromatosis type I patients, it is also important to be vigilant for associated lesions such as neurofibromas and optic nerve gliomas that may arise on follow-up imaging.

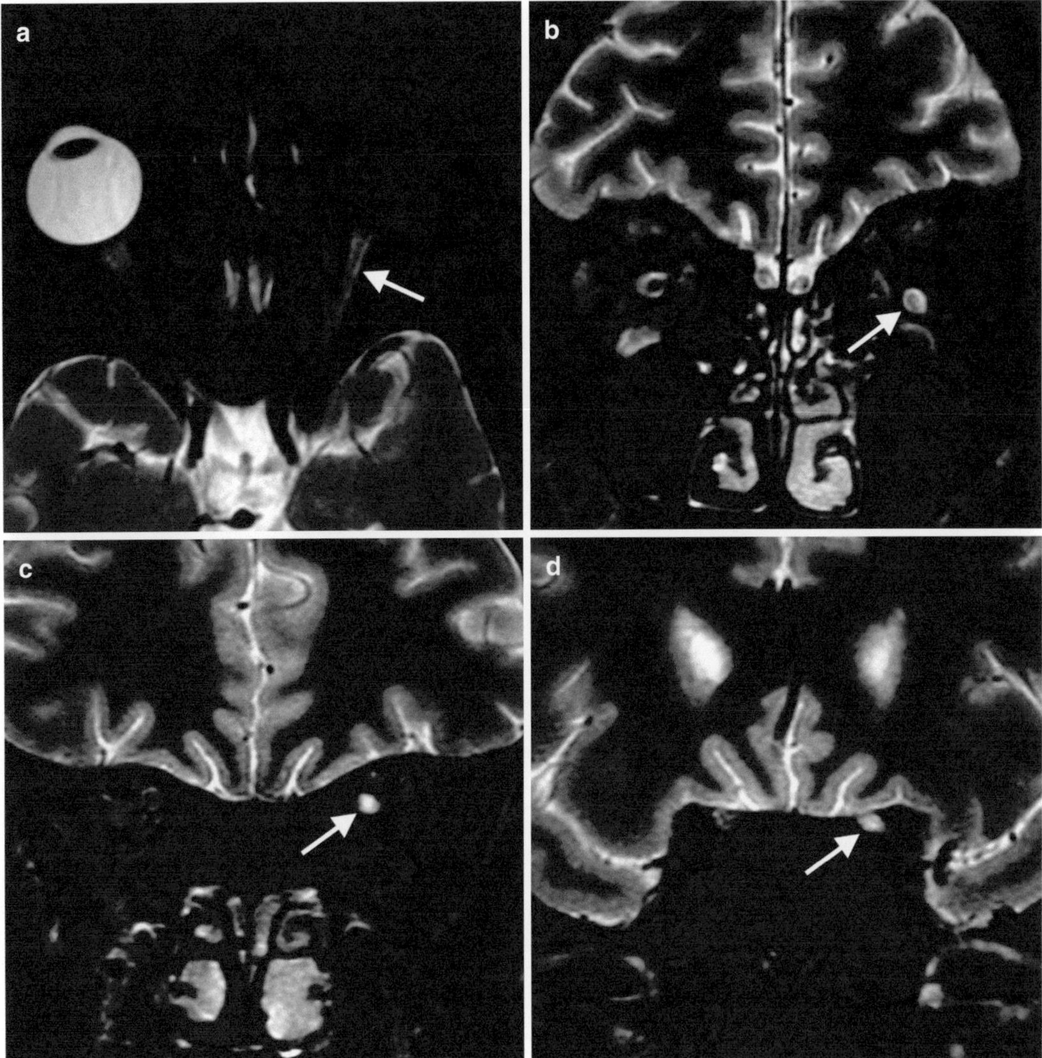

Fig. 5.29 Optic nerve changes after enucleation. Axial (**a**) and coronal (**b–d**) MRI show that the optic nerve ipsilateral to the enucleated eye (*arrows*) is atrophic and displays T2 hyperintense signal compared to the normal contralateral optic nerve, an expected finding after enucleation

5.12 Orbital Augmentation for Enophthalmos

Silent sinus syndrome consists of maxillary sinus atelectasis and orbital enlargement. Patients typically present with cosmetic changes to their facial appearance, including enophthalmos, hypoglobus, and deep upper lid sulcus. This condition can be treated via combined endoscopic antrostomy and/or orbital floor augmentation. Dermis grafts, sheet implants, and wedge implants can be used to restore orbital volume and are apparent on imaging (Fig. 5.63, 5.64, and 5.65). After successful treatment, the orbital floor can be observed to rise to a more normal level with re-expansion of the maxillary sinus. Both CT and MRI can be used in the postoperative setting to evaluate patients with excess or inadequate augmentation or other complications related to surgery, such as hemorrhage or infection. Otherwise, these postoperative changes may be encountered incidentally on imaging performed for other reasons.

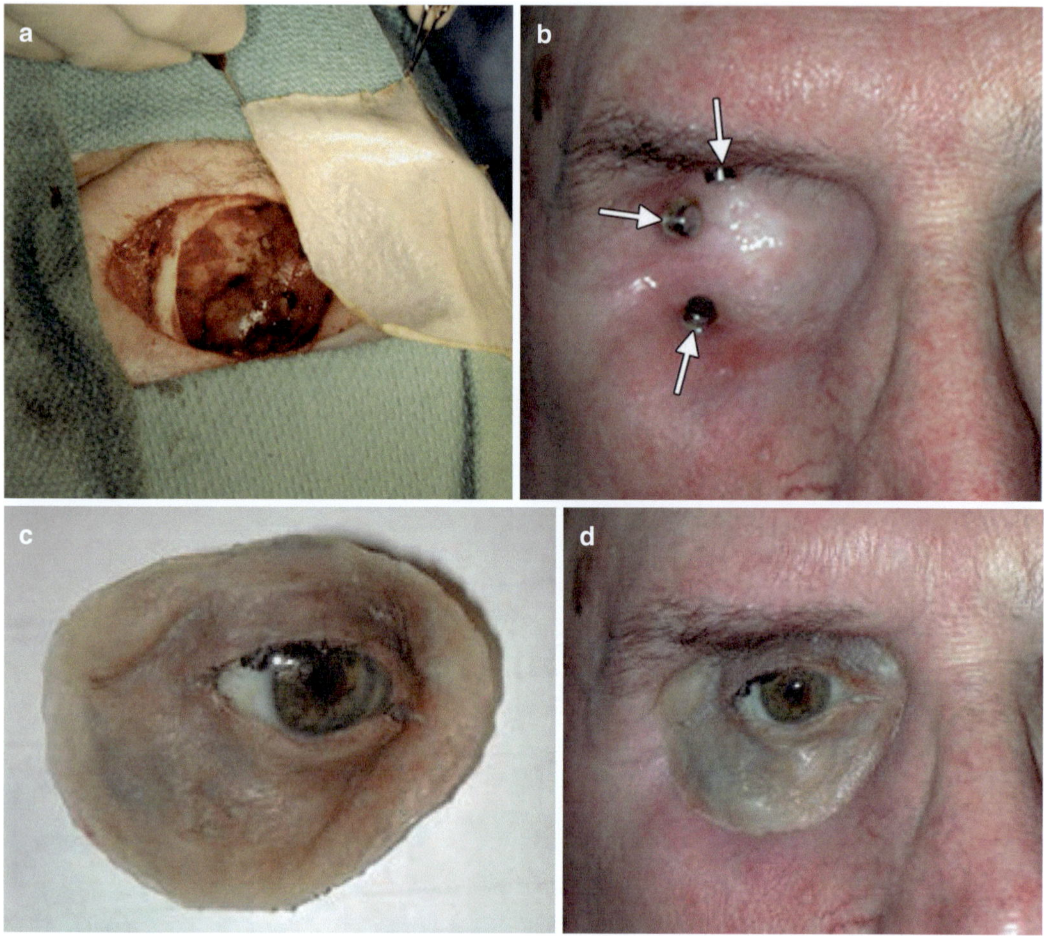

Fig. 5.30 Exenteration procedure with orbital prosthesis. Photograph (**a**) shows entire contents removed from the right orbit with split-thickness skin graft ready for placement. Photograph (**b**) shows the fully healed, skin-covered exenteration socket with endosseous magnetic implants (*arrows*) used to secure the orbital prosthesis. Photograph (**c**) shows the orbital prosthesis consisting of an artificial eye and adnexal structures. Photograph (**d**) demonstrates the orbital prosthesis in position, providing a satisfactory cosmetic result, especially if covered with large-framed spectacles

5.13 Orbital Decompression

The goals of surgical decompression for thyroid orbitopathy include relief of compressive optic neuropathy and reduction of proptosis, leading to improvement in exposure keratopathy and overall periorbital cosmesis. Decompression of any combination of the inferior, medial, and lateral walls may be performed, while the superior orbital wall is rarely decompressed (Fig. 5.66). Fat removal may result in further proptosis reduction. Medial and inferior wall decompression can be performed via a transnasal endoscopic approach or via a variety of external approaches, such as a transcaruncular approach or a swinging eyelid approach. There may be some advantages to an endoscopic approach in cases of compressive optic neuropathy since a more posterior decompression may be possible endoscopically. The risk of postoperative diplopia due to inferior globe displacement can be reduced by preserving the inferomedial strut located at the junction of the maxillary and ethmoid sinuses. Another less commonly used surgical method to improve proptosis is the placement of orbital rim expanders (Fig. 5.67).

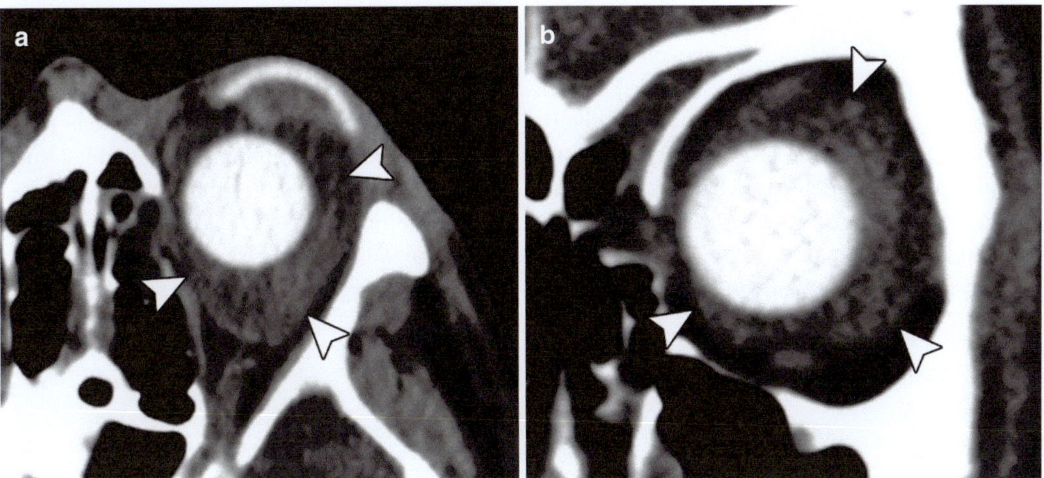

Fig. 5.31 Orbital hemorrhage after enucleation. Axial (**a**) and coronal (**b**) CT images show fluid within orbit surrounding the silicone ocular implant (*arrowheads*)

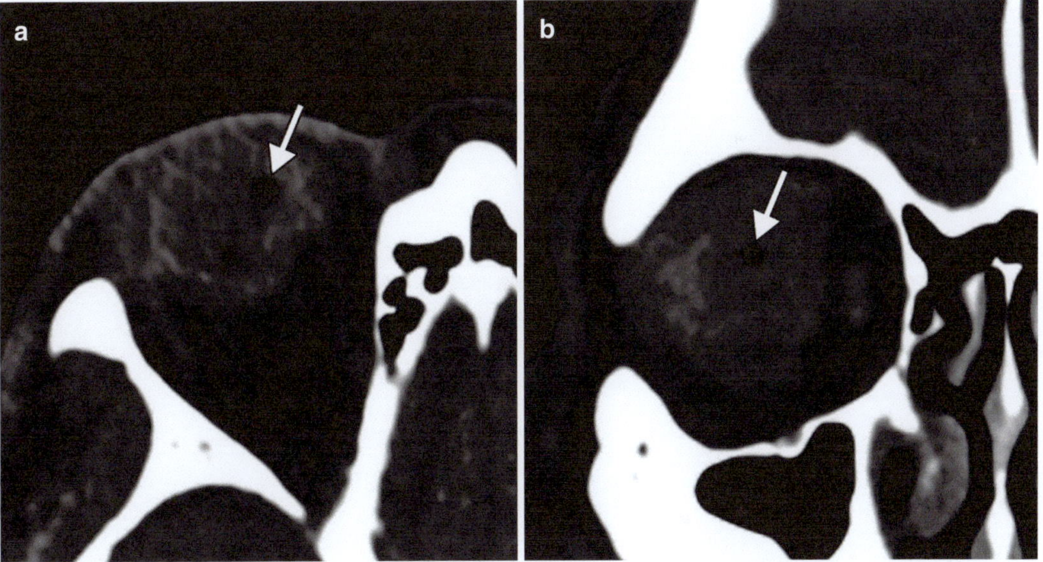

Fig. 5.32 Infection after evisceration. Axial (**a**) and coronal (**b**) CT images show gas (*arrows*) and fluid within the eviscerated right sclera. There is also stranding of the surrounding orbital fat

Diagnostic imaging is sometimes requested following orbital decompression for thyroid orbitopathy, such as for delineation of residual apical crowding in cases of persistent compressive optic neuropathy and for evaluation of complications, such as new-onset strabismus, paranasal sinus obstruction, CSF leak, and nasolacrimal duct obstruction. High-resolution orbital MRI, particularly coronal sequences, provides superior delineation of the optic nerves and extraocular muscles. The administration of intravenous contrast is usually not necessary for delineating the soft tissue anatomy. The disadvantage of MRI is the poor depiction of bony structures. On the other hand, CT displays an excellent view of the bony orbit and paranasal sinuses. Thus, the two modalities may serve complementary functions when planning revision surgery. Persistent optic nerve compression after surgery can result from insufficient decompression of the orbital wall, particularly towards the apex (Fig. 5.68), which can be relatively difficult to access. Alternatively, optic nerve compression after surgery can result from hematomas or displaced bone fragments, which are most conspicuous on CT. In addition, the herniated extraocular muscles may assume new positions within the orbit, leading to diplo-

pia. The herniated orbital contents can sometimes impede the paranasal sinus drainage pathways, leading to accumulation of secretions and mucocele formation (Fig. 5.69). CSF leaks can result from inadvertent disruption of the orbital roof. On imaging, a fluid collection can be delineated within the orbit (Fig. 5.70), in association with an orbital wall defect. Occasionally, a meningocele or meningoencephalocele may form. The

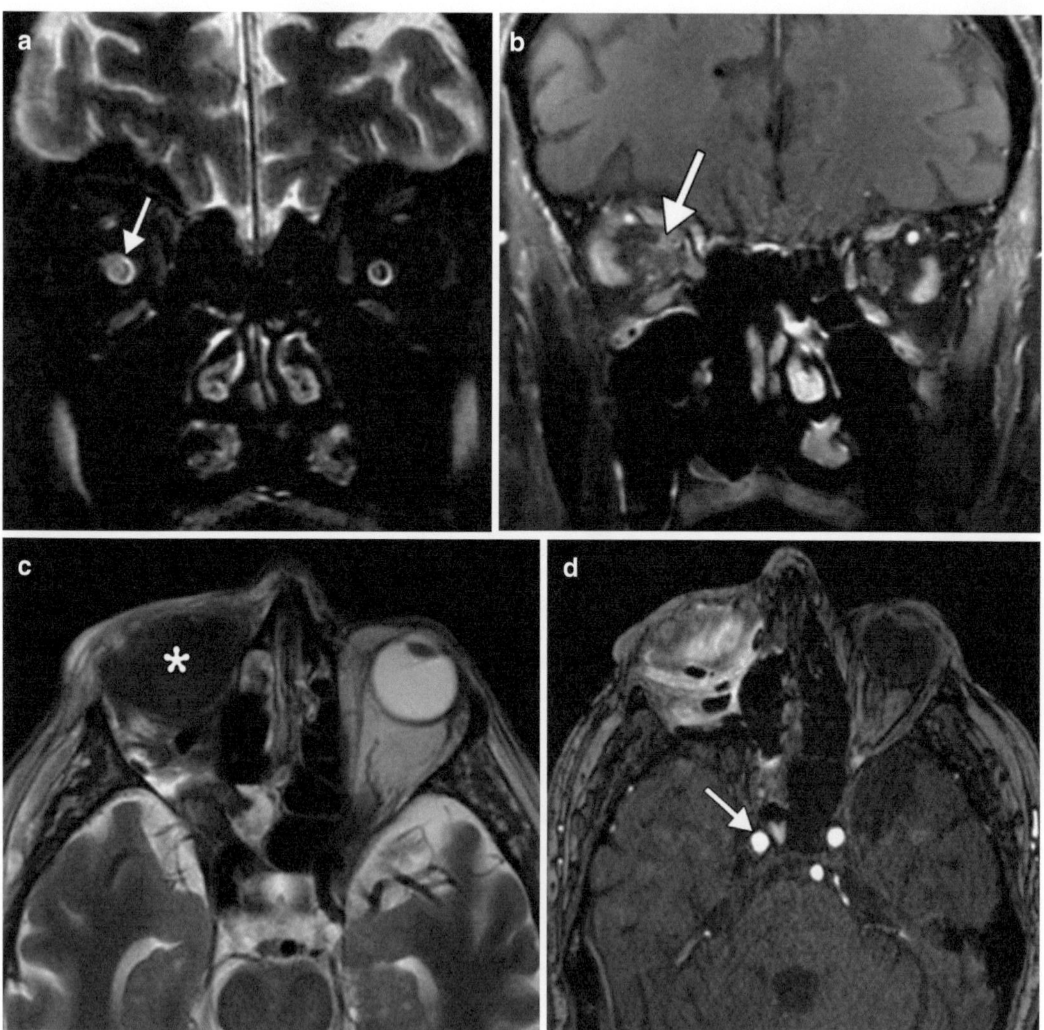

Fig. 5.33 Exenteration for rhino-orbitocerebral mucormycosis. Initial coronal T2-weighted (**a**) and post-contrast T1-weighted (**b**) MR images show abnormal enhancement in the right orbital apex and high T2 signal within the right optic nerve (*arrows*). Initial postoperative axial T2-weighted (**c**) image shows right orbital exenteration with myocutaneous flap (*). The concurrent time-of-flight MRA (**d**) shows that the right carotid artery is still patent (*arrow*). Follow-up axial CTA (**e**) obtained one week later shows opacification of the right sphenoid sinus and new occlusion of the right internal carotid artery (*arrow*). DWI (**f**) shows small areas of acute infarction in the right cerebral hemisphere watershed zones (*arrows*)

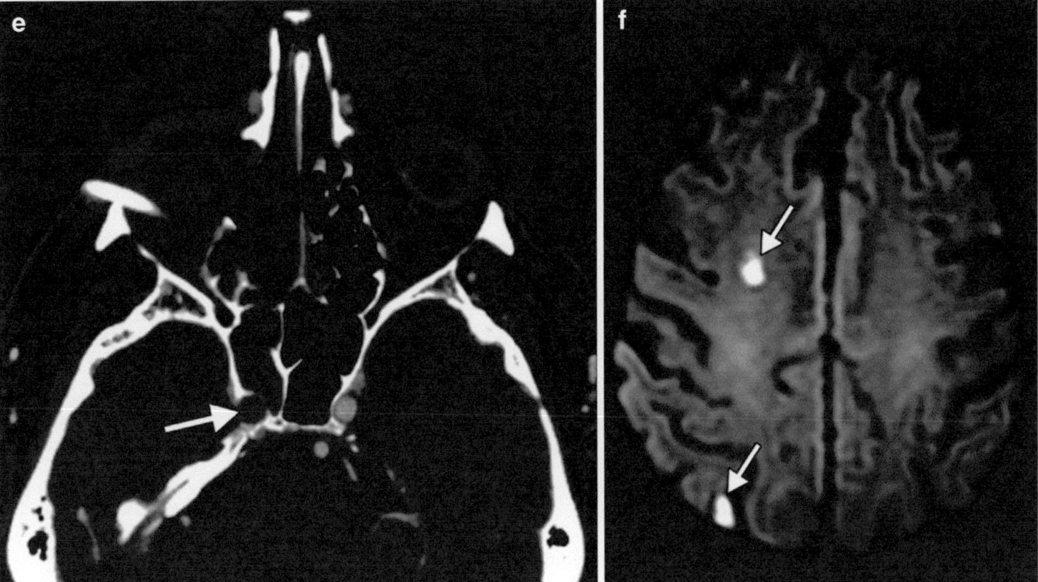

Fig. 5.33 (continued)

possibility of associated intracranial hemorrhage should also be evaluated in the acute setting. Nasolacrimal duct obstruction is an uncommon complication of orbital decompression surgery for thyroid orbitopathy. This complication may have a delayed presentation and likely results from inadvertent damage to the system intraoperatively. The obstruction is typically located distal to the common punctum, which can be delineated via dacryocystography (Fig. 5.71).

5.14 Dacryocystorhinostomy, Conjunctivodacryocystorhinostomy, and Nasolacrimal Tubes

Dacryocystorhinostomy (DCR) is performed for patients with dacryocystitis or epiphoria due to lacrimal sac/duct obstruction if the upper system (canaliculi) is intact. DCR consists of anastomosing the lacrimal sac to the nasal mucosa in an area above the obstruction. If the canaliculi (upper system) are obstructed, conjunctivodac-ryocystorhinostomy is performed, in which a glass Jones tube is inserted to connect the ocular surface (conjunctiva) to the nasal cavity. On CT, a bony defect in the lacrimal fossa is evident following both dacryocystorhinostomy and conjunctivodacryocystorhinostomy (Fig. 5.72). Jones tubes have a flange at the superior end in order to maintain their position and can be delineated on CT as hyperattenuating structures that extend from the medial orbit to the nasal cavity (Fig. 5.73). A portion of the middle turbinate may be resected in order to accommodate the Jones tube (Fig. 5.74). Complications of Jones tubes include extrusion, malposition, obstruction, infection, and pneumo-orbit, which can occur after CPAP usage or sneezing (Figs. 5.75 and 5.76). Although the use of porous polyethylene-coated tubes helps to minimize the risk of extrusion, the coating can irritate the conjunctiva and lead to intolerance or granuloma formation. Recurrent obstruction may present with distension of the lacrimal sac (Fig. 5.77) and can be further evaluated via dacryocystography (Fig. 5.78).

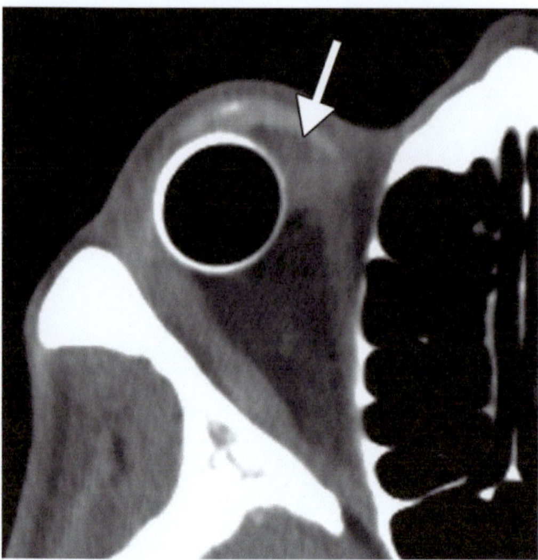

Fig. 5.34 Peri-implant infection. The patient presented with purulent discharge from the right eye socket. Axial CT image shows a fluid collection (*arrow*) between the ocular implant and prosthesis

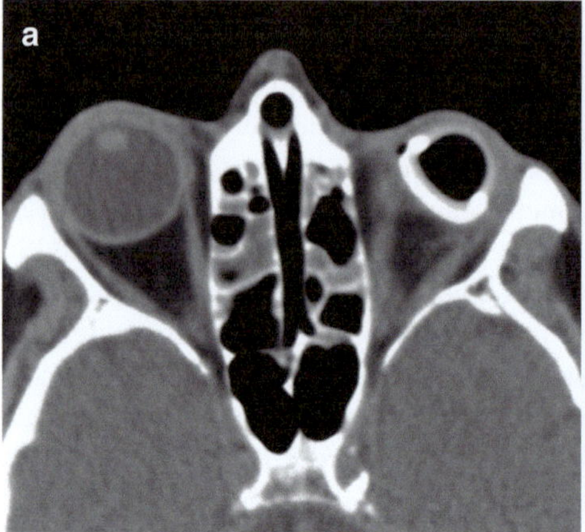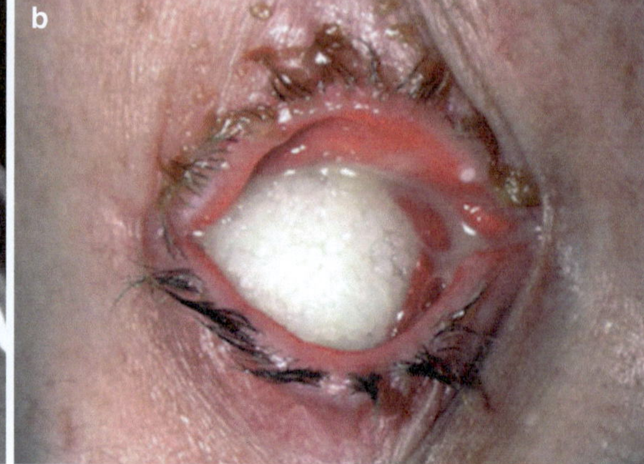

Fig. 5.35 Ocular prosthesis exposure. Axial CT (**a**) shows deficiency of soft tissue anterior to the left ocular prosthesis. Chronic left orbit inflammatory changes are also present. Clinical photograph (**b**) in another patient shows the porous implant exposed through a melted conjunctiva. Although exposure is obvious on clinical exam, radiological imaging can help assess for potential etiologies

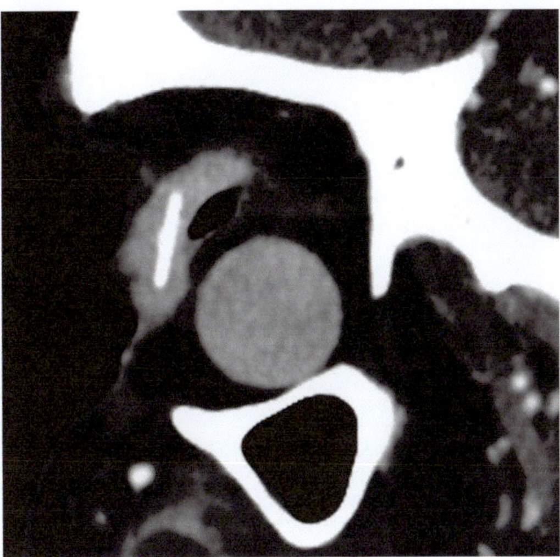

Fig. 5.36 Postenucleation socket with significant orbital volume loss. The sagittal CT image shows enophthalmos, deepening of the superior sulcus, tilting of the prosthesis, and sinking of the implant

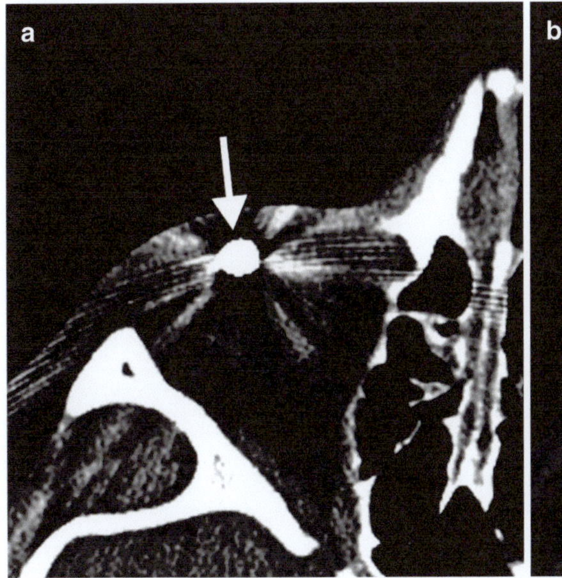

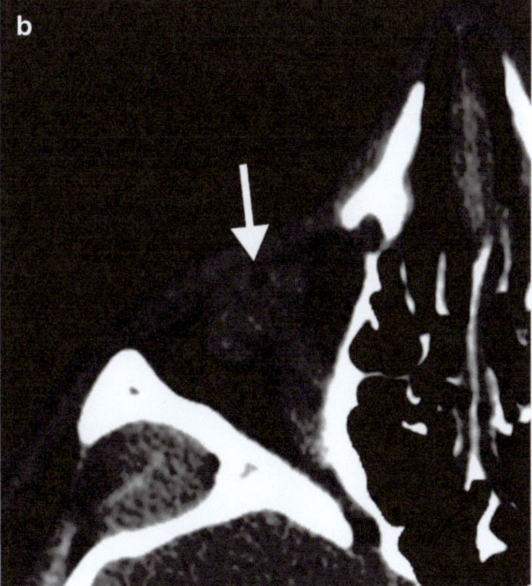

Fig. 5.37 Orbital foreign body removal. Preoperative CT image (**a**) shows a metallic foreign body in the anterior orbit (*arrow*). Postoperative CT image (**b**) shows interval absence of the metallic foreign body with a small amount of residual air (*arrow*)

Table 5.2 Orbital wall reconstruction materials

Material	Properties	Imaging features
Titanium, vitallium, stainless steel	Mesh may be shaped to fit contours of orbit	High attenuation on CT; generally MRI compatible
Medpor	Vascularized via tissue ingrowth may resist infection and movement	Intermediate attenuation between soft tissue and fat on CT; low T1 signal and intermediate to high T2 signal on MRI
Silicone	Smooth and easy to shape and place in orbit; cause fibrous capsule to form within weeks of implantation; do not become stabilized as well as porous implants; may have severe inflammatory reaction to material; at risk for capsular hemorrhage	Attenuation between soft tissue and bone on CT; low signal on MRI
Resorbable	Various biodegradable materials, including polydioxanone sulfate	Nearly soft tissue attenuation on CT and low signal on MRI; the materials become less discernible over the course of months due to resorption
Glass bioceramic	Individually prefabricated using computer-assisted design and manufacturing	Hyperattenuating on CT; low signal on all MRI sequences
Composite	Porous polyethylene implants with embedded titanium provide a newer alternative for orbital reconstruction with a profile that combines several advantages of porous polyethylene and titanium implants	Different imaging characteristics for the components of the implant

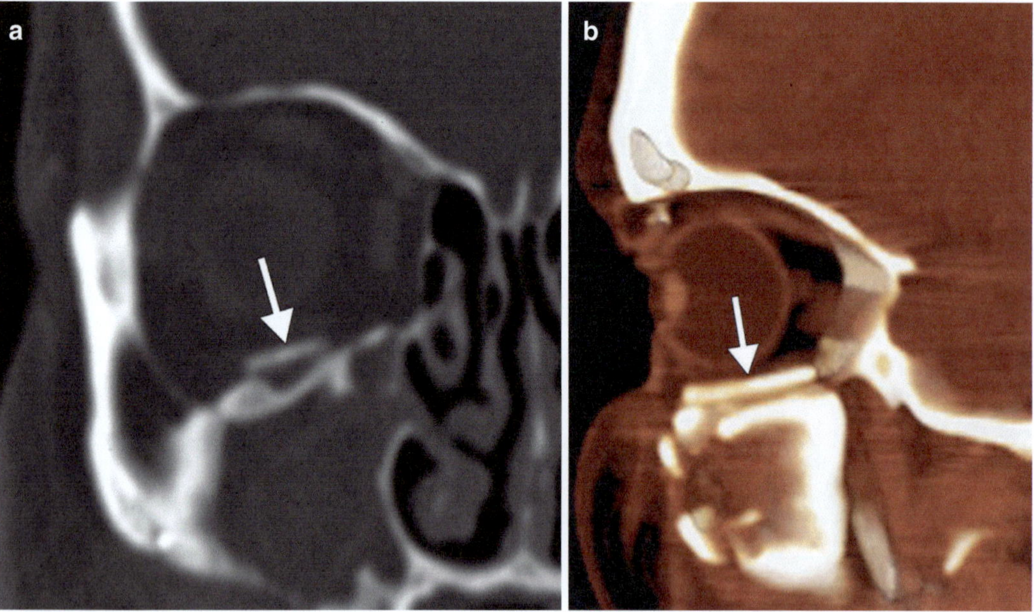

Fig. 5.38 Bone graft. Coronal CT image in the bone window (**a**) and colorized sagittal maximum intensity projection CT image (**b**) show bone positioned along the orbital floor (*arrows*)

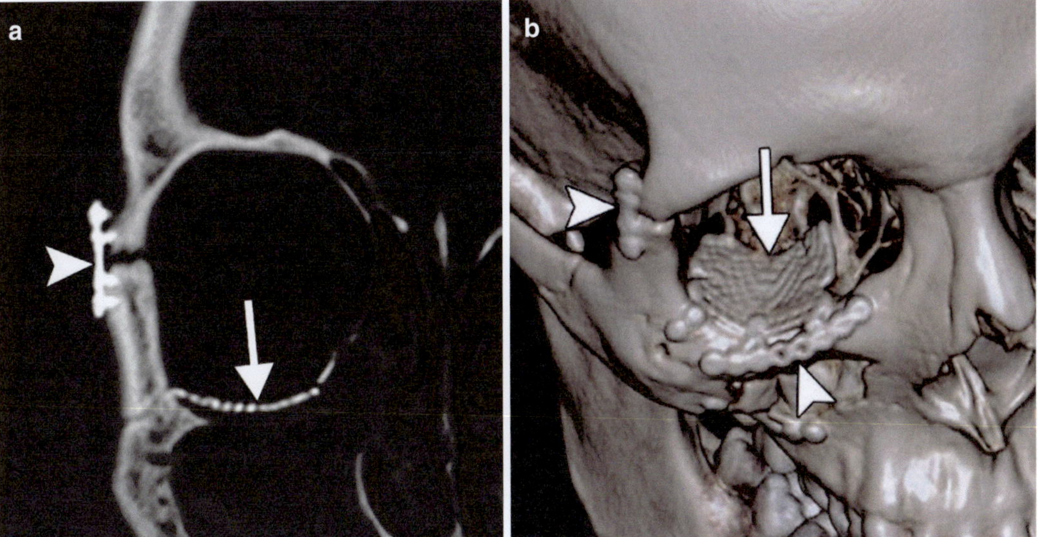

Fig. 5.39 Titanium mesh plate. Coronal (**a**) and 3D volume-rendered CT (**b**) images show the mesh positioned along the floor of the right orbit (*arrows*). Miniplates and screws secure the orbital rim fractures (*arrowheads*)

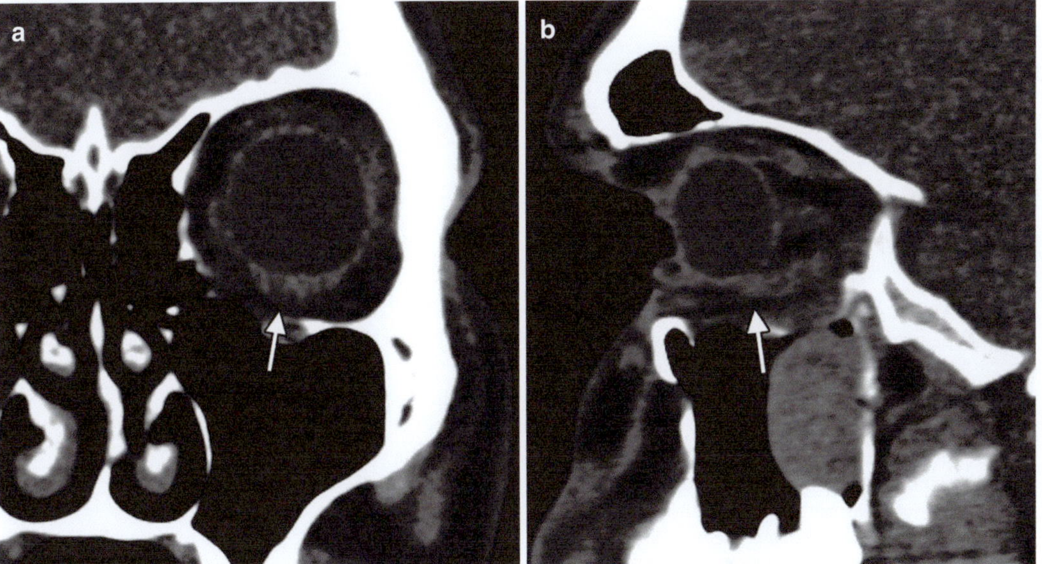

Fig. 5.40 Medpor implant. Coronal (**a**) and sagittal (**b**) CT images show that the inferior orbital wall implant appears as a thin sheet with intermediate attenuation between soft tissue and fat (*arrows*)

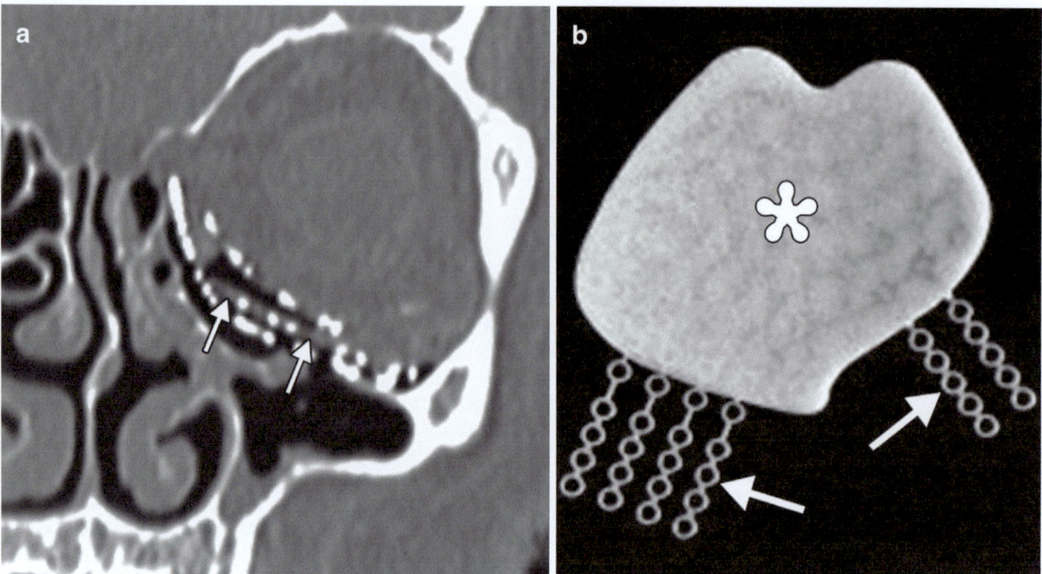

Fig. 5.41 Medpor Titan implant. Coronal CT image (**a**) shows stacked layers of metallic mesh and lower attenuation Medpor component (*arrows*). Photograph (**b**) of a Medpor Titan implant comprising a sheet of Medpor (*) with partially embedded titanium strips (*arrows*)

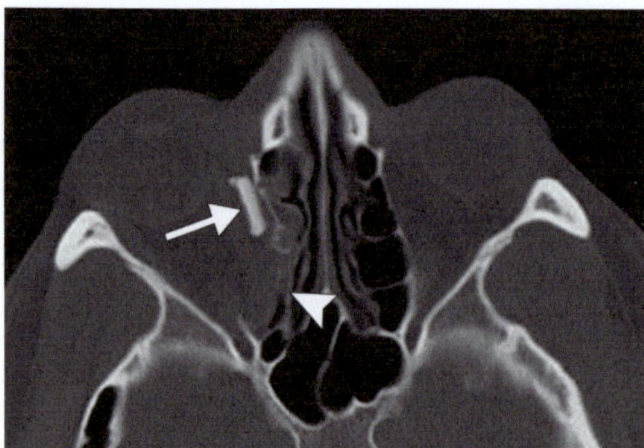

Fig. 5.42 Medial orbital wall fracture repair. Axial CT image shows a medial right orbital wall fracture with a poorly positioned and overly thick bone graft (*arrow*) along the anterior aspect of the fracture. The posterior portion of the fracture remains uncovered, and there is associated herniation of orbital contents (*arrowhead*)

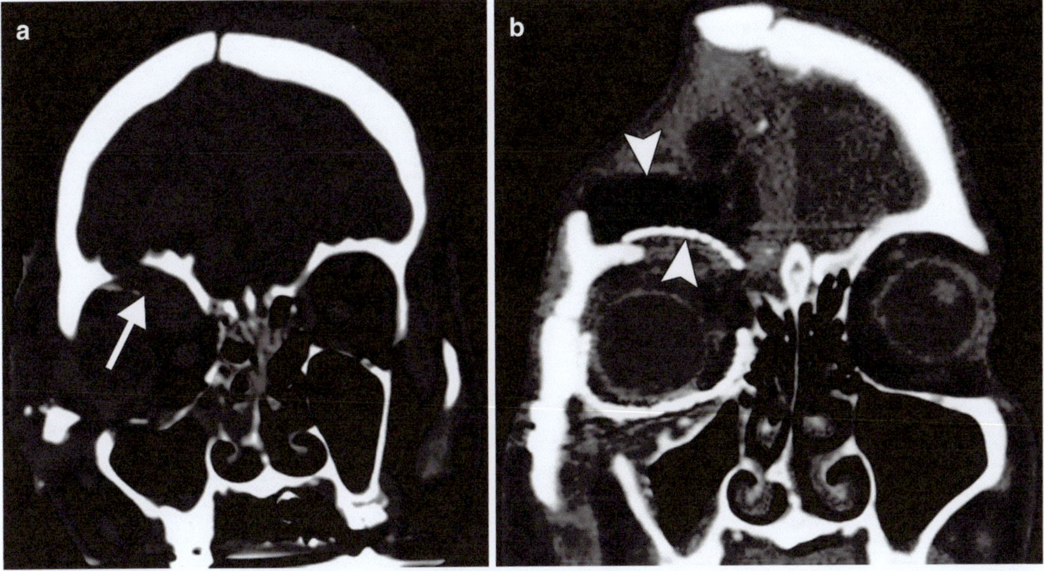

Fig. 5.43 Orbital roof fracture repair with CSF leak. Initial coronal CT image (**a**) shows right orbital wall fractures, including a displaced orbital roof fracture associated with hemorrhage as well as herniation of brain tissue and CSF into the orbit (*arrow*). Postoperative coronal CT image (**b**) shows interval right frontal craniectomy and orbital roof repair with titanium mesh and overlying fat graft (*arrowheads*)

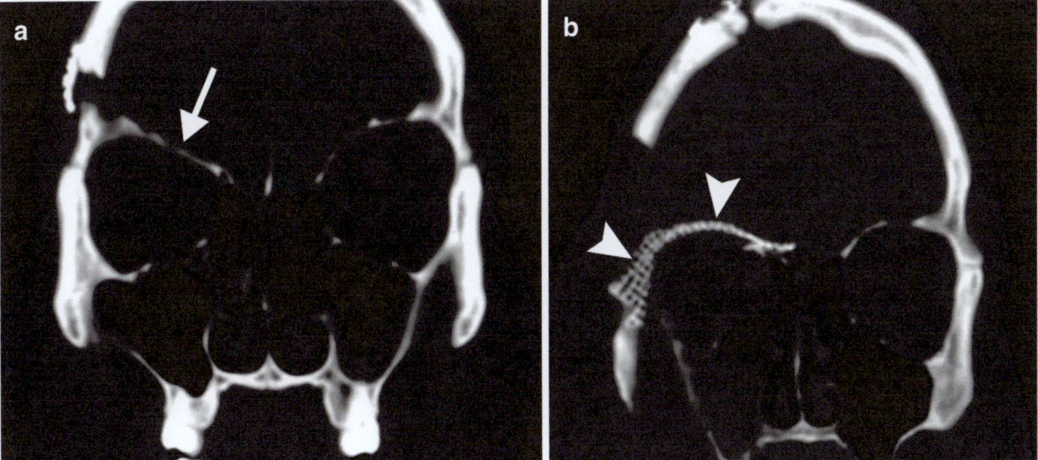

Fig. 5.44 Flattened orbital roof after reconstruction. Coronal CT (**a**) after right orbital roof repair via an intracranial approach shows a flattened configuration of the orbital roof (*arrow*) resulting in exophthalmos. Another patient with the same problem underwent corrective surgery using a custom fit titanium mesh (*arrowheads*) as shown on the coronal CT (**b**)

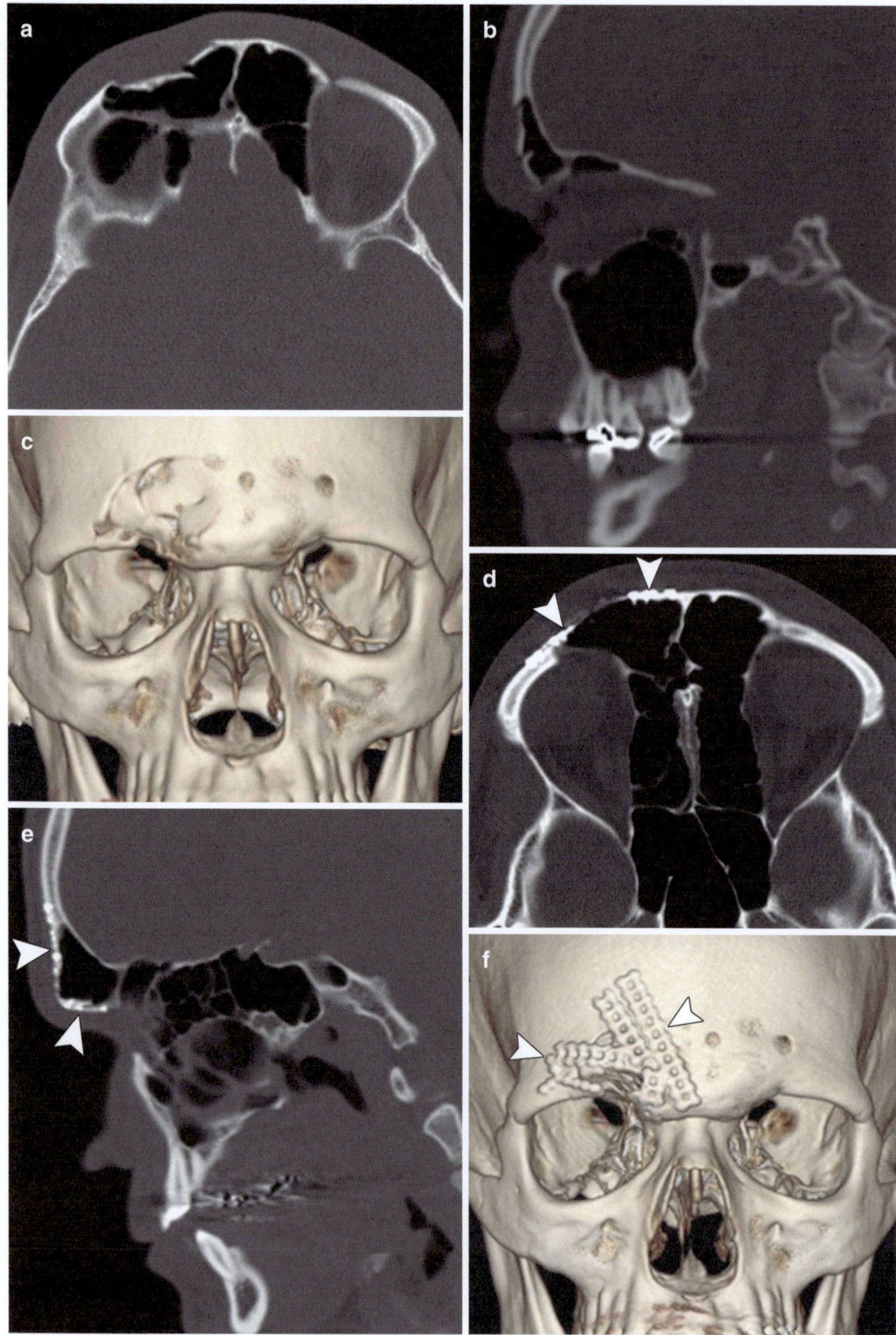

Fig. 5.45 Superior orbital rim fracture repair. Preoperative axial (**a**), sagittal (**b**), and 3D volume-rendered (**c**) CT images show a comminuted, depressed fracture of the right superior orbital rim and frontal sinus. Postoperative axial (**d**), sagittal (**e**), and 3D volume-rendered (**f**) CT images show interval improved alignment of the fracture fragments using strips of low-profile titanium mesh (*arrowheads*)

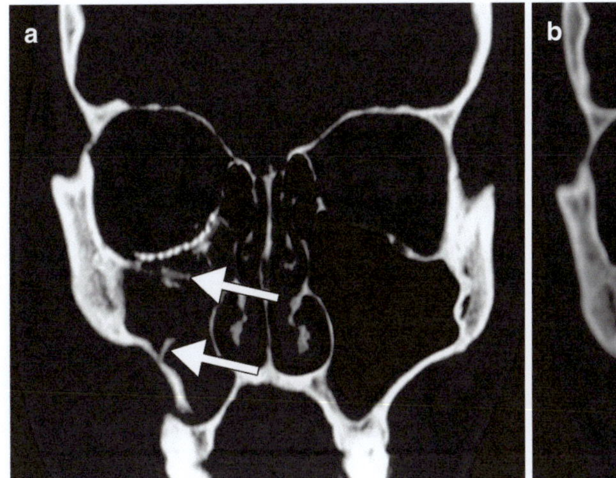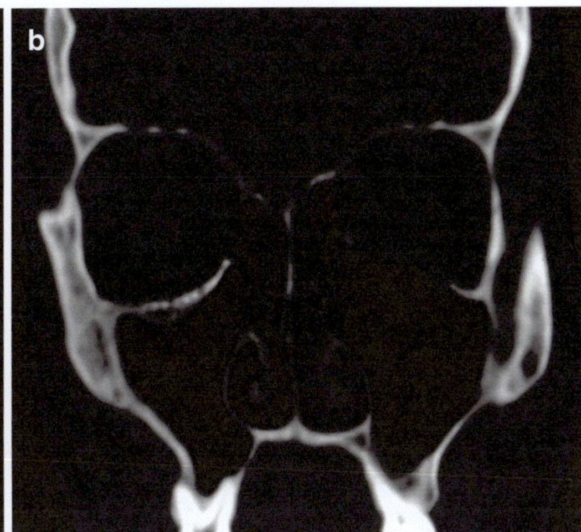

Fig. 5.46 Evolution of orbital floor fracture after repair. Initial postoperative coronal CT image (**a**) shows satisfactory repair of the right orbital floor fracture with titanium mesh. There are residual bone fragments within the maxillary sinus (*arrows*), which is completely opacified. Follow-up coronal CT image (**b**) obtained several months later shows resorption of the bone fragments, resolution of the maxillary sinus opacification, and healing at the fracture site

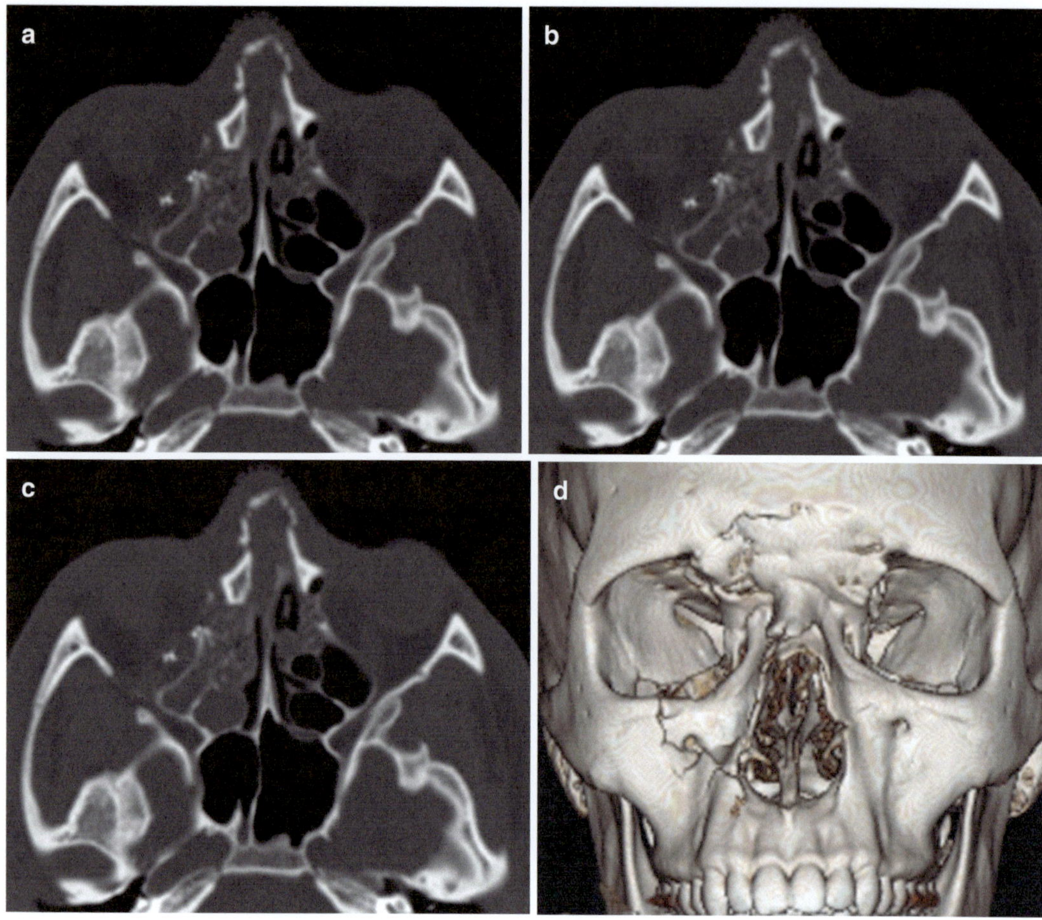

Fig. 5.47 Nasoorbitoethmoid fracture repair. Preoperative axial and 3D CT images (**a–d**) show comminuted fractures of the frontal sinus walls, bilateral lamina papyracea, nasal bones, frontal processes of the maxilla, and right inferior orbital rim and wall. Postoperative axial, coronal, and 3D CT images (**e–h**) show interval obliteration of the frontal sinuses and frontoethmoid recesses using bone chips and fat graft (*arrows*) with near-anatomic reduction of the fractures using abundant mesh and fixation plates

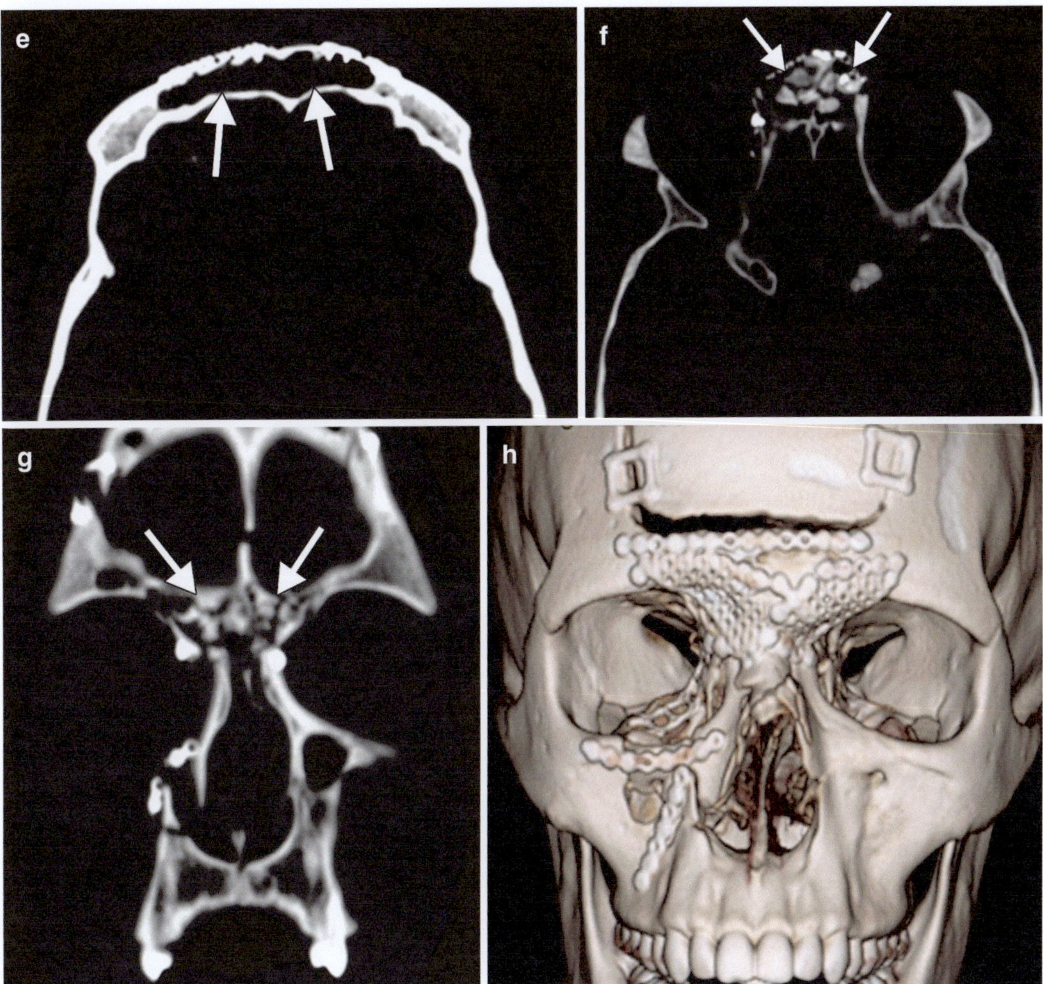

Fig. 5.47 (continued)

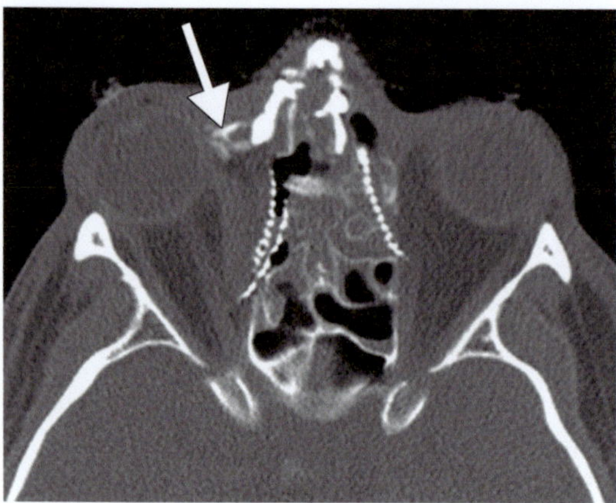

Fig. 5.48 Persistent telecanthus after nasoorbitoethmoid fracture repair. Axial CT image shows a laterally displaced fracture fragment at the site of medial canthal tendon attachment (*arrow*)

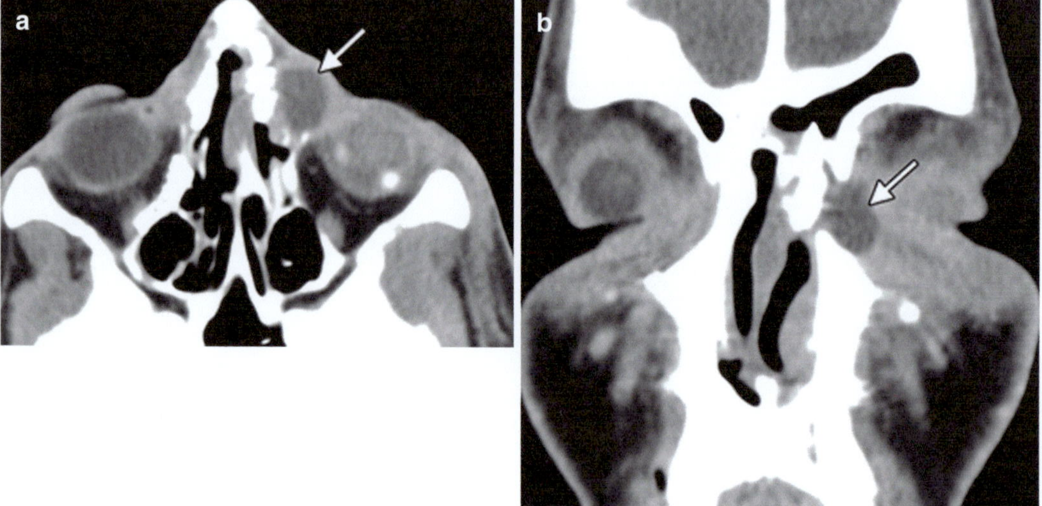

Fig. 5.49 Dacryocystocele after nasoorbitoethmoid fracture repair. Axial (**a**) and coronal (**b**) CT images show a fluid collection in the expected location of the left lacrimal sac (*arrows*)

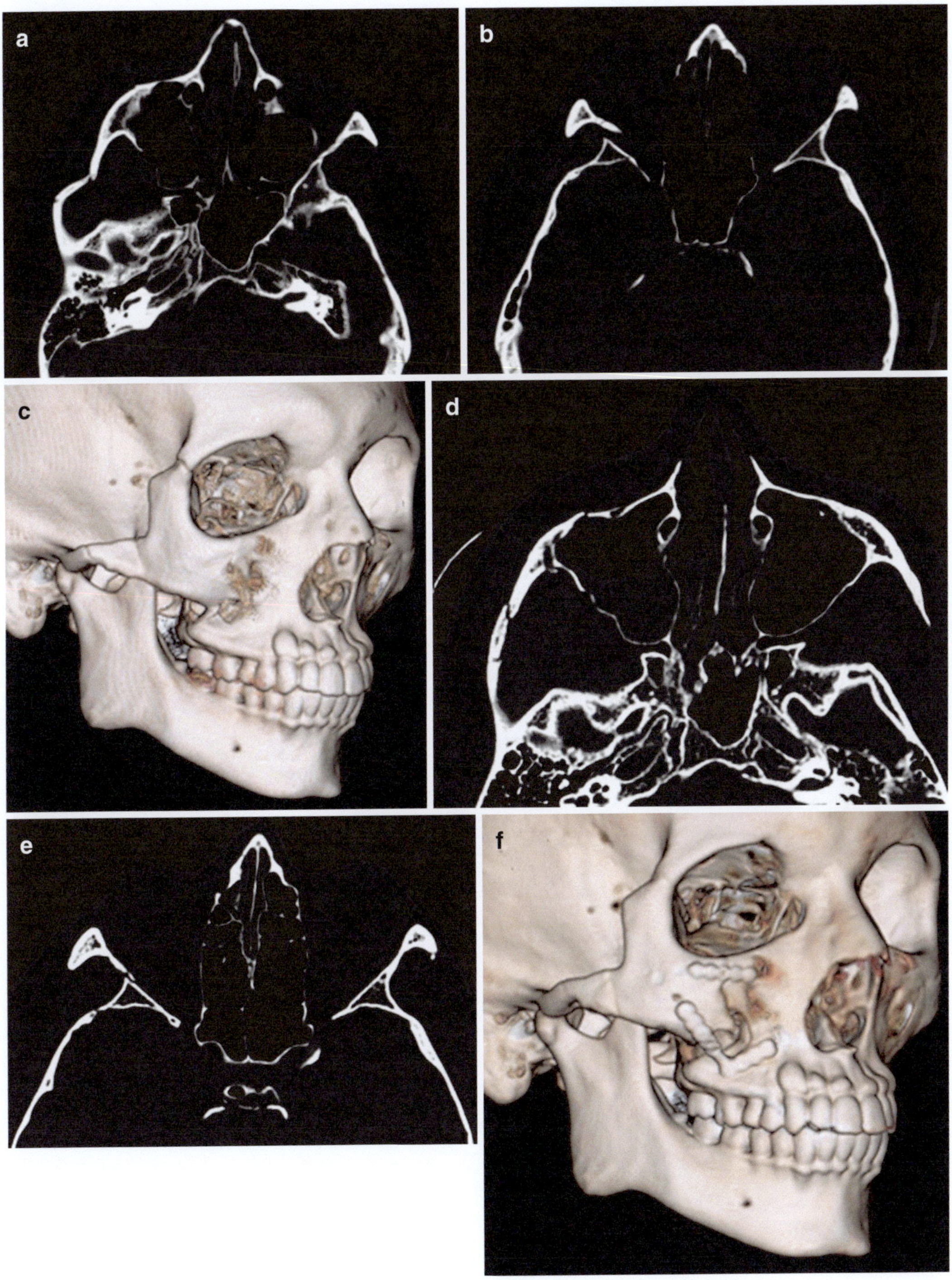

Fig. 5.50 Zygomaticomaxillary complex fracture repair. Preoperative axial (**a** and **b**) and 3D (**c**) CT images show displaced fractures of the right lateral orbital wall, inferior orbital rim, and zygomatic arch with concern for bony impingement on the right lateral rectus muscle. Postoperative axial (**d** and **e**) and 3D (**f**) CT images show interval reduction of the lateral orbital wall and zygomatic arch fractures. There has been fixation of the *upper* transverse maxillary and lateral maxillary buttresses with miniplates and screws

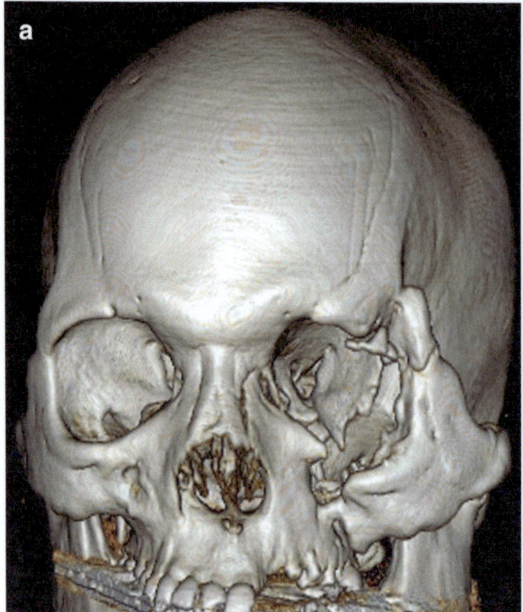
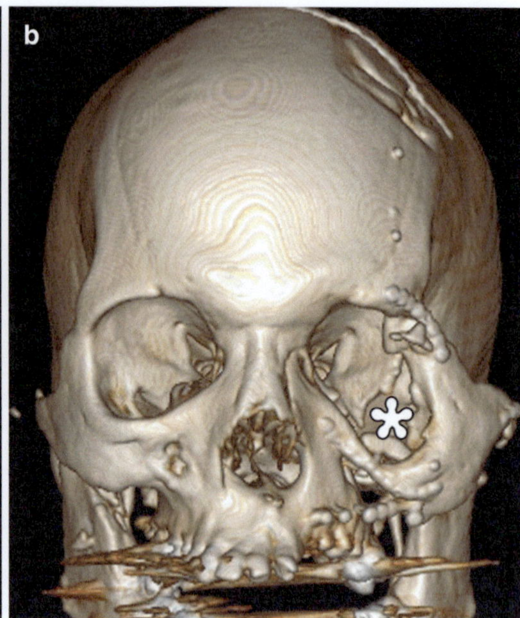

Fig. 5.51 Persistent orbital deformity after zygomatico-maxillary complex fracture repair. Preoperative 3D volume-rendered CT image (**a**) shows inferolateral displacement of the left inferior and lateral orbital walls as part of the ZMC fracture. Postoperative 3D volume-rendered CT image (**b**) shows improved alignment of the fracture fragments, but the left orbit is excessively voluminous inferiorly (*)

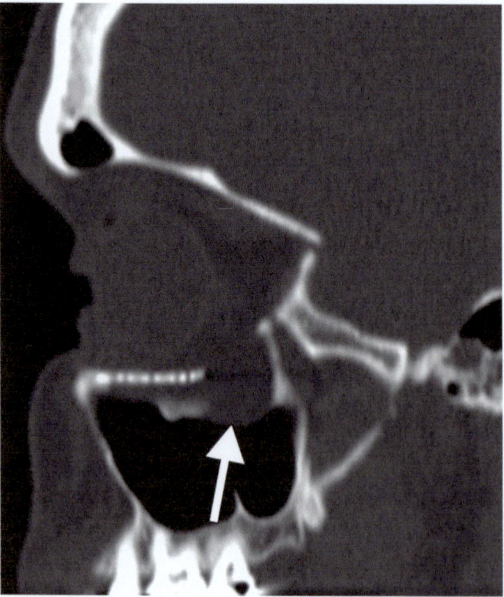

Fig. 5.52 Orbital blow out fracture repair with malpositioned mesh. Sagittal CT image shows a nearly horizontal orientation of the left orbital floor titanium mesh (*arrow*), which is directed inferior to the posterior bony ledge and of inadequate length

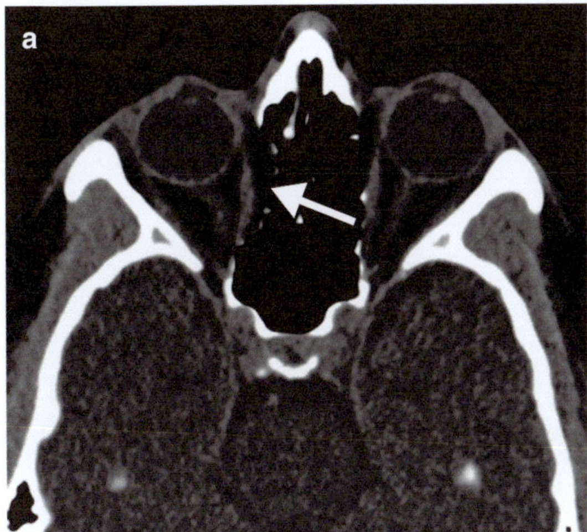
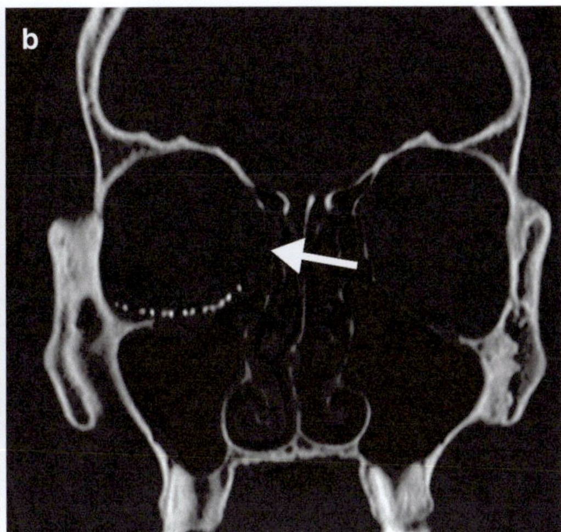

Fig. 5.53 Insufficient orbital wall fracture repair. Axial (**a**) and coronal (**b**) CT images show inadequate repair of a right orbital floor and medial orbital wall fracture with titanium mesh. There is residual right enophthalmos due to herniation of the orbital contents medially (*arrows*)

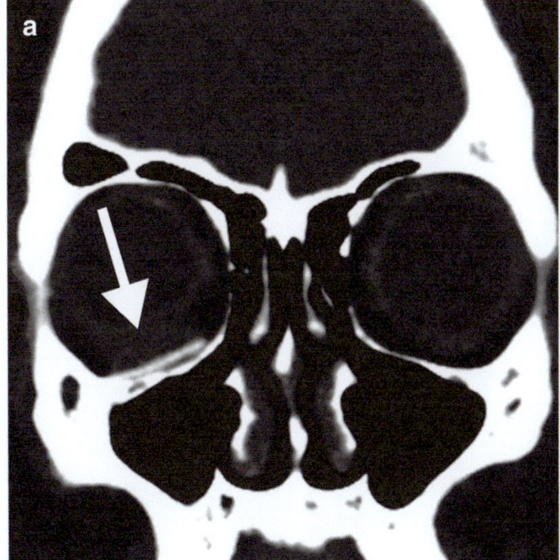
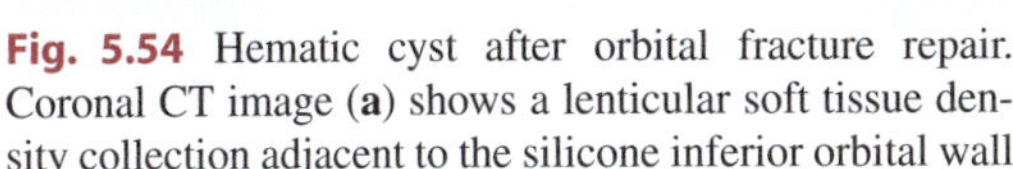
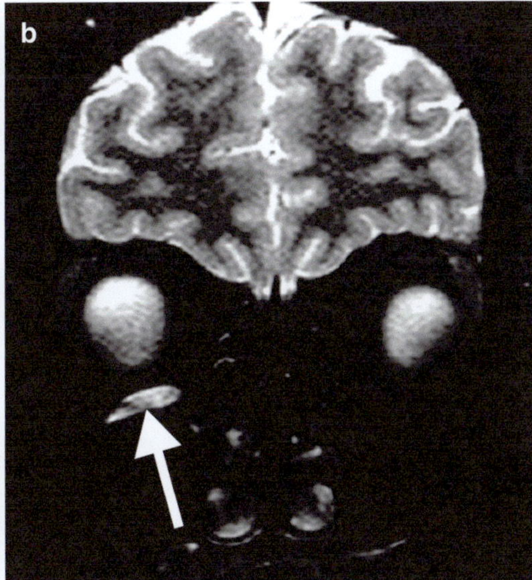

Fig. 5.54 Hematic cyst after orbital fracture repair. Coronal CT image (**a**) shows a lenticular soft tissue density collection adjacent to the silicone inferior orbital wall plate (*arrow*).Coronal T2-weighted MRI (**b**) shows the high signal within the hematic cyst (*arrow*)

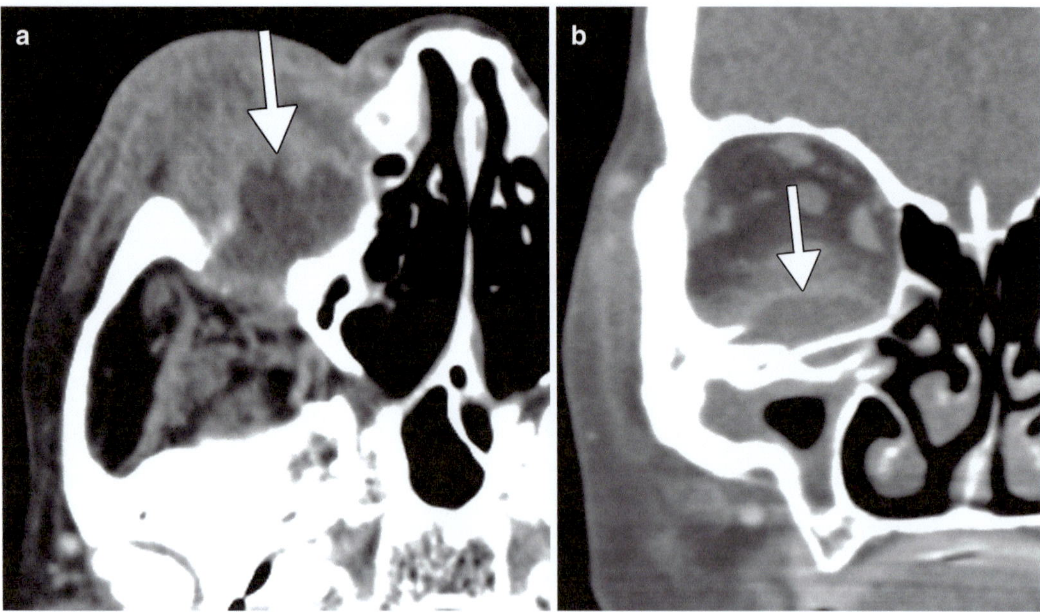

Fig. 5.55 Peri-implant abscess. Axial (**a**) and coronal (**b**) post-contrast CT images show a peripherally enhancing fluid collection surrounding the right orbital floor implant (*arrow*) with associated fat stranding in the preseptal and postseptal spaces, compatible with orbital cellulitis

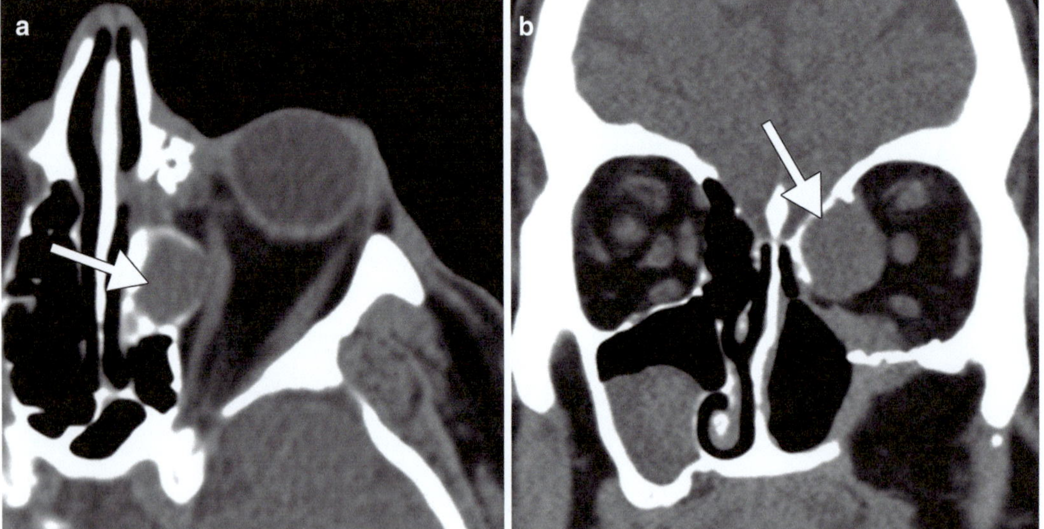

Fig. 5.56 Mucocele after orbital fracture repair. Axial (**a**) and coronal (**b**) CT images show an opacified and expanded left ethmoid air cell that bulges into the left orbit causing lateral displacement of the medial rectus muscle (*arrow*)

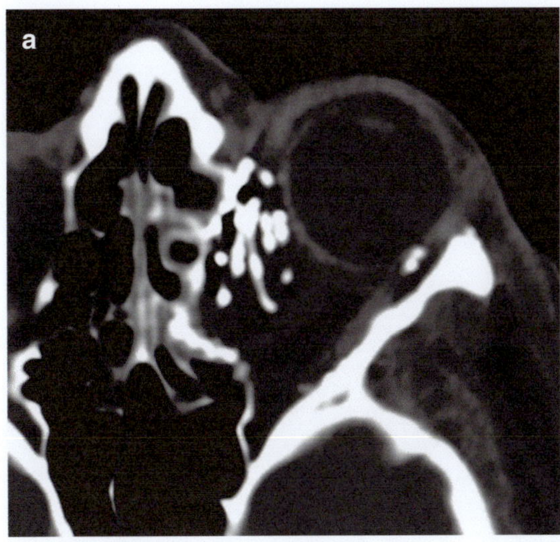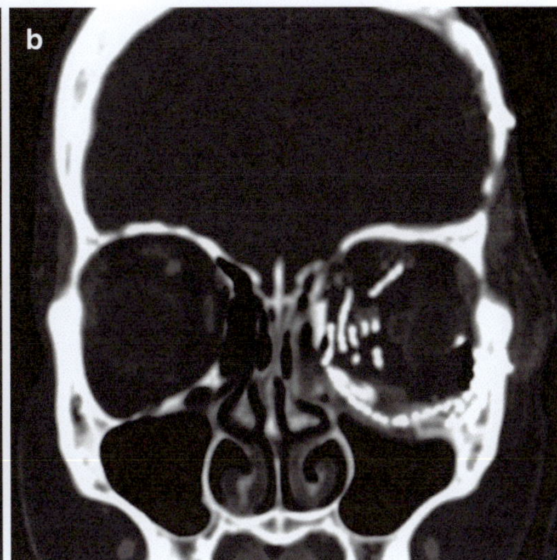

Fig. 5.57 Optic nerve impingement. Axial (**a**) and coronal (**b**) CT images show multiple overlapping mesh implants in the medial left orbit that were used to augment the orbital volume after inferior and medial orbital wall fractures in which the wraparound mesh buckled medially. These resulted in impingement of the optic nerve, globe, and extraocular muscles

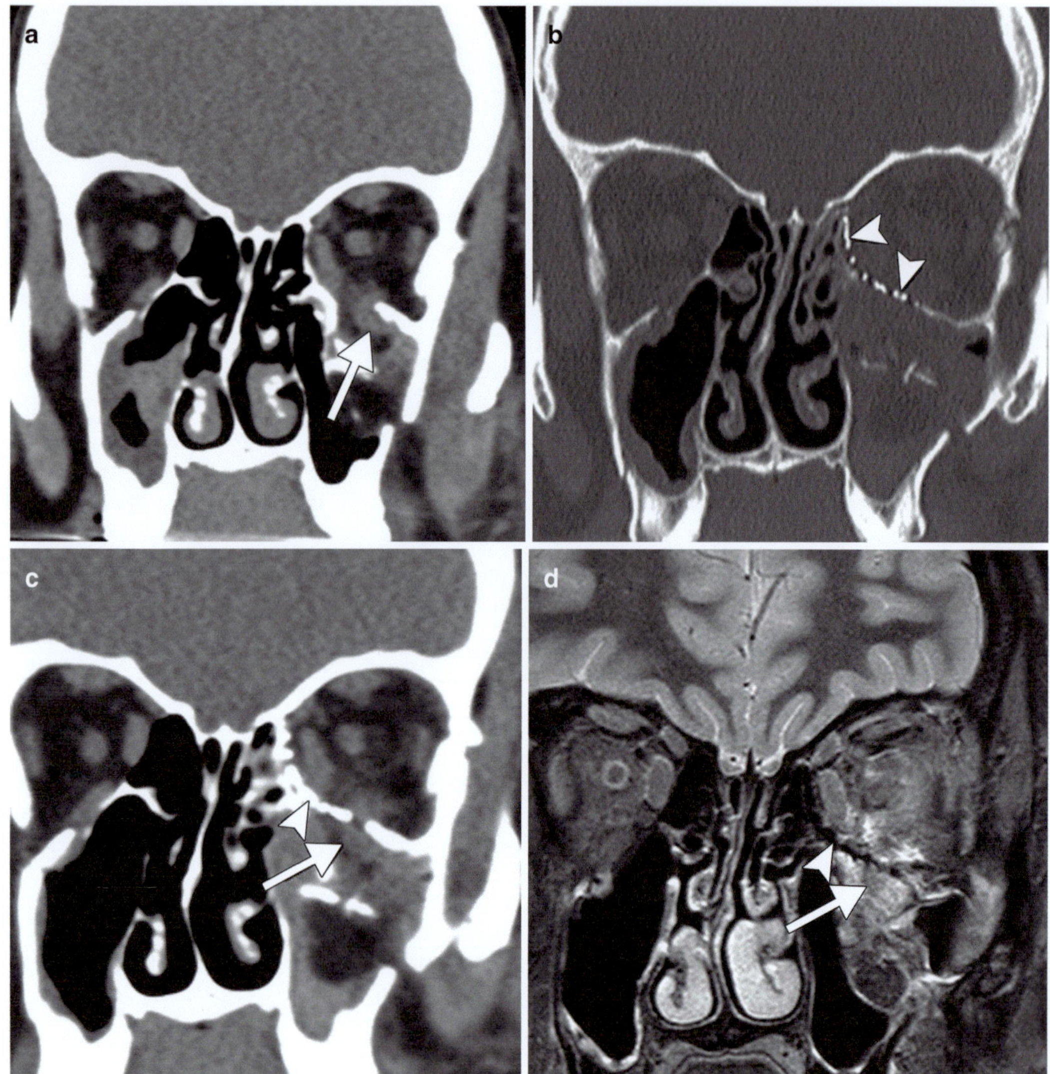

Fig. 5.58 Postoperative rectus muscle entrapment. The patient presented with esotropia following left orbital floor fracture repair. Initial preoperative coronal CT image (**a**) shows a left orbital floor fracture with herniation of a portion of the orbital contents. Postoperative coronal CT images (**b**, **c**) and coronal and sagittal MRI sequences (**d–f**) show interval insertion of a titanium orbital wall implant (*arrowheads*) that closely approximates the natural contours of the orbit. However, there is persistent inferior herniation of the orbital contents, including a portion of the inferior rectus muscle (*arrow*)

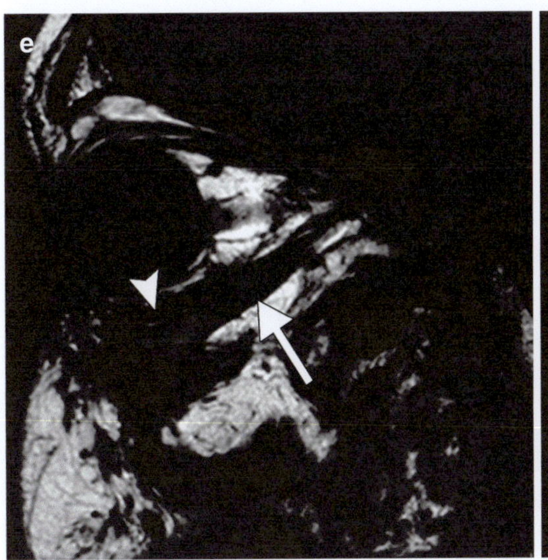
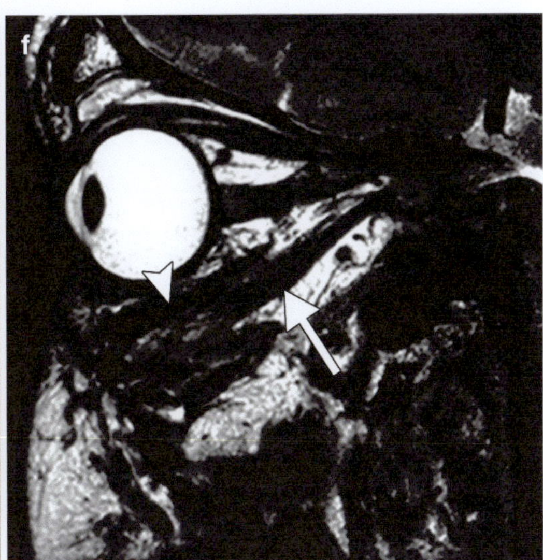

Fig. 5.58 (continued)

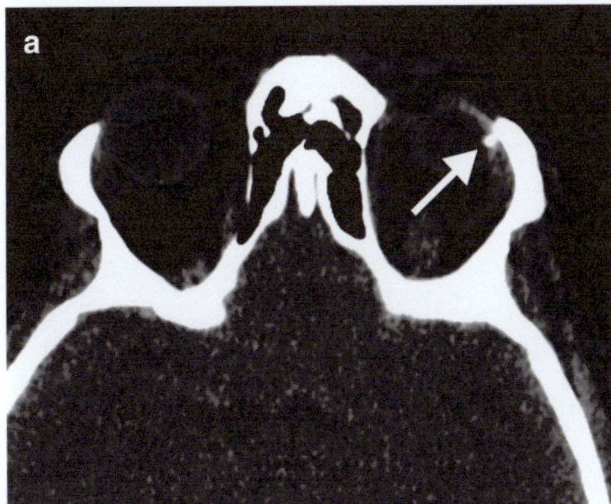
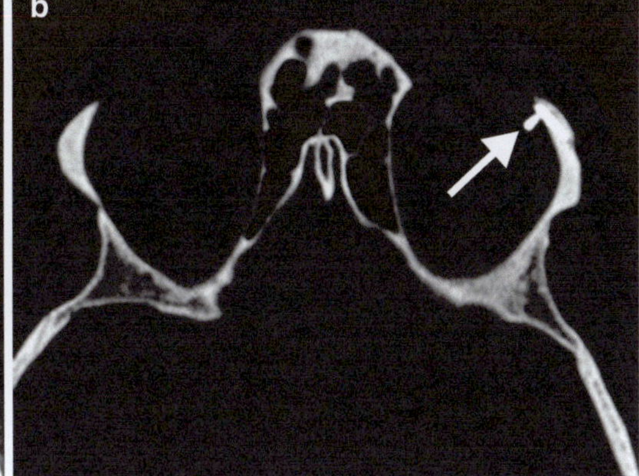

Fig. 5.59 Globe impingement by screws. The patient experienced restrictive ocular dysmotility OS following superior orbital wall and rim fracture repair. Axial CT images in the soft tissue (**a**) and bone (**b**) windows show a fixation screw projecting in close proximity to the left globe (*arrows*)

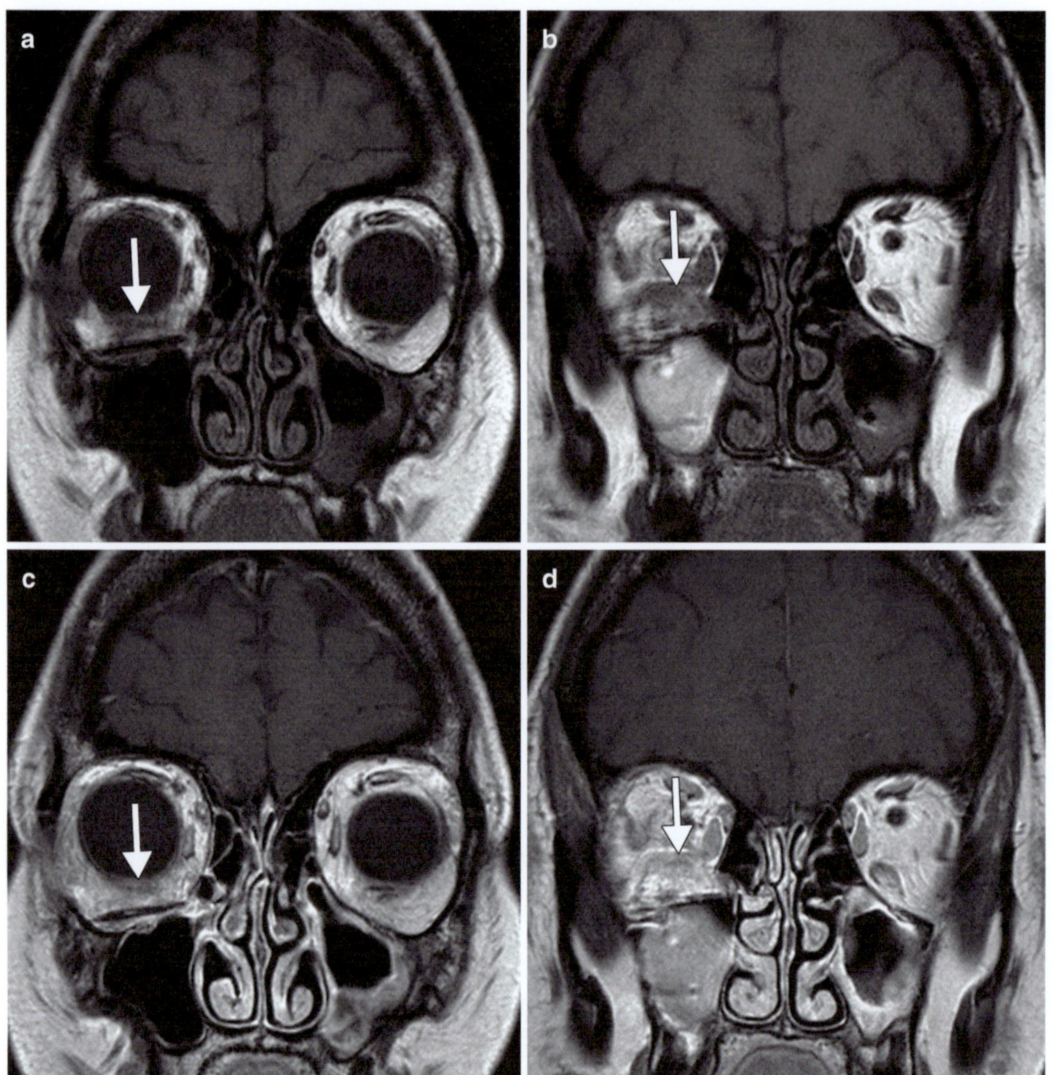

Fig. 5.60 Scar tissue. The patient experienced strabismus following right orbital floor fracture repair. Coronal T1-weighted (**a**, **b**), post-contrast T1-weighted (**c**, **d**), and T2-weighted (**e**, **f**) MR images show extensive, diffuse, ill-defined soft tissue (*arrows*) in the inferior orbit between the irregular inferior rectus and the implant

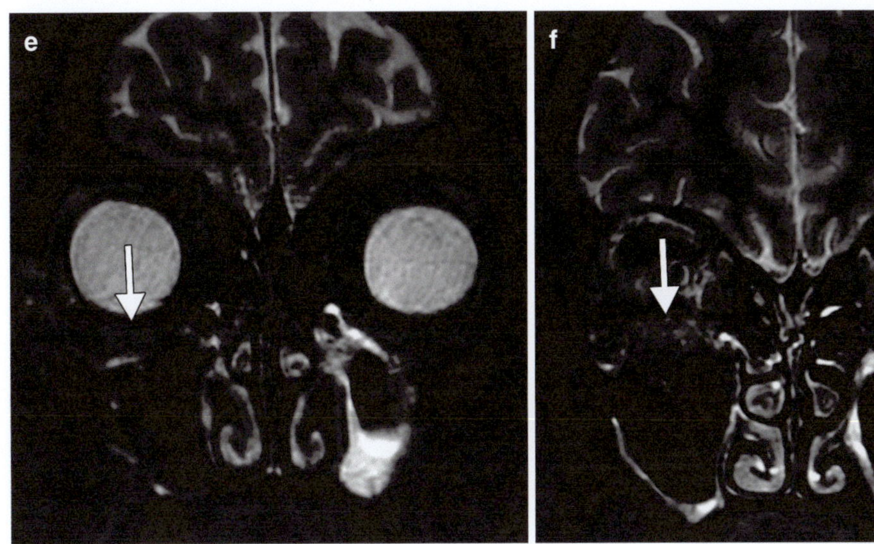

Fig. 5.60 (continued)

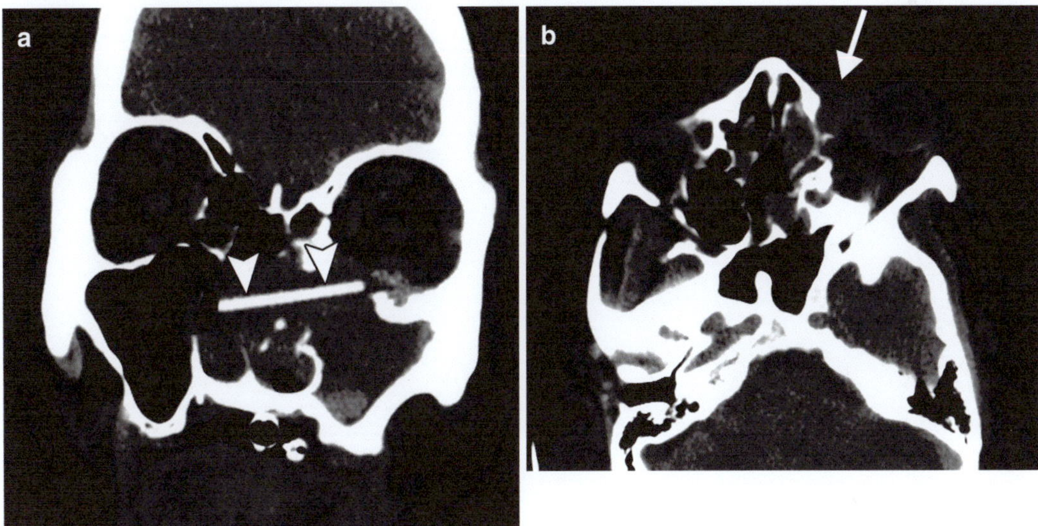

Fig. 5.61 Implant displacement. Coronal CT image (**a**) shows inferior and medial displacement of the silastic orbital floor reconstruction plate into the nasal cavity (*arrowheads*).There is opacification of the left maxillary sinus and nasal cavity surrounding the implant. In addition, the axial CT image (**b**) shows associated dilatation of the lacrimal sac (*arrow*) due to obstruction of the nasolacrimal duct system

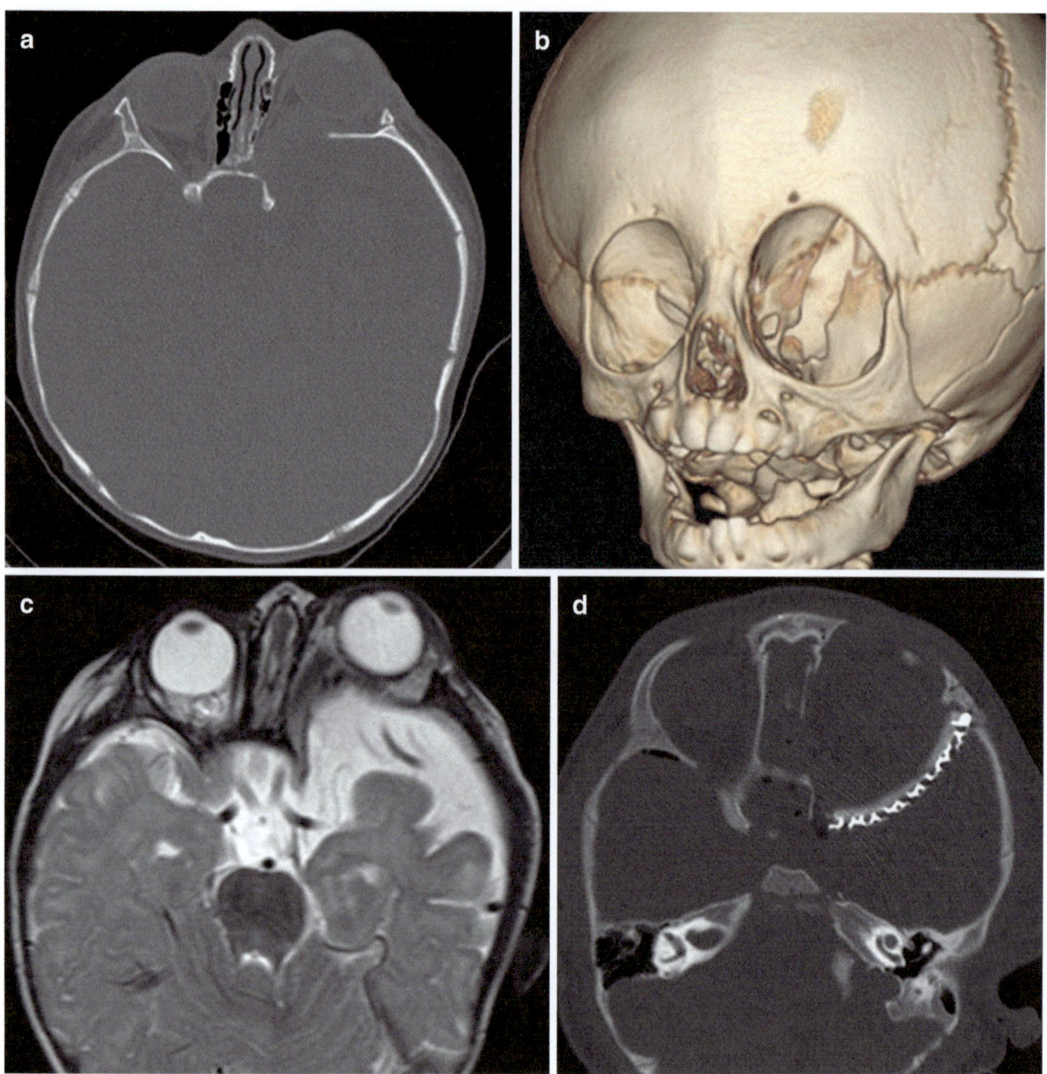

Fig. 5.62 Sphenoid wing dysplasia repair. Preoperative axial CT (**a**), 3D CT (**b**), and axial T2-weighted MRI (**c**) show left sphenoid wing dysplasia with associated meningocele and exophthalmos. Postoperative axial CT (**d**), coronal CT (**e**), 3D CT (**f**), axial T2-weighted (**g**), and coronal T2-weighted (**h**) MR images show reconstruction of the superolateral orbital wall defect using combined bone graft and titanium mesh. The bone graft was harvested from the calvarium (*arrow*) adjacent to the frontal craniotomy performed for orbitofrontal advancement. A plexiform neurofibroma (*arrows*) has grown within the left orbit in the intervening period

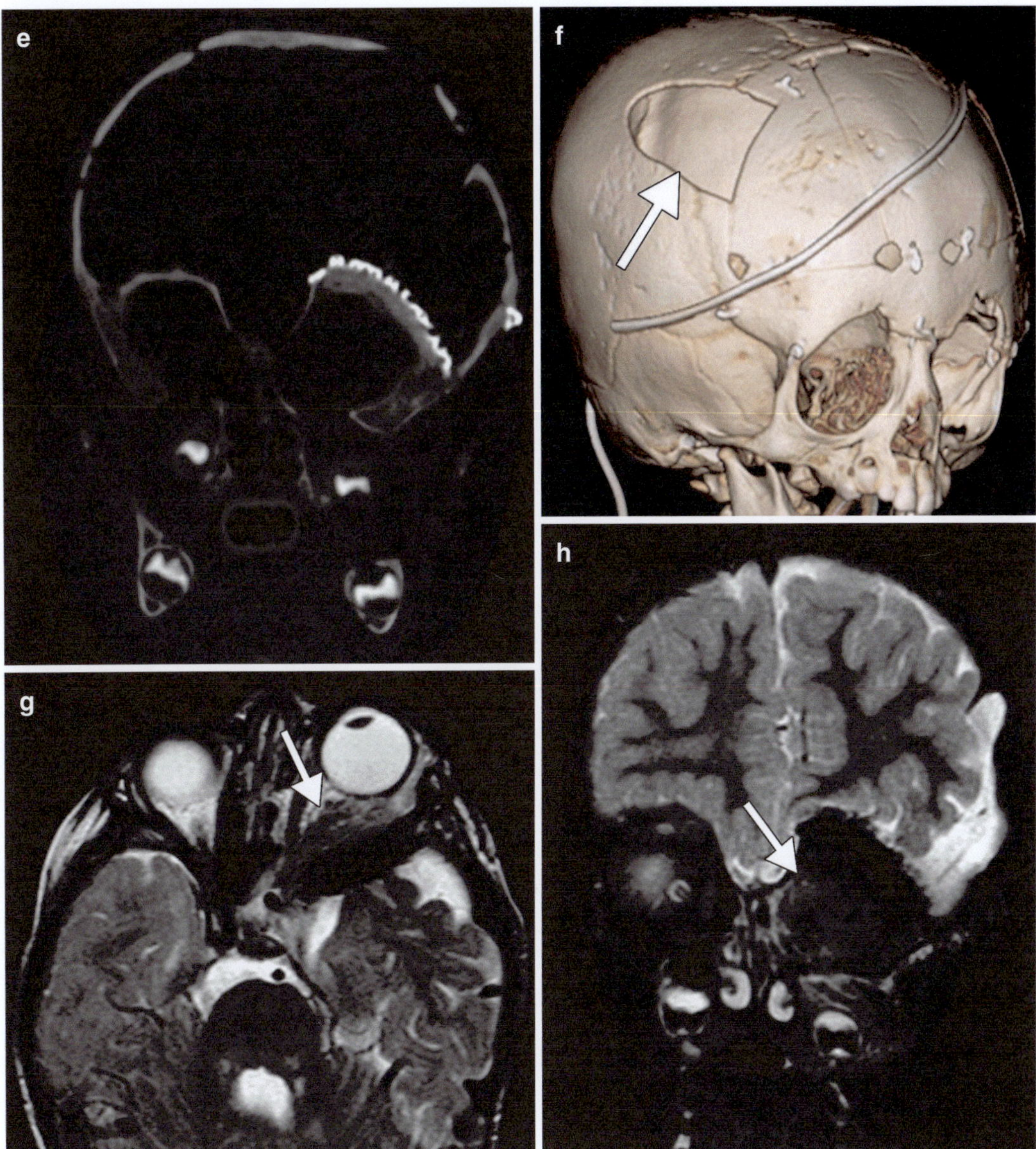

Fig. 5.62 (continued)

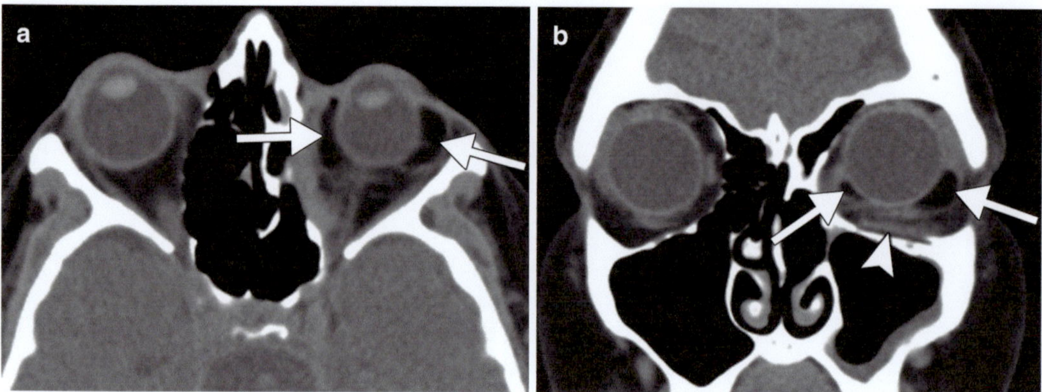

Fig. 5.63 Fat graft augmentation for correction of post-traumatic enophthalmos. Axial (**a**) and coronal (**b**) CT images show fat graft within the left orbit (*arrows*). A wedge implant is also present (*arrowhead*)

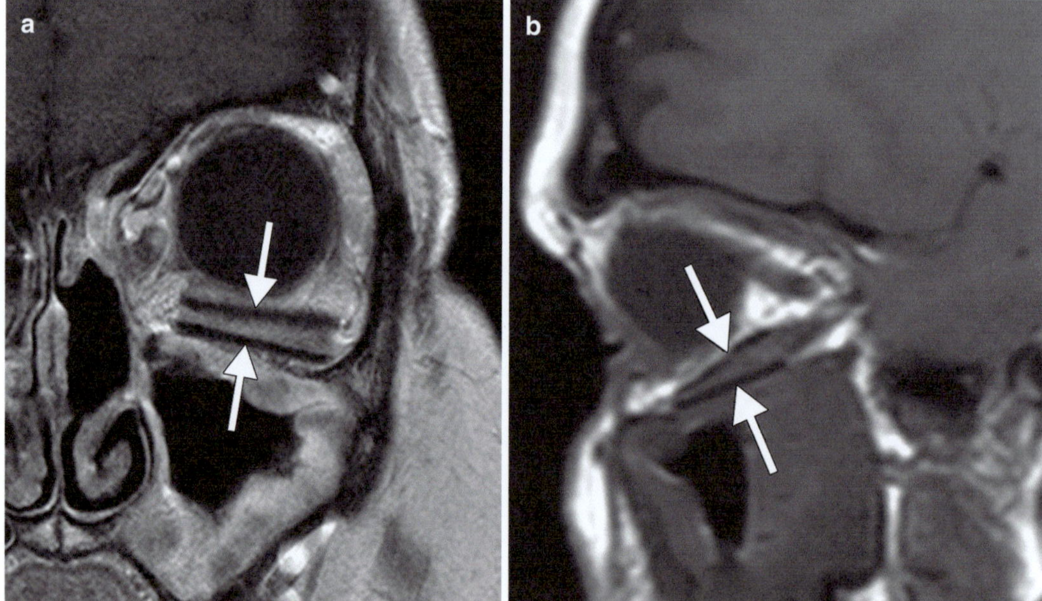

Fig. 5.64 Wedge implant for correction of post-traumatic enophthalmos. Coronal (**a**) and sagittal (**b**) T1-weighted (**b**) MR images show the two leaflets of the implant (*arrows*) within the inferior orbit

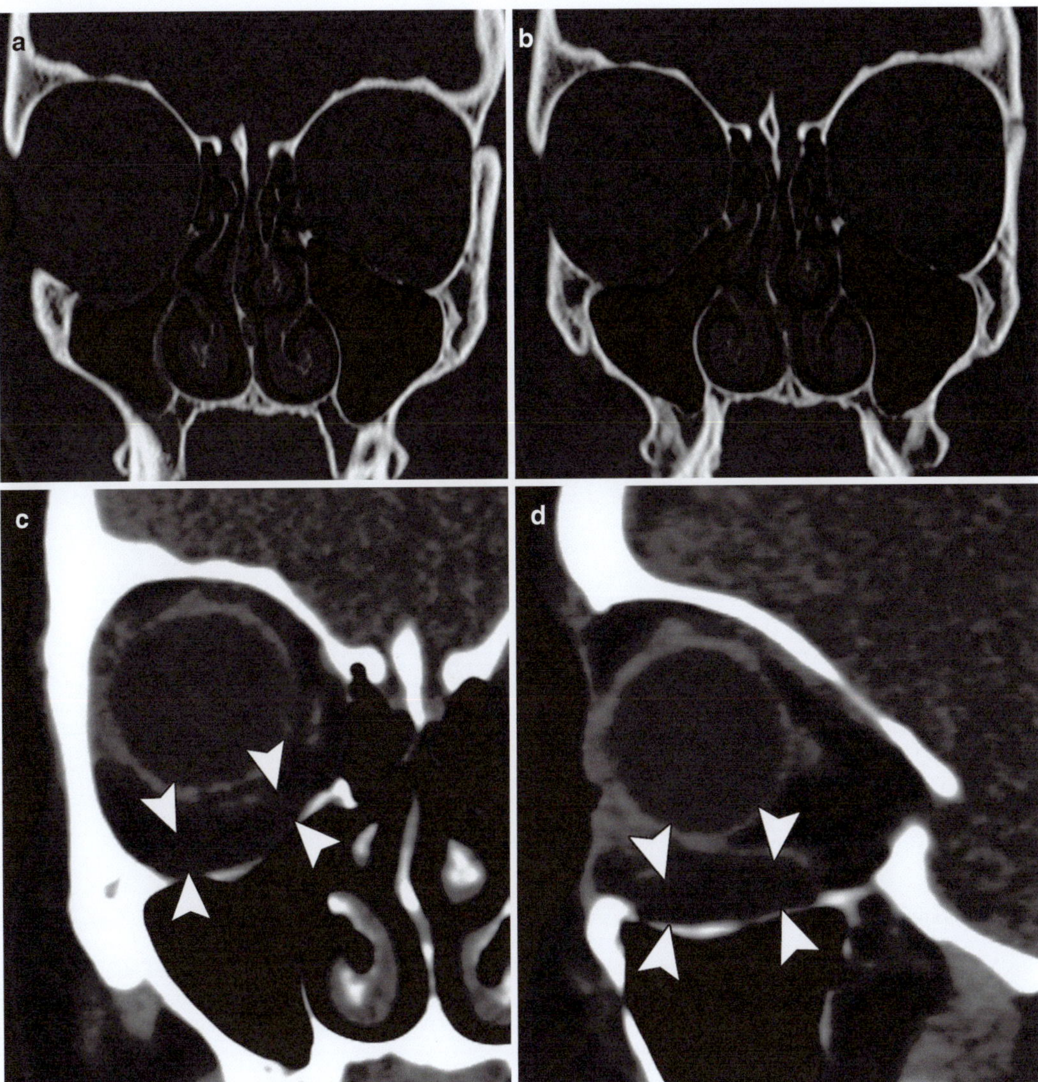

Fig. 5.65 Uncinectomy and orbital augmentation for silent sinus syndrome. Preoperative coronal CT image (**a**) shows a low-lying right orbital floor, which contacts the uncinate process and obliterates the infundibulum. Postoperative coronal CT in the bone window (**b**) shows interval resection of the right uncinate and decreased inferior bowing of the right orbital floor. Coronal (**c**) and sagittal (**d**) CT images in the soft tissue windows show the Medpor implant in the right orbit extraconal space (*arrowheads*)

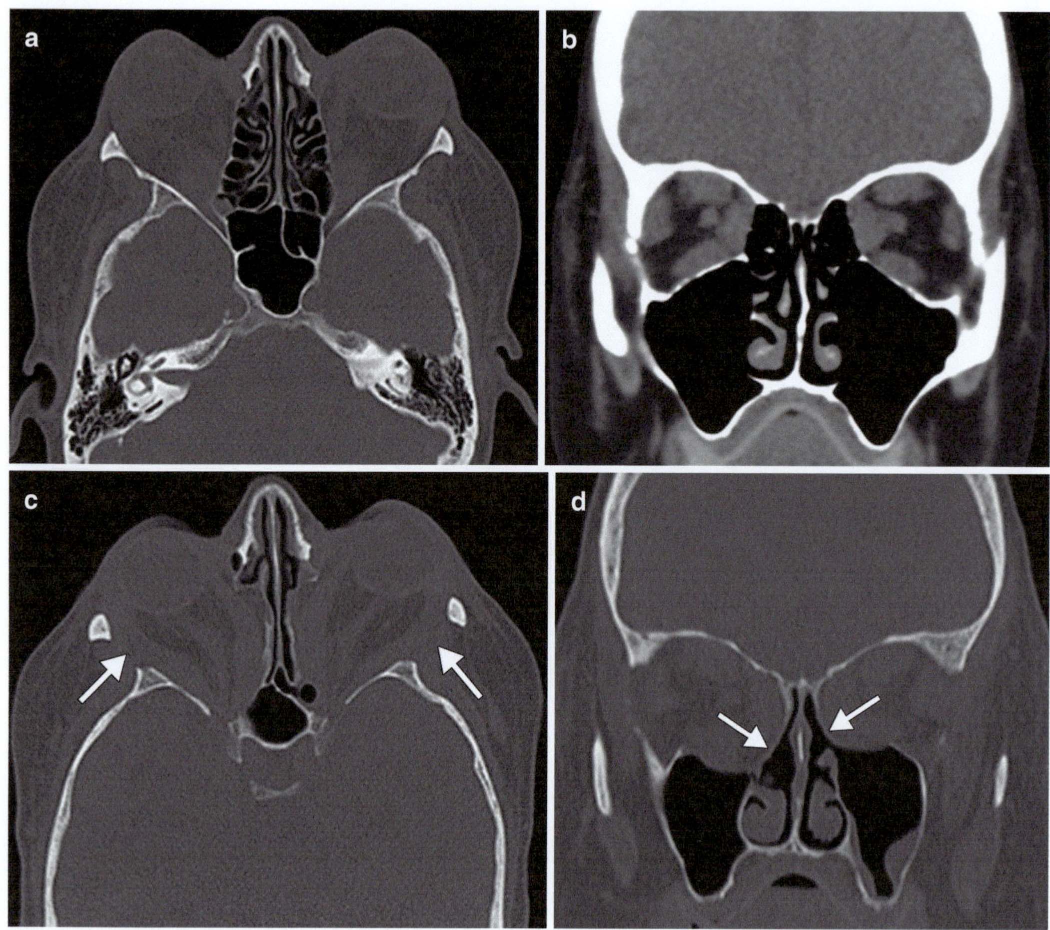

Fig. 5.66 Three-wall orbital decompression. Preoperative axial (**a**) and coronal (**b**) CT images show marked bilateral proptosis and extraocular muscle enlargement in a patient with thyroid orbitopathy. Axial (**c**) and coronal (**d**) postoperative CT images show bilateral inferior, lateral, and medial orbital wall decompression with herniation of orbital contents into the adjacent sinuses (*arrows*)

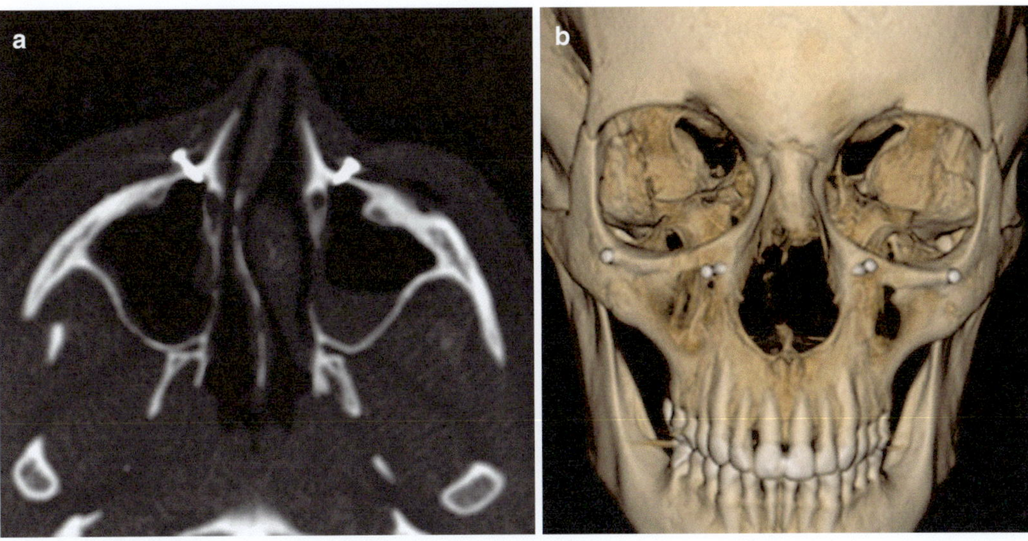

Fig. 5.67 Eyelid retraction repair. Axial (**a**) and 3D (**b**) CT images show bilateral inferior orbital rim metallic screws for attachment of Medpor implants, which are otherwise not conspicuous on these images

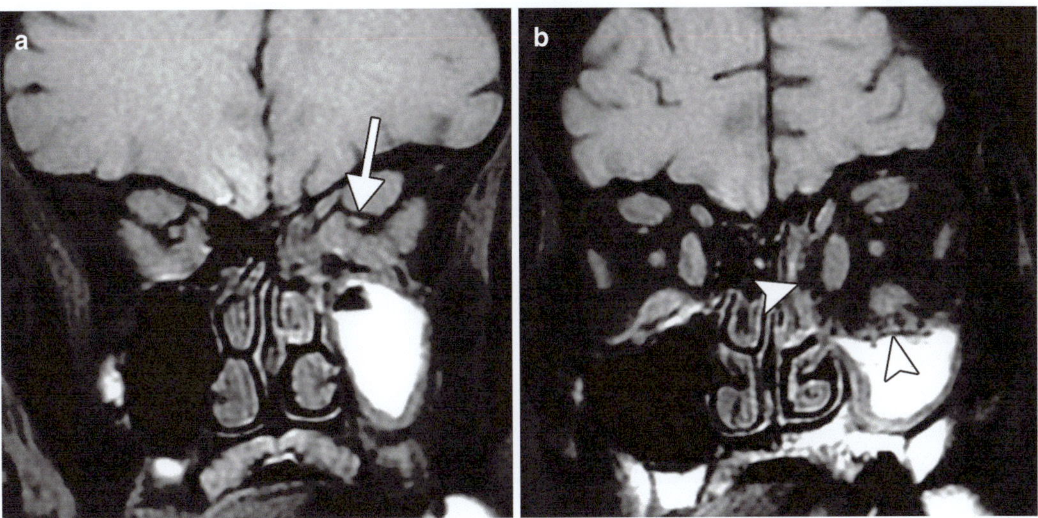

Fig. 5.68 Persistent optic nerve compression following orbital wall decompression. Coronal fat-suppressed T1-weighted MR images of the orbit show that enlarged extraocular muscles compress the optic nerve (*arrow*) in the orbital apex (**a**), while more anteriorly the medial and inferior orbital walls have been decompressed (*arrowheads*) (**b**)

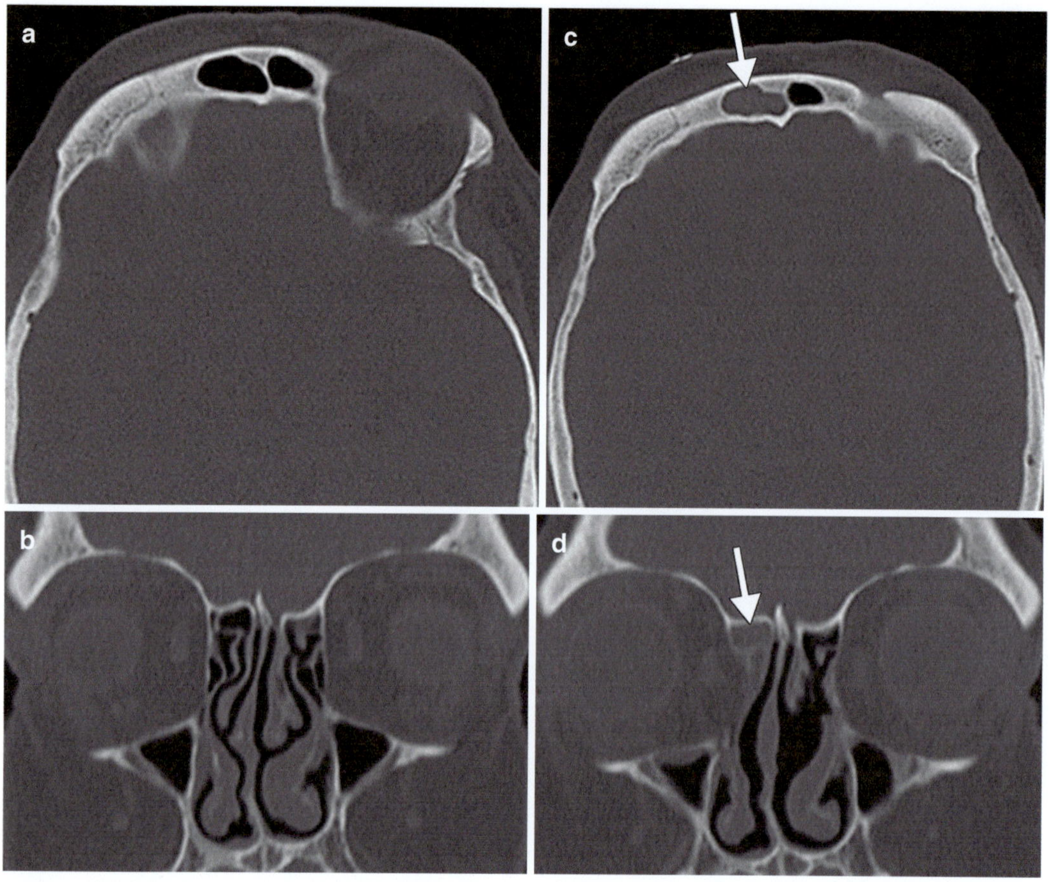

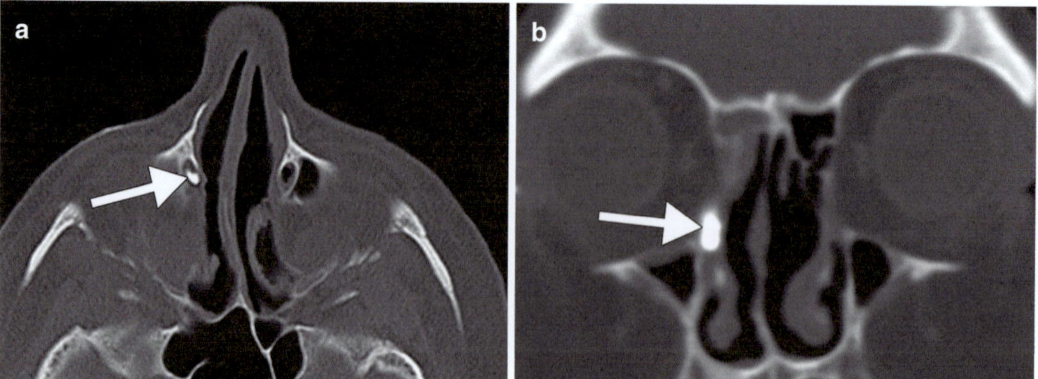

Fig. 5.69 Sinus obstruction after orbital decompression. Preoperative axial (**a**) and coronal (**b**) CT images show clear paranasal sinuses. Postoperative axial (**c**) and coronal (**d**) CT images show interval bilateral medial wall decompression, in which there is greater herniation of orbital contents on the right side, with new opacification of the right ethmoid and frontal sinuses (*arrows*)

Fig. 5.70 Nasolacrimal duct obstruction after orbital wall decompression. Axial (**a**) and coronal (**b**) CT dacryocystogram images show bilateral medial wall decompressions. Contrast did not progress beyond the midportion of the nasolacrimal duct (*arrows*)

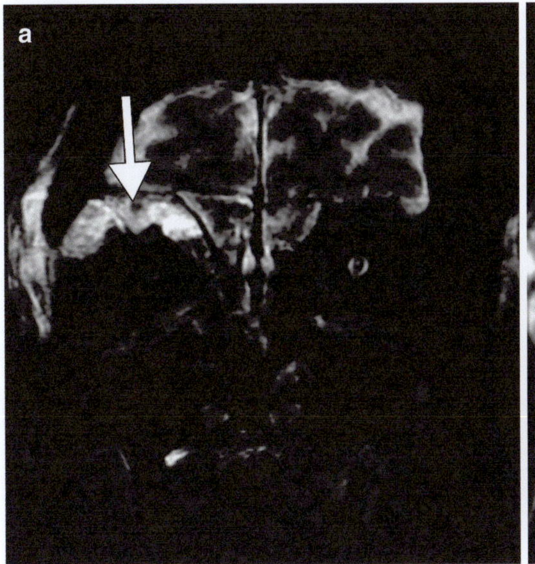
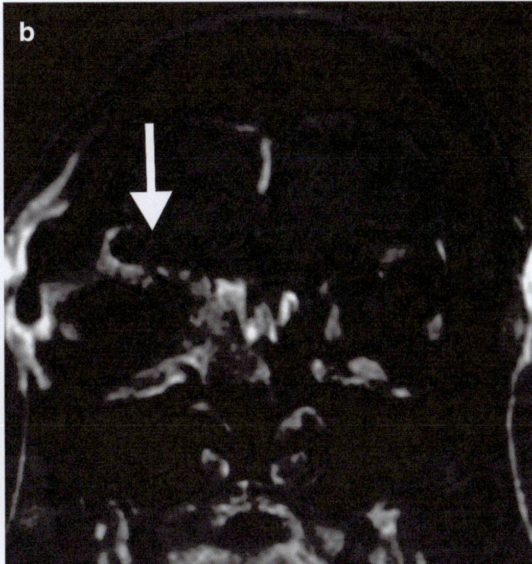

Fig. 5.71 CSF leak after orbital decompression. The patient presented with right eye pain and progressive proptosis following medial and lateral bony orbital decompression. Coronal T2-weighted (**a**) and post-contrast T1-weighted (**b**) MR images show a fluid collection in the superior right orbit (*arrows*). The images are degraded by patient motion, due to seizure activity

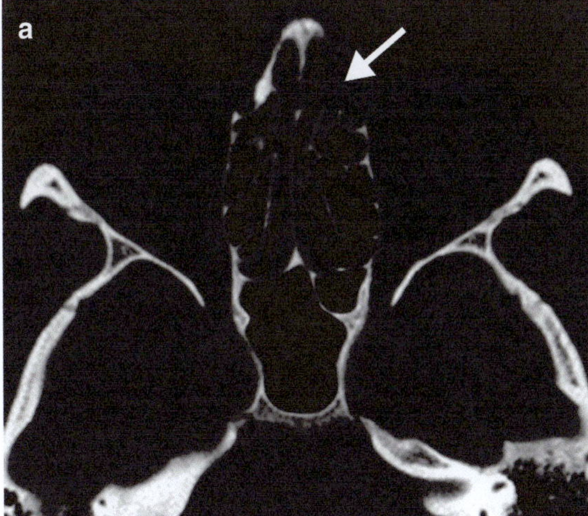
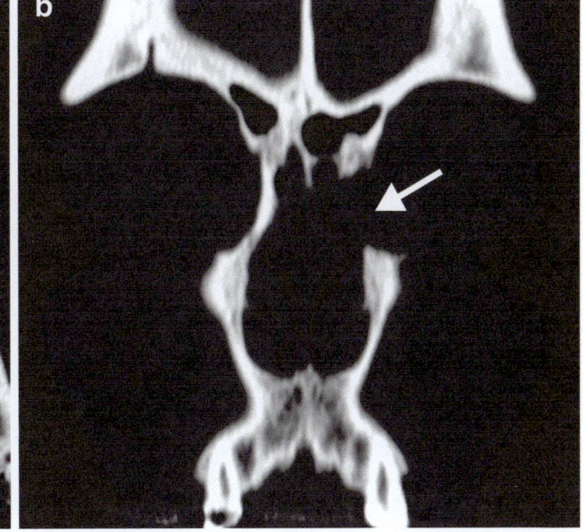

Fig. 5.72 Dacryocystorhinostomy. Axial (**a**) and coronal (**b**) CT images show a defect in the left lacrimal bone and frontal process of the maxilla, allowing a direct communication between the lacrimal sac and middle meatus of the nose (*arrows*)

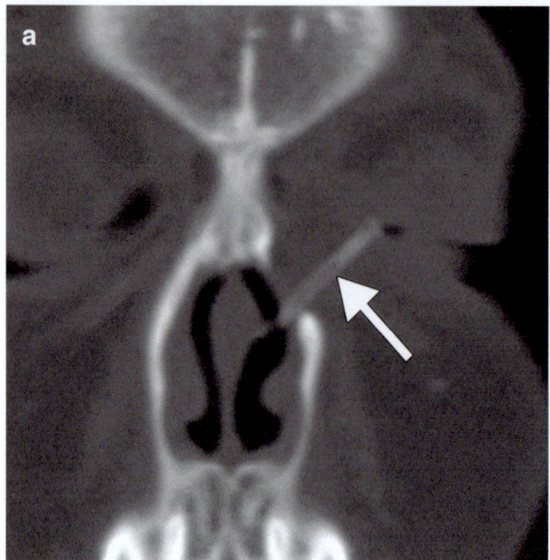
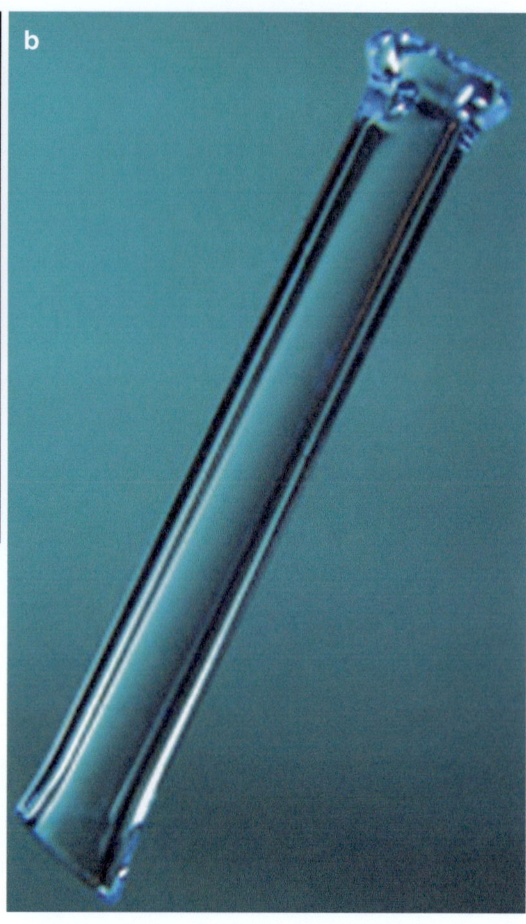

Fig. 5.73 Jones tube. Coronal CT image (**a**) demonstrates a Jones tube (*arrow*) that extends from the ocular surface conjunctiva to the nasal cavity via a surgically created osseous defect. Photograph courtesy of Gunther Weiss Scientific Glass Blowing Company (**b**)

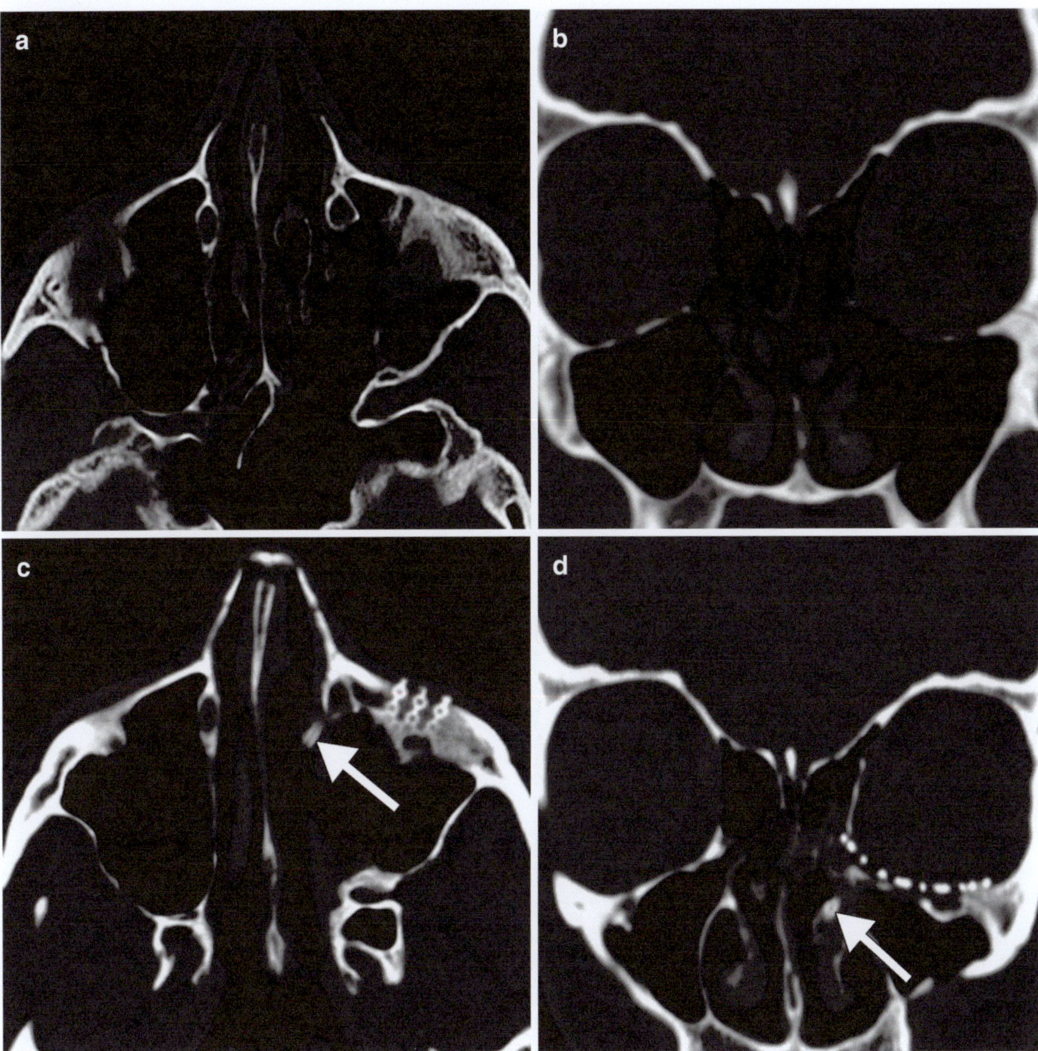

Fig. 5.74 Conjunctivodacryocystorhinostomy with partial middle turbinectomy. The patient suffered a prior left orbital wall fracture that was repaired with titanium mesh with associated nasolacrimal duct stenosis. Axial (**a**) and coronal (**b**) CT images obtained before conjunctivodacryocystorhinostomy show an intact left middle turbinate. Postoperative axial (**c**) and coronal (**d**) CT images show interval resection of a portion of the left middle turbinate to accommodate the Jones tube (*arrows*)

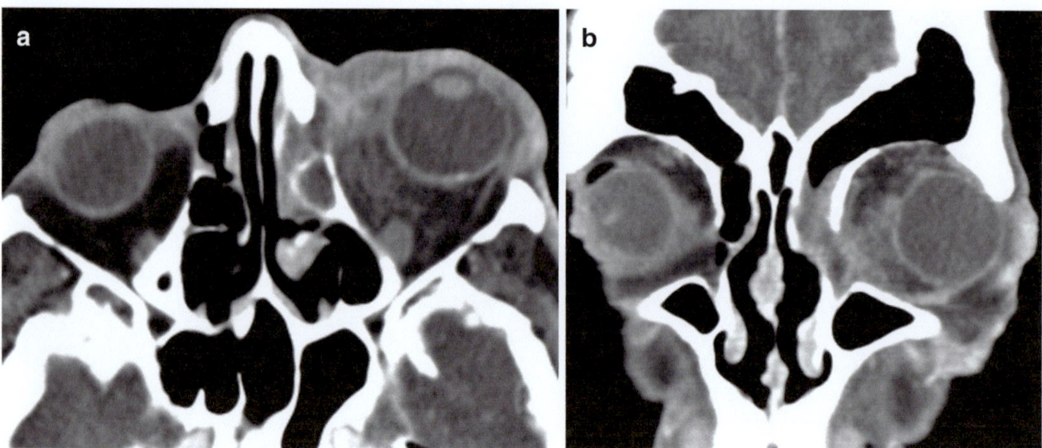

Fig. 5.75 Infection after dacryocystorhinostomy. Axial (**a**) and coronal (**b**) CT images show proptosis and left orbital fat stranding surrounding the surgical site

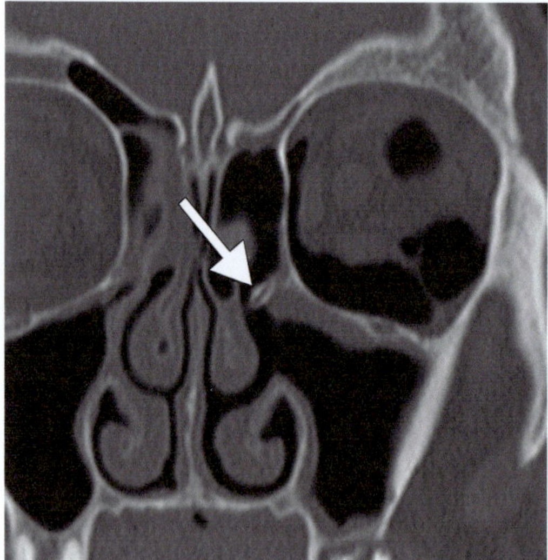

Fig. 5.76 Orbital emphysema related to Jones. Axial CT image show extensive left pneumo-orbit and a Jones tube in position (*arrow*)

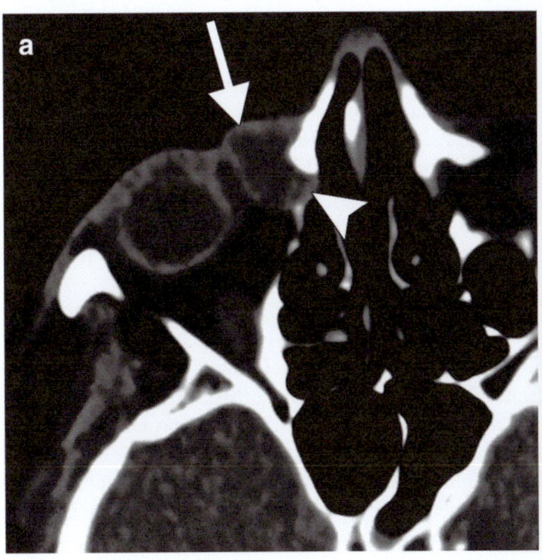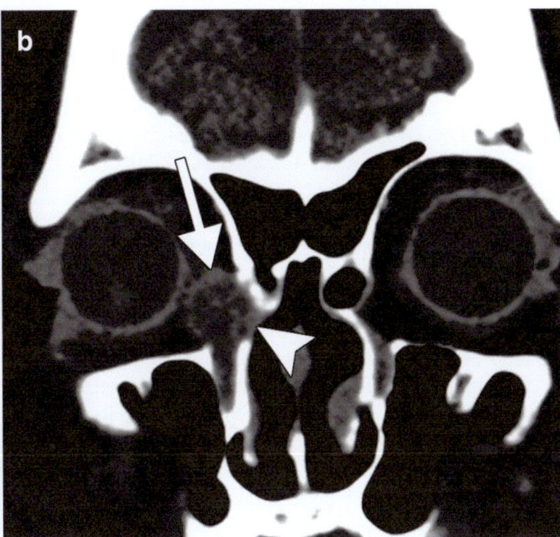

Fig. 5.77 Recurrent nasolacrimal duct obstruction after dacryocystorhinostomy. Axial (**a**) and coronal (**b**) CT images show a markedly distended right lacrimal sac (*arrows*) despite right dacryocystorhinostomy defect (*arrowheads*)

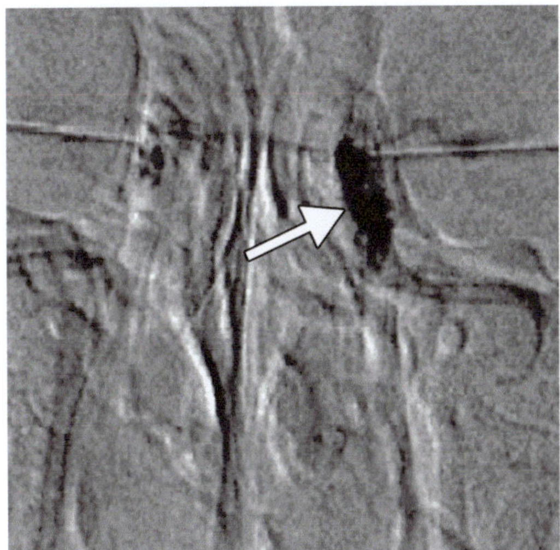

Fig. 5.78 Obstructed nasolacrimal system after dacryocystorhinostomy depicted on dacryocystography. Digital subtraction dacryocystogram image shows accumulation of contrast (*arrow*) within the proximal left nasolacrimal duct but without free spillage into the nasal cavity

Further Reading

Abdulhafez M, Elgazayerli E, Mansour T, Khalaf MA. A new modification in the porous polyethylene-coated lester jones tube. Orbit. 2009;28(1):25–8.

Alsuhaibani AH, Carter KD, Policeni B, Nerad JA. Effect of orbital bony decompression for Graves' orbitopathy on the volume of extraocular muscles. Br J Ophthalmol. 2011;95(9):1255–8.

Badilla J, Dolman PJ. Cerebrospinal fluid leaks complicating orbital or oculoplastic surgery. Arch Ophthalmol. 2007;125(12):1631–4.

Baino F. Biomaterials and implants for orbital floor repair. Acta Biomater. 2011;7(9):3248–66.

Baxter SA, Laibson PR. Punctal plugs in the management of dry eyes. Ocul Surf. 2004;2(4):255–65.

Behbehani R, Vacareza N, Bilyk JR, Rubin PA, Pribitkin EA. Simultaneous endoscopic antrostomy and orbital reconstruction in silent sinus syndrome. Orbit. 2006;25(2):97–101.

Bladen JC, Norris JH, Malhotra R. Indications and outcomes for revision of gold weight implants in upper eyelid loading. Br J Ophthalmol. 2012;96(4):485–9.

Bourkiza R, Lee V. A review of the complications of lacrimal occlusion with punctal and canalicular plugs. Orbit. 2012;31(2):86–93.

Bratton EM, Durairaj VD. Orbital implants for fracture repair. Curr Opin Ophthalmol. 2011;22(5):400–6.

Brown AE, Banks P. Late extrusion of alloplastic orbital floor implants. Br J Oral Maxillofac Surg. 1993;31(3):154–7.

Brucoli M, Arcuri F, Cavenaghi R, Benech A. Analysis of complications after surgical repair of orbital fractures. J Craniofac Surg. 2011;22(4):1387–90.

Caesar RH, Friebel J, McNab AA. Upper lid loading with gold weights in paralytic lagophthalmos: a modified technique to maximize the long-term functional and cosmetic success. Orbit. 2004;23(1):27–32.

Choi HY, Hong SE, Lew JM. Long-term comparison of a newly designed gold implant with the conventional implant in facial nerve paralysis. Plast Reconstr Surg. 1999;104(6):1624–34.

Chu EA, Miller NR, Lane AP. Selective endoscopic decompression of the orbital apex for dysthyroid optic neuropathy. Laryngoscope. 2009;119(6):1236–40.

Custer PL, Trinkaus KM. Porous implant exposure: incidence, management, and morbidity. Ophthal Plast Reconstr Surg. 2007;23(1):1–7.

Custer PL, Kennedy RH, Woog JJ, Kaltreider SA, Meyer DR. Orbital implants in enucleation surgery: a report by the American Academy of Ophthalmology. Ophthalmology. 2003;110(10):2054–61.

Onerci M. Dacryocystorhinostomy. Diagnosis and treatment of nasolacrimal canal obstructions. Rhinology. 2002;40(2):49–65.

Dailey RA, Tower RN. Frosted jones pyrex tubes. Ophthal Plast Reconstr Surg. 2005;21(3):185–7.

Demirci H, Frueh BR. Palpebral spring in the management of lagophthalmos and exposure keratopathy secondary to facial nerve palsy. Ophthal Plast Reconstr Surg. 2009;25(4):270–5.

Dunaway DJ, David DJ. Intraorbital tissue expansion in the management of congenital anophthalmos. Br J Plast Surg. 1996;49(8):529–35.

Dusart A, Duprez T, Van Snick S, Godfraind C, Sindic C. Fatal rhinocerebralmucormycosis with intracavernous carotid aneurysm and thrombosis: a late complication of transsphenoidal surgery? Acta Neurol Belg. 2013;113:179–84.

Eckstein A, Schittkowski M, Esser J. Surgical treatment of Graves' ophthalmopathy. Best Pract Res Clin Endocrinol Metab. 2012;26(3):339–58.

European Group on Graves' Orbitopathy (EUGOGO), Mourits MP, Bijl H, Altea MA, Baldeschi L, Boboridis K, Currò N, Dickinson AJ, Eckstein A, Freidel M, Guastella C, Kahaly GJ, Kalmann R, Krassas GE, Lane CM, Lareida J, Marcocci C, Marino M, Nardi M, Mohr C, Neoh C, Pinchera A, Orgiazzi J, Pitz S, Saeed P, Salvi M, Sellari-Franceschini S, Stahl M, von Arx G, Wiersinga WM. Outcome of orbital decompression for disfiguring proptosis in patients with Graves' orbitopathy using various surgical procedures. Br J Ophthalmol. 2009;93(11):1518–23.

Fay A, Santiago YM. A modified levine palpebral spring for the treatment of myogenic ptosis. Ophthal Plast Reconstr Surg. 2012;28(5):372–5.

Finn JC, Cox S. Fillers in the periorbital complex. Facial Plast Surg Clin North Am. 2007;15(1):123–32, viii.

Friedrich RE, Heiland M, Kehler U, Schmelzle R. Reconstruction of sphenoid wing dysplasia with pulsating exophthalmos in a case of neurofibromatosis type 1 supported by intraoperative navigation using a new skull reference system. Skull Base. 2003;13(4):211–7.

Galluzzi P, De Francesco S, Giacalone G, Cerase A, Monti L, Vallone IM, Lazzeretti L, Venturi C, Hadjistilianou T. Contrast-enhanced magnetic resonance imaging of fibrovascular tissue ingrowth within synthetic hydroxyapatite orbital implants in children. Eur J Ophthalmol. 2011;21(5):521–8.

Garibaldi DC, Iliff NT, Grant MP, Merbs SL. Use of porous polyethylene with embedded titanium in orbital reconstruction: a review of 106 patients. Ophthal Plast Reconstr Surg. 2007;23(6):439–44.

Gierloff M, Seeck NG, Springer I, Becker S, Kandzia C, Wiltfang J. Orbital floor reconstruction with resorbable polydioxanone implants. J Craniofac Surg. 2012;23(1):161–4.

Gilhotra JS, McNab AA, McKelvie P, O'Donnell BA. Late orbital haemorrhage around alloplastic orbital floor implants: a case series and review. Clin Experiment Ophthalmol. 2002;30(5):352–5.

Ginat DT, Freitag SK. Orbital Emphysema Complicating Jones Tube Placement in a Patient Treated With Continuous Positive Airway Pressure. Ophthal Plast Reconstr Surg. 2014, Oct 1.

Ginat DT, Schatz CJ. Imaging features of midface injectable fillers and associated complications. AJNR Am J Neuroradiol. 2013;34(8):1488–95.

Ginat DT, Bhama P, Cunnane ME, Hadlock TA. Facial reanimation procedures depicted on radiologic imaging. AJNR Am J Neuroradiol. 2014;35(9):1662–6.

Glavas I, Lissauer B, Hornblass A. Chronic subperiosteal hematic cyst formation twelve years after orbital fracture repair with alloplastic orbital floor implant. Orbit. 2005;24(1):47–9.

Hardman J, Halpin SF, Hourihan MD, Mars S, Lane C. MRI of the anterior optic pathways following enucleation. Neuroradiology. 1997;39(11):815–7.

Harrisberg BP, Singh RP, Croxson GR, Taylor RF, McCluskey PJ. Long-term outcome of gold eyelid weights in patients with facial nerve palsy. Otol Neurotol. 2001;22(3):397–400.

Heiland M, Schulze D, Rother U, Schmelzle R. Postoperative imaging of zygomaticomaxillary complex fractures using digital volume tomography. J Oral Maxillofac Surg. 2004;62(11):1387–91.

Ho VH, Wilson MW, Fleming JC, Haik BG. Retained intraorbital metallic foreign bodies. Ophthal Plast Reconstr Surg. 2004;20(3):232–6.

Holds JB, Anderson RL. Medial canthotomy and cantholysis in eyelid reconstruction. Am J Ophthalmol. 1993;116(2):218–23.

Hui JI. Outcomes of orbital implants after evisceration and enucleation in patients with endophthalmitis. Curr Opin Ophthalmol. 2010;21(5):375–9.

Hunter PD, Baker SS. The treatment of enophthalmos by orbital injection of fat autograft. Arch Otolaryngol Head Neck Surg. 1994;120(8):835–9.

Jamal BT, Pfahler SM, Lane KA, Bilyk JR, Pribitkin EA, Diecidue RJ, Taub DI. Ophthalmic injuries in patients with zygomaticomaxillary complex fractures requiring surgical repair. J Oral Maxillofac Surg. 2009;67(5):986–9.

Kashkouli MB, Pakdel F, Sasani L, Hodjat P, Kaghazkanani R, Heirati A. High-density porous polyethylene wedge implant in correction of enophthalmos and hypoglobus in seeing eyes. Orbit. 2011;30(3):123–30.

Klein M, Glatzer C. Individual CAD/CAM fabricated glass-bioceramic implants in reconstructive surgery of the bony orbital floor. Plast Reconstr Surg. 2006;117(2):565–70.

Kosins AM, Kohan E, Shajan J, Jaffurs D, Wirth G, Paydar K. Fixation of the medial canthal tendon using the Mitek anchor system. Plast Reconstr Surg. 2010;126(6):309e–10.

Kotlus BS, Dryden RM. Correction of anophthalmic enophthalmos with injectable calcium hydroxylapatite (Radiesse). Ophthal Plast Reconstr Surg. 2007;23(4):313–4.

Lari AR, Kanjoor JR, Vulvoda M, Katchy KC, Khan ZU. Orbital reconstruction following sino-nasal mucormycosis. Br J Plast Surg. 2002;55(1):72–5.

Lee HB, Nunery WR. Orbital adherence syndrome secondary to titanium implant material. Ophthal Plast Reconstr Surg. 2009;25(1):33–6.

Lee DH, Joo YE, Lim SC. Migrated orbital silastic sheet implant mimicking bilateral sinusitis. J Craniofac Surg. 2011;22(6):2158–9.

Lim C, Martin P, Benger R, Kourt G, Ghabrial R. Lacrimal canalicular bypass surgery with the Lester Jones tube. Am J Ophthalmol. 2004;137(1):101–8.

Mauriello Jr JA. Inferior rectus muscle entrapped by Teflon implant after orbital floor fracture repair. Ophthal Plast Reconstr Surg. 1990;6(3):218–20.

Mauriello Jr JA, Lee HJ, Nguyen L. CT of soft tissue injury and orbital fractures. Radiol Clin North Am. 1999;37(1):241–52, xii.

Mazzoli RA, Raymond 4th WR, Ainbinder DJ, Hansen EA. Use of self-expanding, hydrophilic osmotic expanders (hydrogel) in the reconstruction of congenital clinical anophthalmos. Curr Opin Ophthalmol. 2004;15(5):426–31.

Meslemani D, Kellman RM. Zygomaticomaxillary complex fractures. Arch Facial Plast Surg. 2012;14(1):62–6.

Mihora LD, Holck DE. Hematic cyst in a barrier-covered porous polyethylene/titanium mesh orbital floor implant. Ophthal Plast Reconstr Surg. 2011;27(5):e117–8.

Montes JR. Volumetric considerations for lower eyelid and midface rejuvenation. Curr Opin Ophthalmol. 2012;23(5):443–9.

Nasr AM, Haik BG, Fleming JC, Al-Hussain HM, Karcioglu ZA. Penetrating orbital injury with organic foreign bodies. Ophthalmology. 1999;106(3):523–32.

Nazzi V, Marras C, Broggi G. Upper eyelid gold weight implants in patients with facial nerve palsy. Surgical technique. J Neurosurg Sci. 2006;50(4):107–10.

Nguyen M, Koshy JC, Hollier Jr LH. Pearls of nasoorbitoethmoid trauma management. Semin Plast Surg. 2010;24(4):383–8.

Nunery WR, Tao JP, Johl S. Nylon foil "wraparound" repair of combined orbital floor and medial wall fractures. Ophthal Plast Reconstr Surg. 2008;24(4):271–5.

Oester Jr AE, Fowler BT, Fleming JC. Inferior orbital septum release compared with lateral canthotomy and cantholysis in the management of orbital compartment syndrome. Ophthal Plast Reconstr Surg. 2012;28(1):40–3.

Okazaki M, Akizuki T, Ohmori K. Medical canthoplasty with the Mitek anchor system. Ann Plast Surg. 1997;38(2):124–8.

Ozturk S, Sengezer M, Isik S, Turegun M, Deveci M, Cil Y. Long-term outcomes of ultra-thin porous polyethylene implants used for reconstruction of orbital floor defects. J Craniofac Surg. 2005;16(6):973–7.

Papay FA, Zins JE, Hahn JF. Split calvarial bone graft in cranio-orbital sphenoid wing reconstruction. J Craniofac Surg. 1996;7(2):133–9.

Park DJ, Garibaldi DC, Iliff NT, Grant MP, Merbs SL. Smooth nylon foil (SupraFOIL) orbital implants in orbital fractures: a case series of 181 patients. Ophthal Plast Reconstr Surg. 2008;24(4):266–70.

Pinto A, Brunese L, Daniele S, Faggian A, Guarnieri G, Muto M, Romano L. Role of computed tomography in the assessment of intraorbital foreign bodies. Semin Ultrasound CT MR. 2012;33(5):392–5.

Quaranta-Leoni FM. Treatment of the anophthalmic socket. Curr Opin Ophthalmol. 2008;19(5):422–7.

Rabensteiner DF, Boldin I, Klein A, Horwath-Winter J. Collared silicone punctal plugs compared to intracanalicular plugs for the treatment of dry eye. Curr Eye Res. 2013;38(5):521–5.

Rapidis AD. Orbitomaxillarymucormycosis (zygomycosis) and the surgical approach to treatment: perspectives from a maxillofacial surgeon. Clin Microbiol Infect. 2009;15 Suppl 5:98–102.

Raschke GF, Rieger UM, Bader RD, Schaefer O, Guentsch A, Hagemeister C, Schultze-Mosgau S. The zygomaticomaxillary complex fracture – An anthropometric appraisal of surgical outcomes. J Craniomaxillofac Surg. 2013;41:331–7.

Schrom T, Bloching M, Wernecke K, Scherer H. Measurement of upper eyelid implants curvature by ultrasound. Laryngoscope. 2005;115(5):884–8.

Seiff SR, Shorr N. Nasolacrimal drainage system obstruction after orbital decompression. Am J Ophthalmol. 1988;106(2):204–9.

Sellari-Franceschini S, Muscatello L, Seccia V, Lenzi R, Santoro A, Nardi M, Mazzi B, Pinchera A, Marcocci C. Reasons for revision surgery after orbital decompression for Graves' orbitopathy. Clin Ophthalmol. 2008;2(2):283–90.

Steele EA, Dailey RA. Conjunctivodacryocystorhinostomy with the frosted jones pyrex tube. Ophthal Plast Reconstr Surg. 2009;25(1):42–3.

Stewart MG, Patrinely JR, Appling WD, Jordan DR. Late proptosis following orbital floor fracture repair. Arch Otolaryngol Head Neck Surg. 1995;121(6):649–52.

Sundaram H, Kiripolsky M. Nonsurgical rejuvenation of the upper eyelid and brow. Clin Plast Surg. 2013;40(1):55–76.

Tai MC, Cosar CB, Cohen EJ, Rapuano CJ, Laibson PR. The clinical efficacy of silicone punctal plug therapy. Cornea. 2002;21(2):135–9.

Thomas RD, Graham SM, Carter KD, Nerad JA. Management of the orbital floor in silent sinus syndrome. Am J Rhinol. 2003;17(2):97–100.

Trotter WL, Meyer DR. Endoscopic conjunctivodacryocystorhinostomy with Jones tube placement. Ophthalmology. 2000;107(6):1206–9.

Tse DT, Abdulhafez M, Orozco MA, Tse JD, Azab AO, Pinchuk L. Evaluation of an integrated orbital tissue expander in congenital anophthalmos: report of preliminary clinical experience. Am J Ophthalmol. 2011;151(3):470–82.e1.

Vagefi MR, McMullan TF, Burroughs JR, Georgescu D, McCann JD, Anderson RL. Orbital augmentation with injectable calcium hydroxylapatite for correction of postenucleation/evisceration socket syndrome. Ophthal Plast Reconstr Surg. 2011;27(2):90–4.

Vassallo S, Hartstein M, Howard D, Stetz J. Traumatic retrobulbar hemorrhage: emergent decompression by lateral canthotomy and cantholysis. J Emerg Med. 2002;22(3):251–6.

Wiener E, Kolk A, Neff A, Settles M, Rummeny E. Evaluation of reconstructed orbital wall fractures: high-resolution MRI using a microscopy surface coil versus 16-slice MSCT. Eur Radiol. 2005;15(6):1250–5.

Wu CT, Lee ST, Chen JF, Lin KL, Yen SH. Computer-aided design for three-dimensional titanium mesh used for repairing skull base bone defect in pediatric neurofibromatosis type 1. A novel approach combining biomodeling and neuronavigation. Pediatr Neurosurg. 2008;44(2):133–9.

Xu JJ, Teng L, Jin XL, Ji Y, Lu JJ, Zhang B. Porous polyethylene implants in orbital blow-out fractures and enophthalmos reconstruction. J Craniofac Surg. 2009;20(3):918–20.

Yüce S, Akal A, Doğan M, Uysal IO, Müderris S. Results of endoscopic endonasal dacryocystorhinostomy. J Craniofac Surg. 2013;24(1):e11–2.

Zilelioğlu G, Gündüz K. Conjunctivodacryocystorhinostomy with Jones tube. A 10-year study. Doc Ophthalmol. 1996–1997;92(2):97–105.

Imaging of Strabismus and Craniofacial Malformation Surgery

6

Daniel Thomas Ginat, Mohammad Ali Sadiq, and Linda R. Dagi

6.1 Part I: Strabismus Surgery and Postoperative Imaging

6.1.1 Overview

The term strabismus is derived from the Greek word "strabismos – to squint, to look obliquely, or askance." Thus, strabismus consists of ocular misalignment caused by any of a wide range of abnormalities of binocular vision; extraocular muscle development; third, fourth, or sixth cranial nerve palsies; myasthenia gravis; orbital masses; orbital trauma; or inflammatory disorders, such as Graves' orbitopathy or orbital pseudotumor. Strabismus surgery plays an important role in visual development in pediatric and adult patients by restoring the normal alignment of the eye and in some cases, improving binocular function, resolving double vision, or reducing torticollis. Different types of strabismus surgery are performed depending upon the etiology of the strabismus. The scope includes weakening procedures such as recessions, myotomies, and tenotomies; strengthening procedures such as resections, plications, and tucks; and mus-

cle transposition procedures designed to change the vector force of the muscle. High spatial resolution orbital MRI can help delineate pertinent anatomy prior to intervention and can be particularly useful when records detailing previous surgical procedures are unavailable. Furthermore, imaging can help the strabismus surgeon with preoperative surgical planning after complications including lost or slipped extraocular muscles, torn muscles, inclusion cysts, and hardware migration from prior craniofacial or orbital repair. High spatial resolution MRI, coupled with quantitative morphometric analysis, can demonstrate the size and contractility of muscles, and surface coils enhance image quality.

6.1.2 Muscle Weakening Procedures

Myectomy, myotomy, tenotomy, and recession surgery. Myectomy involves removal of a portion of the muscle, while myotomy is the partial or complete surgical division of the muscle. Tenotomy is the transection of the extraocular tendon. In all cases, the remaining muscle passively inserts on the globe. Extraocular muscle recession involves detaching the distal muscle tendon and resecuring this tendon to the globe with suture (Fig. 6.1). These techniques exploit the principle of the Starling length tension curve in which the force generated by a muscle is directly related to the amount of tension in the muscle. The location of the recessed, myotomized, myectomized or tenotomized muscle

D.T. Ginat, MD, MS (✉)
Director of Head and Neck Imaging,
Department of Radiology, University of Chicago,
5841 S Maryland Avenue, Chicago, IL 60637, USA
e-mail: ginatd01@gmail.com

M.A. Sadiq, MD, MBBS • L.R. Dagi, MD
Department of Ophthalmology, Boston Children's
Hospital, Boston, MA, USA

D.T. Ginat, S.K. Freitag (eds.), *Post-treatment Imaging of the Orbit*,
DOI 10.1007/978-3-662-44023-0_6, © Springer-Verlag Berlin Heidelberg 2015

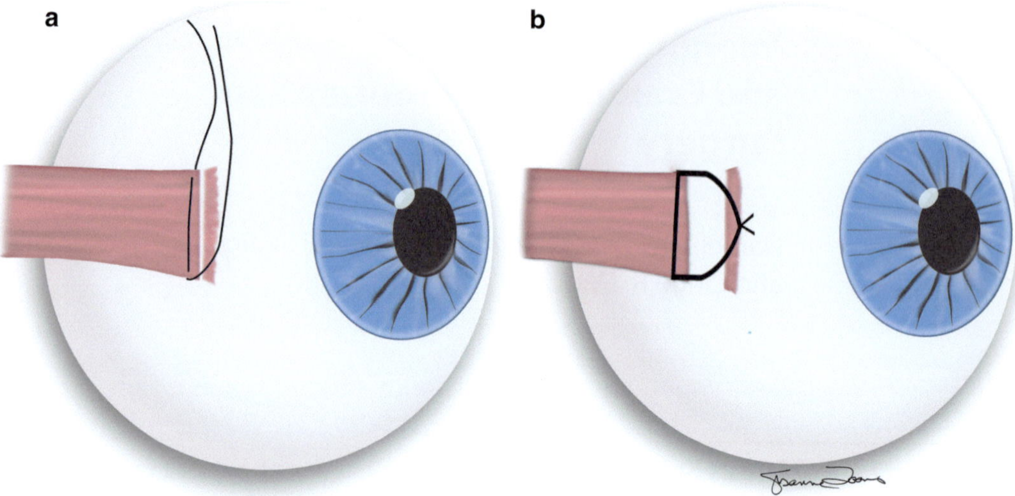

Fig. 6.1 Illustration of recession surgery. The lateral rectus, after being secured with suture is detached from the insertion site (**a**) and reattached at a proximal site by partial thickness scleral bites (**b**)

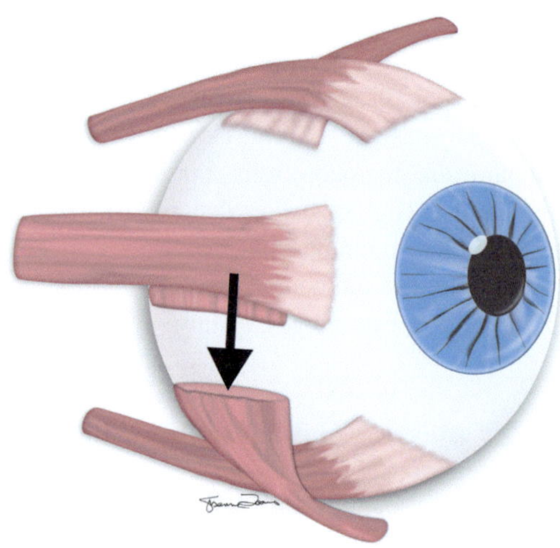

Fig. 6.2 Illustration of inferior oblique myectomy. The Inferior oblique muscle is hooked in the region between the lateral and inferior rectus muscles. A portion of the muscle is excised (myectomy) and the two ends allowed to passively reinsert on the globe. The distal end retracts to the anatomical insertion and the proximal end typically reinserts close to the lateral border of the inferior rectus, well posterior to its insertion (*arrow*)

effectively shortens the course of the muscle, and muscle tone becomes more lax. Since the Starling length curve is nonlinear, the effect of shortening a muscle can vary considerably (Fig. 6.2).

The muscle slack resulting from the recession, myotomy, and tenotomy procedures can be depicted on imaging as increased maximum transverse diameter of the involved muscle belly

(Fig. 6.3). Otherwise, it is difficult to appreciate the actual degree of recession as current imaging techniques cannot accurately identify the site of an extraocular muscle insertion when it is anterior to the equator of the eye (the most typical location), unless surface coils are used.

6.1.3 Muscle Strengthening Procedures

Resection and, Tuck/Plication. Muscle action can be augmented via tightening or shortening. Muscle shortening involves removing a specific length of muscle ("resection") and reimplanting the foreshortened muscle on the globe (Fig. 6.4). Alternatively, a muscle tuck or plication procedure can provide equivalent shortening while preserving the anterior ciliary circulation by creating a redundancy in the muscle (Fig. 6.5). The effects of such procedures can be very subtle or not directly apparent even on high spatial resolution MRI. Nevertheless, MRI can be useful for delineating the postoperative anatomy, particularly when further surgery is contemplated (Figs. 6.6 and 6.7).

6.1.4 Muscle Transposition

Transposition procedures are typically employed when loss of innervation to one or more of the

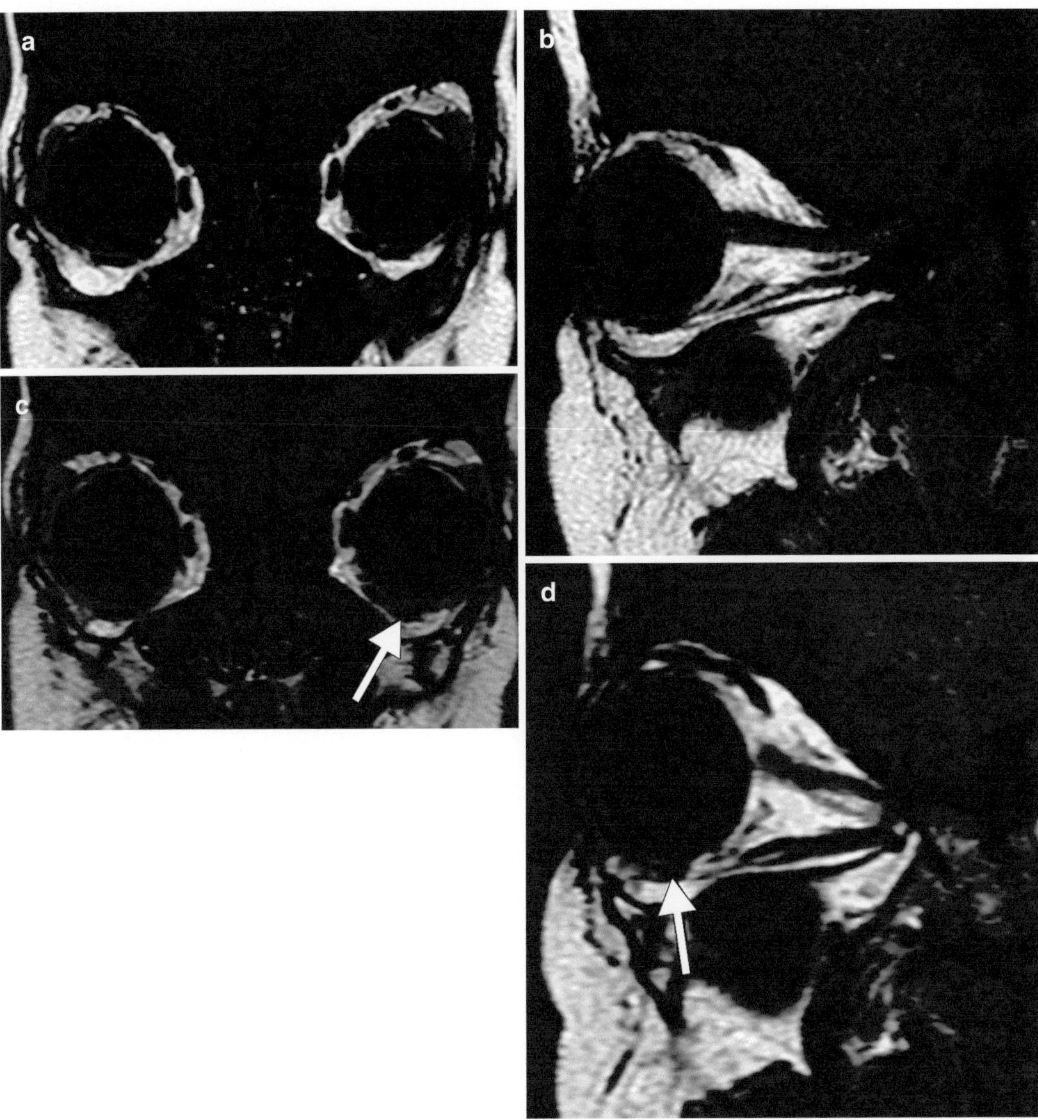

Fig. 6.3 MRI of inferior oblique myectomy with a residual band (*top arrow*). Coronal and sagittal T1-weighted MR images before (**a**, **b**) and after (**c**, **d**) surgery show that the left inferior oblique muscle belly has shifted slightly medially and has a larger cross-sectional diameter (*arrows*)

extraocular muscles, or traumatic loss of an extraocular muscle, limits options to remediate the misalignment. Extraocular muscle transposition consists of disinserting and reattaching all or part of the muscle to the globe at a site remote from the original path of the muscle (Fig. 6.8). The purpose of this procedure is to alter the direction of the force vector and therefore, the action that the extraocular muscle exerts on the globe. For example, if the superior rectus is disinserted from the globe and reattached near the anatomical insertion of the lateral rectus muscle, it will lose some ability to elevate the eye and gain capacity to abduct or outwardly pull the eye. Transposition of the superior rectus with or without transposition of the inferior rectus to the region adjacent to the lateral rectus muscle is one option used to restore abduction in patients with sixth nerve palsy. In addition, botulinum toxin A can be injected into the medial rectus, or it can be recessed in order to limit its action. Splitting the lateral rectus into superior and inferior halves and transposing each nasally to a

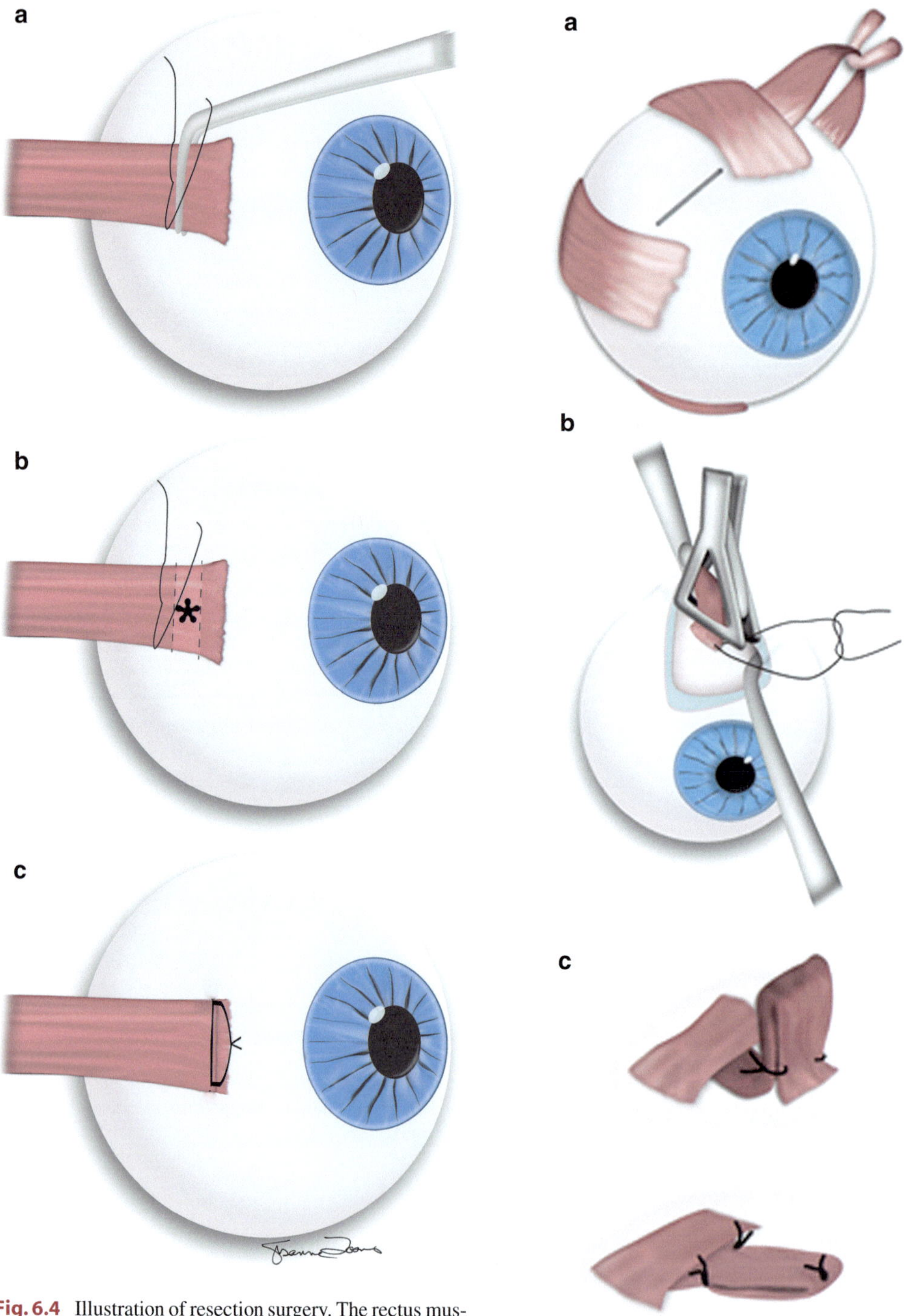

Fig. 6.4 Illustration of resection surgery. The rectus muscle is secured with sutures at a measured site distal to the muscle insertion. The muscle is then clamped and cut proximal to the sutures (**a**). The muscle stump (*) is then removed (**b**) and the shortened (resected) muscle is advanced and secured at the anatomical insertion site (**c**)

Fig. 6.5 Illustration of superior oblique tuck. Superior oblique is identified and secured with a hook (**a**). Superior oblique is lifted from the orbit, folded onto itself; folded muscle is secured with suture (**b**). Final configuration of the oblique tuck nasal to the superior rectus muscle (**c**)

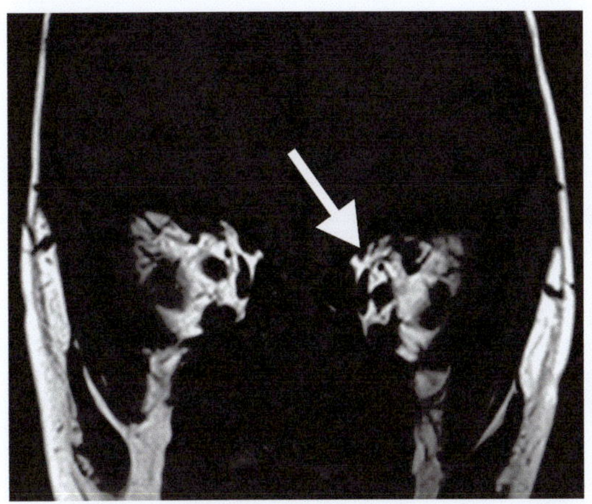

Fig. 6.6 Superior oblique tuck. The patient presented with persistent symptoms of left superior oblique palsy after superior oblique tuck. Coronal high spatial resolution T1-weighted MRI shows an asymmetrically small left superior oblique (*arrow*)

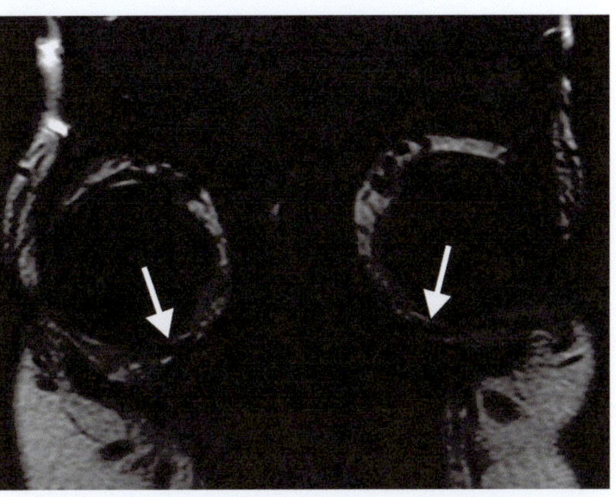

Fig. 6.7 Bilateral inferior oblique myectomy. Coronal high spatial resolution T1-weighted MRI shows the residual portions of the bilateral inferior oblique muscles (*arrows*)

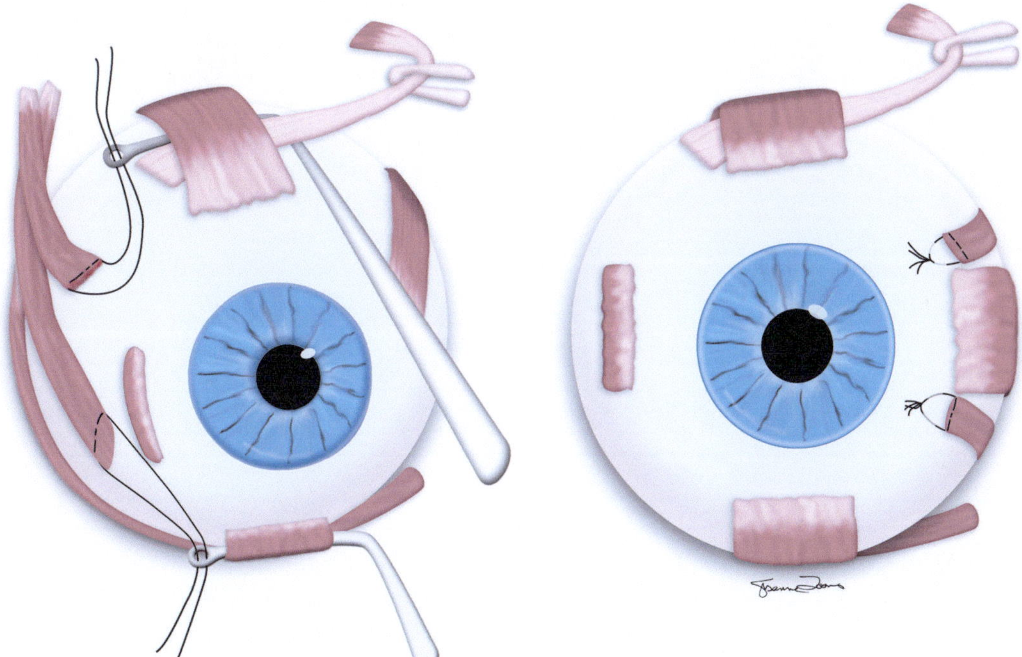

Fig. 6.8 Adjustable medial transposition of the split lateral rectus is one surgical option used to treat misalignment from complete third nerve palsy (Adapted with permission from Shah et al. (2014))

location adjacent to the medial rectus effectively pulls the eye medially and can remediate much of the misalignment created by complete third nerve palsy. High-resolution T1-weighted images can often adequately depict the path and morphology of transposed extraocular muscles (Fig. 6.9).

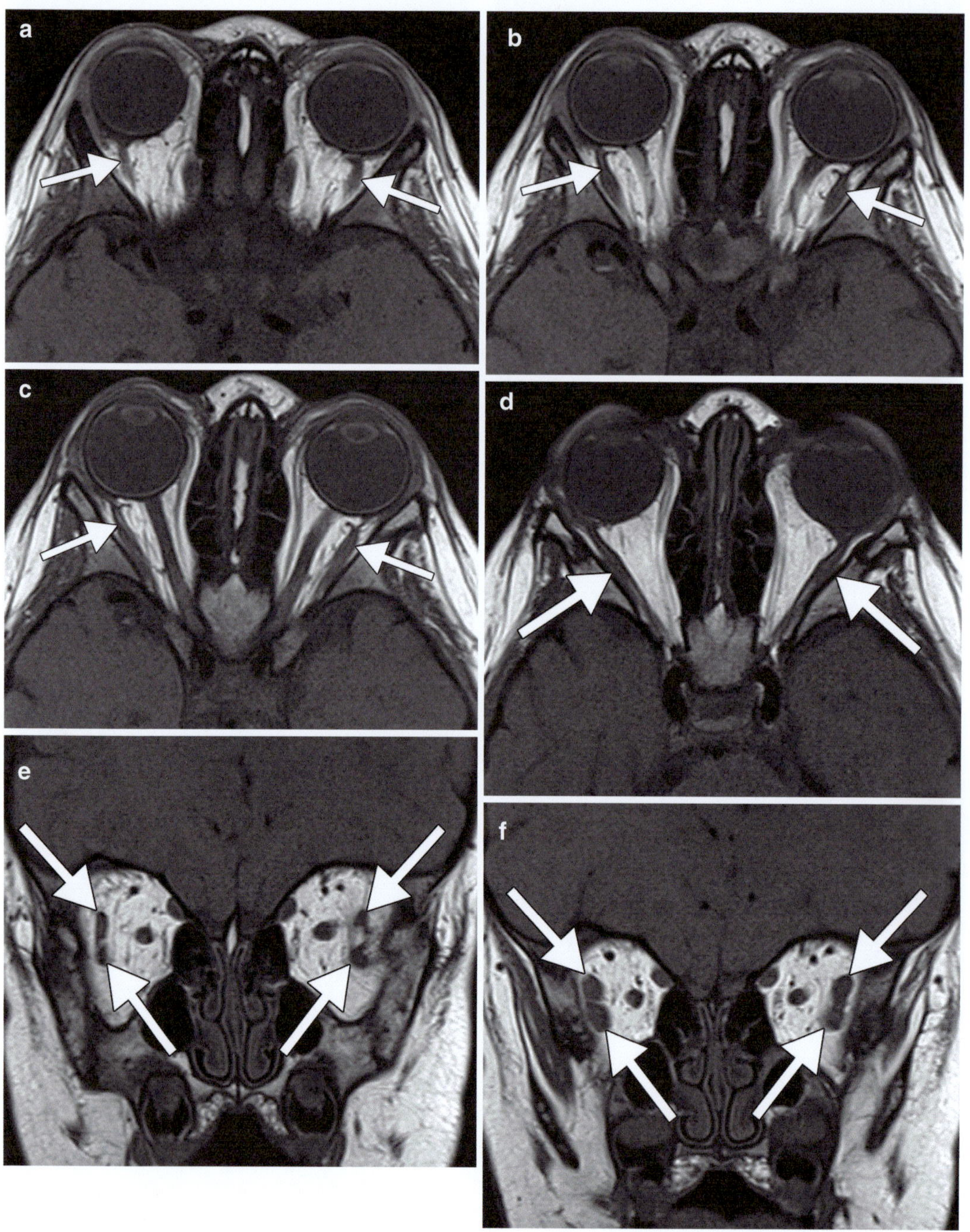

Fig. 6.9 Y splitting of the lateral rectus with medial transposition. The patient is a 19-month-old with bilateral third nerve palsy. Sequential axial (**a–d**) and coronal (**e–h**) T1-weighted MR images show splitting and thickening of both lateral rectus muscles distally (*arrows*) (Adapted with permission from Shah et al. (2014))

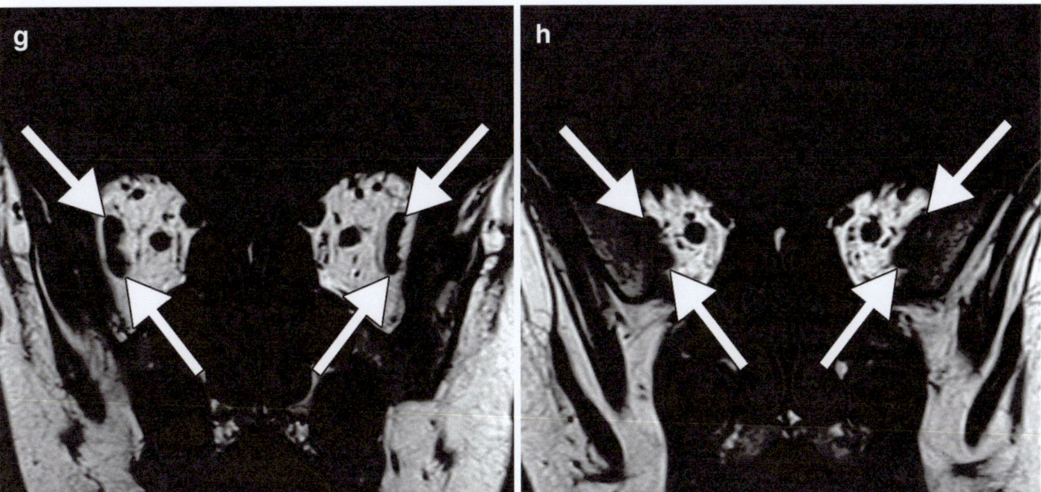

Fig. 6.9 (continued)

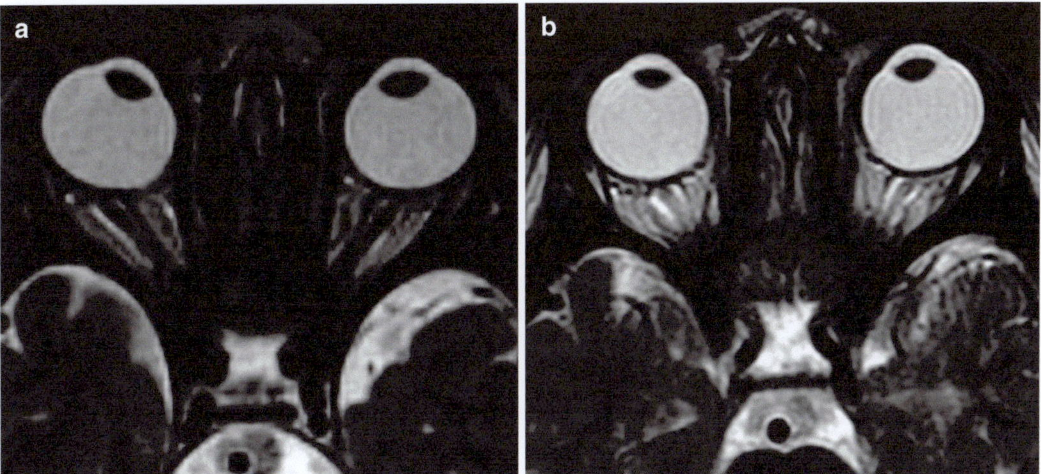

Fig. 6.10 Botulinum toxin. The patient has a history of complete sixth nerve palsy with medial rectus contracture, and is status post inferior rectus and superior rectus full tendon transposition to the lateral rectus of the right eye. The axial T2-weighted MR images obtained before (**a**) and after (**b**) botulinum toxin treatment to the right medial rectus muscle show improved alignment of the right globe

6.1.5   Chemosurgery

Botulinum toxin injection. Botulinum is a potent neurotoxin produced by the bacterium *Clostridium botulinum.* It interferes with neural transmission by blocking the release of acetylcholine, thereby resulting in muscle paralysis. Botulinum toxin administration or chemodenervation is a reasonable alternative to recession or other surgical weakening procedures in select cases. Although no structural changes in the muscle are discernable on imaging after chemodenervation, the improved ocular alignment can be appreciated (Fig. 6.10).

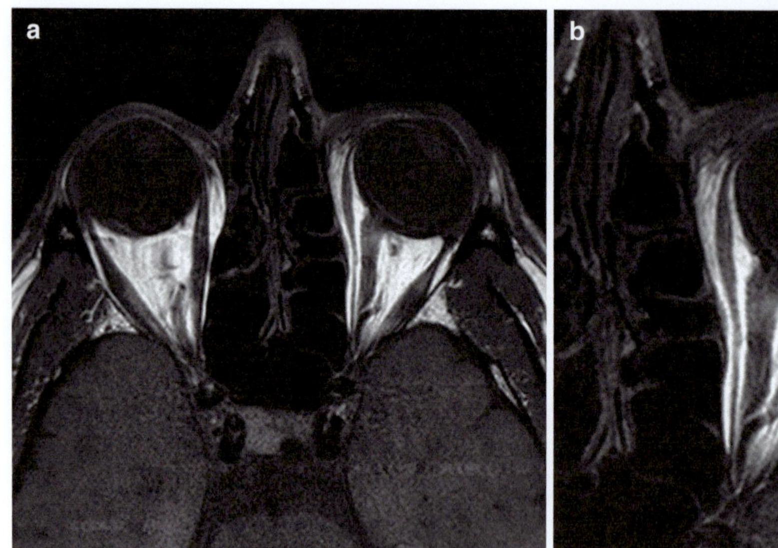

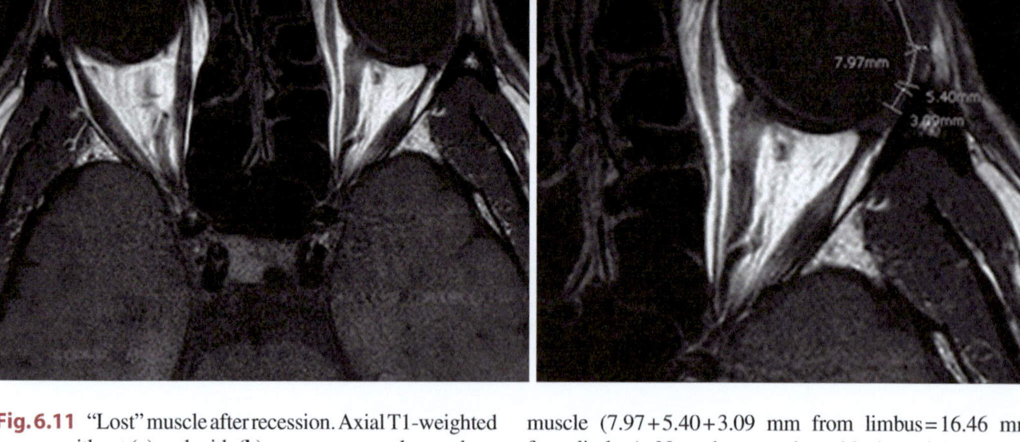

Fig. 6.11 "Lost" muscle after recession. Axial T1-weighted images without (**a**) and with (**b**) measurements drawn show the degree of posterior retraction of the left lateral rectus muscle (7.97 + 5.40 + 3.09 mm from limbus = 16.46 mm from limbus). Note the posterior widening of the muscle belly secondary to this extreme recession

6.1.6 Complications of Strabismus Surgery

Slipped muscles. Extraocular muscles can "slip" from their intended insertion during strabismus surgery when the muscle capsule (external coat) is mistaken for muscle tendon or belly; the capsule, rather than the muscle, is sutured to the globe allowing the muscle to slide back within this capsular sheath, causing a more-than-planned recession effect. Slipped muscles can be retrieved by following the thin avascular muscle capsule posteriorly until the muscle is identified. In addition, muscle slippage or "loss" can occur if the suture securing the muscle to the sclera gives way, allowing the muscle to slip back or recess excessively, sometimes well behind the equator, and even off the globe. This is often called a "lost muscle." In reality, residual check ligaments called "pulleys" and other connective tissue attachments typically approximate the muscle to the globe, thereby facilitating surgical recovery and repair. MRI can often depict the approximate location of the muscle insertion in cases of slipped or "lost" muscles, thereby facilitating recovery (Fig. 6.11).

Torn muscle/Pulled-in-two syndrome. Torn extraocular muscles from strabismus surgery can lead to pulled-in-two syndrome. Pulled-in-two syndrome describes the subtype of "lost muscle" that occurs when there is an unplanned horizontal transection of the muscle. This atypical transection can occur during strabismus surgery in cases of extreme muscle tension (e.g., with thyroid orbitopathy) or when the muscle is weakened by disease or prior surgical trauma. Orbital hardware such as an encircling band used to repair retinal detachment can predispose a muscle to such rupture. Unfortunately, the transection typically occurs at the tendon–muscle junction, approximately 10 mm from the muscle insertion, making recovery of the muscle challenging as the foreshortened muscle readily retracts behind the equator. MRI can be used to localize the distal ruptured muscle in anticipation of retrieval if recovery has not proven feasible during the initial surgical procedure (Fig. 6.12).

Giant conjunctival cyst. Inclusion cysts are rare complications of strabismus surgery that usually occur from months to years after strabismus surgery. The cyst wall is usually composed of non-keratinized epithelial cells. The

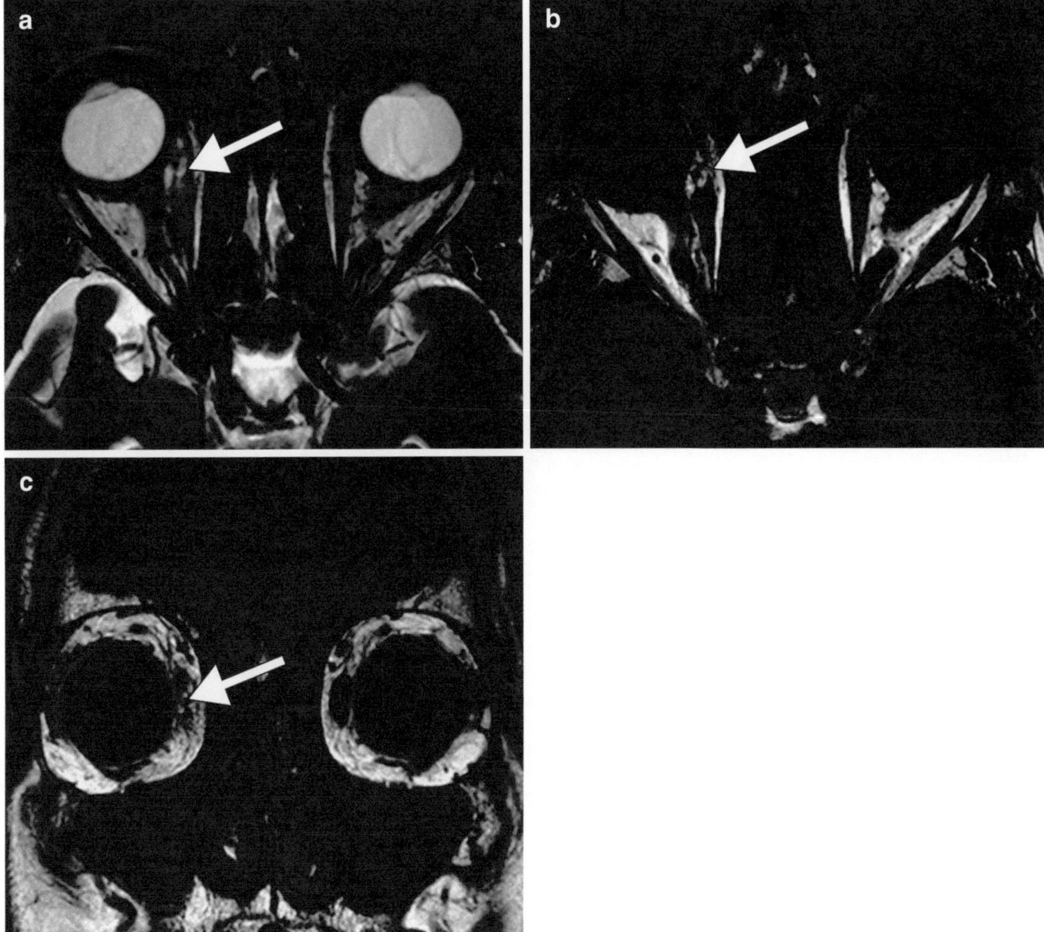

Fig. 6.12 Torn muscle. The patient underwent a recent bilateral medial rectus shortening procedure. Axial T2-weighted (**a**), axial T1-weighted (**b**), and coronal T1-weighted (**c**) MR images show a defect in the belly of the right medial rectus muscle (*arrows*). The right globe is externally rotated. Both medial rectus muscles are otherwise edematous from recent surgery

cysts have a tendency to enlarge over time. Small cysts present as little more than cosmetic deformities. Larger cysts can sometimes become the de facto insertion for the adjacent muscle to the globe; as the cyst enlarges, the insertion of the muscle falls back resulting in a "slipped" or over-recessed muscle. If the extraocular muscle is attached to the cyst rather than directly to the globe "loss" of the muscle may occur during attempted excision of the cyst. Pre-operative imaging can help delineate the relationship of the cyst to the affected extraocular muscle and provide the surgeon with

information needed to prevent this complication. On ultrasound biomicroscopy, inclusion cysts appear as well-circumscribed lesions with low internal reflectivity and hyperechoic components. CT and MRI can be useful for evaluating the posterior extension of the cyst. These lesions typically appear as well-defined fluid attenuation ovoid masses on CT and as non-enhancing T1 hypointense and T2 hyperintense on MRI (Fig. 6.13).

Acquired Brown syndrome. Brown syndrome is a limitation of elevation in adduction due to an abnormality of the superior oblique tendon

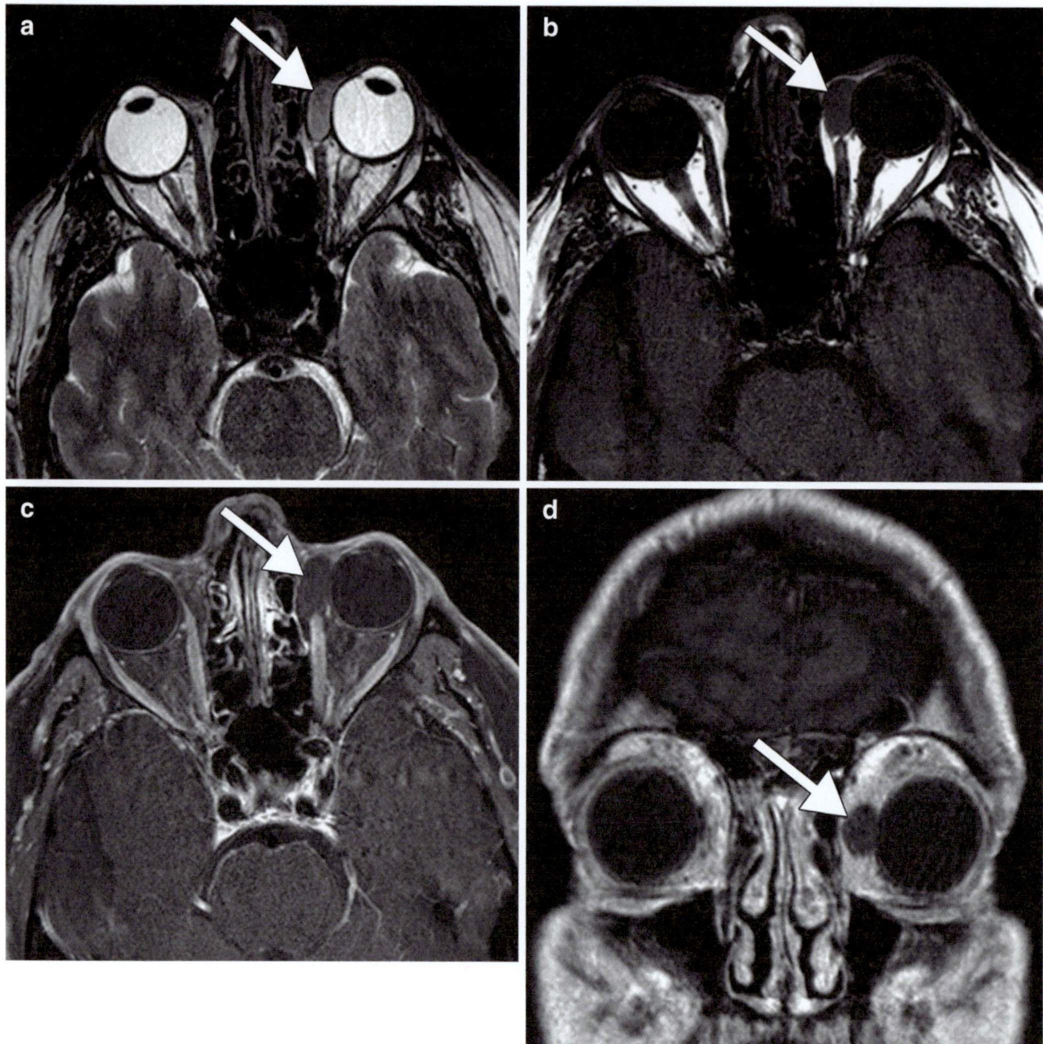

Fig. 6.13 Postoperative conjunctival inclusion cyst. Axial T2-weighted (**a**), axial T1-weighted (**b**), axial post-contrast fat-suppressed T1-weighted (**c**), and coronal post-contrast T1-weighted (**d**) MR images show an oval fluid-filled lesion (*arrows*) posteriorly displacing the insertion of the left medial rectus muscle (Adapted with permission from Mehendale et al. (2012))

sheath complex. This condition can result from superior oblique tuck, or from a cyst or mass in the location of the trochlea. If secondary to a tuck or localized inflammation, thickening of the tendon can be observed on CT or MRI. In particular, abnormal hyperintensity on fat-suppressed T2-weighted sequences and enhancement on post-contrast T1-weighted sequences in and around the superior oblique can be observed on MRI, which is suggestive of an inflammatory process (Fig. 6.14).

6.2 Part II: Orbital Imaging Following Surgery for Craniofacial Malformations

6.2.1 Overview

Craniosynostosis is the premature fusion of sutures in the infant skull. This condition affects 1 in 2,500 births and is syndromic in 15–40 % of cases. Due to the premature fusion the skull

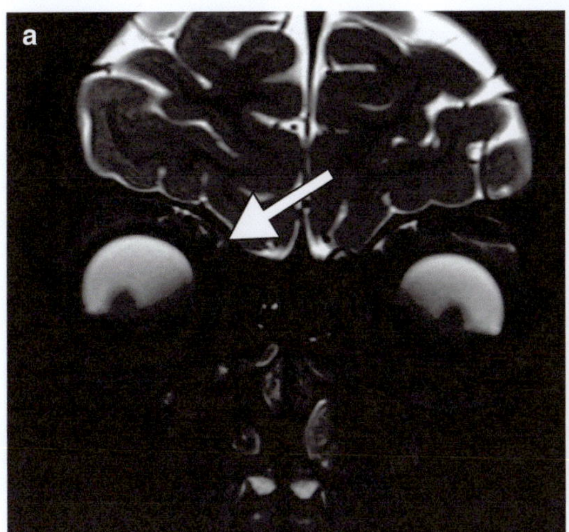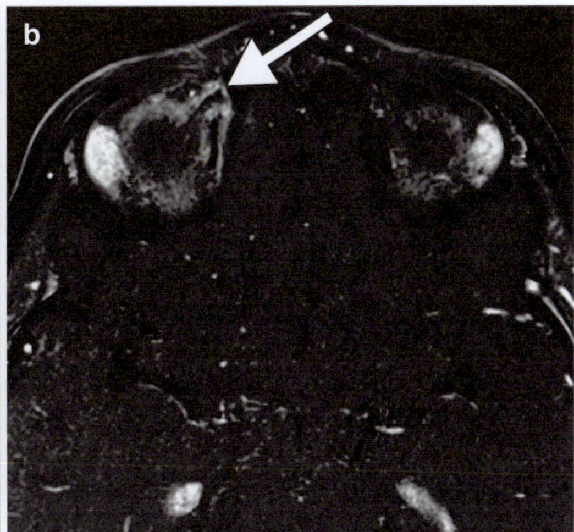

Fig. 6.14 Acquired Brown syndrome. Coronal fat-suppressed T2-weighted (**a**) and axial fat-suppressed post-contrast T1-weighted (**b**) MR images show T2 hyperintensity and enhancement involving the right superior oblique tendon (*arrows*)

acquires an abnormal shape as it grows, and this can potentially restrict cerebral growth and venous or cerebrospinal fluid drainage and a secondary increase in intracranial pressure can ensue. Strabismus occurs in 60–70 % of patients with craniosynostosis. V pattern strabismus is the most common variety. This may be due to excyclorotation of the extraocular muscles, aberrant insertions of extraocular muscles, abnormal extraocular muscle development, and anomalous localization of the superior oblique tendon. Furthermore, orbital depth is decreased in some variants, including Apert, Crouzon, and Pfeiffer syndromes, resulting in exorbitism and often more exaggerated strabismus. Endoscopic strip craniectomy is a procedure designed to directly open prematurely fused sutures and is typically performed between 2 and 4 months of age. Direct calvarial vault expansion is usually delayed until 9–12 months of life. There are a variety of procedures included in the category of calvarial vault expansion including orbitofrontal advancement, distraction osteogenesis, and orbital rim augmentation. These surgeries are complex, may be performed in a staged manner, and sometimes include the use of distraction devices. In addition, some affected patients have associated midface hypoplasia or retrusion, which can be addressed via LeFort osteotomy,

typically later in childhood. Imaging aids initial assessment by providing detailed information on the degree of premature fusion of the sutures and indicators of possible elevation in intracranial pressure (copper-beaten bone, increased ventricular size, and jugular venous stenosis and emissary vein formation). Imaging can be performed after calvarial expansion to assess the evolution of the calvarial morphology, and to help with pre-operative planning of strabismus surgery by determining the degree of excyclorotation of the involved extraocular muscles and aberrancy in the path of the superior oblique. Otherwise, diagnostic imaging is mainly reserved for the evaluation of suspected postoperative complications or to follow cranial and ventricular growth. Advances in CT post-processing techniques such as iterative reconstruction have enabled scanning patients at a considerably lower dose than via standard CT without compromising image quality. Low-dose CT techniques with high spatial resolution can be useful for delineating the osseous structures, while MRI is suitable for imaging the globe and extraocular muscles. Besides craniosynostosis surgery, imaging may occasionally be performed after frontoethmoid encephalocele repair. The purpose of CT or MRI may be to verify complete reduction of the encephalocele, intactness of the surgical

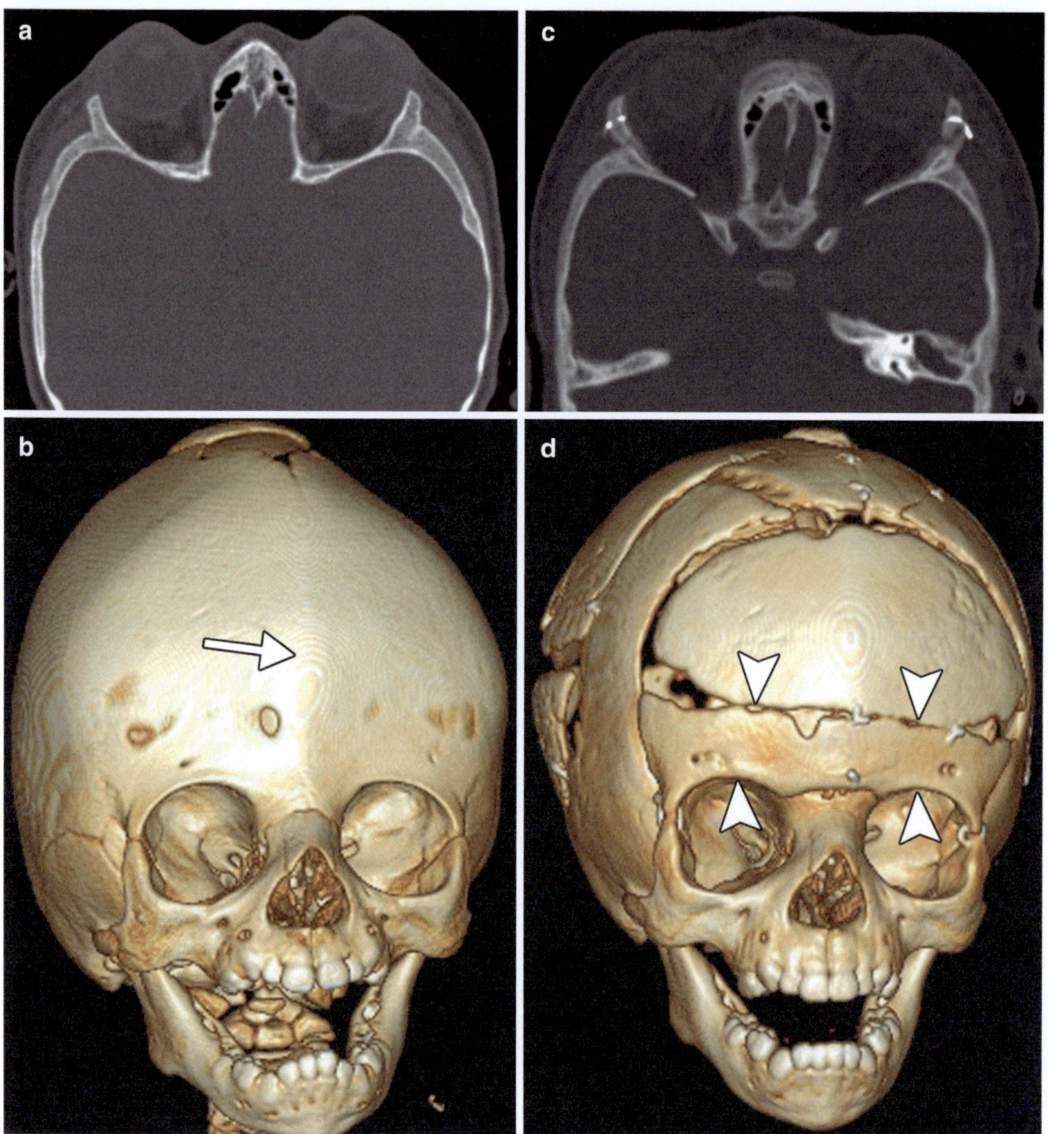

Fig. 6.15 Orbitofrontal advancement. The patient has a history of trigonocephaly. Preoperative axial (**a**) and 3D volume rendered (**b**) CT images show metopic synostosis with a prominent frontal ridge (*arrow*), shallow orbits, and hypotelorism. Postoperative axial (**c**) and 3D volume rendered CT (**d**) images show interval improvement of the contours of the frontal calvarium and less shallow orbital cavities with anterior translation of the orbital bandeau (*arrowheads*)

repair, and to evaluate potential complications, such as CSF leakage.

6.2.2 Orbitofrontal Advancement

Orbitofrontal (fronto-orbital) advancement is performed for metopic, unicoronal, or bicoronal synostosis. The procedure essentially consists of bicoronal craniotomy and anterior translation of the reshaped frontal bone and supraorbital bar after completion of lateral orbital wall osteotomies. The procedure reduces or eliminates the prominent frontal ridge at the metopic suture and deepens the orbital cavities (Fig. 6.15). Postoperative volumetric changes in the orbits can be quantified on CT. Orbit expansion does not fully restore normal orbital volume, but is generally effective for mitigating preoperative symptoms, such as exophthalmos, and corneal erosion.

6.2.3 Barrel Stave Cranial Vault Remodeling

Barrel stave osteotomies can be performed as part of craniosynostosis surgery for the treatment of dolichocephaly and turricephaly. The maneuver consists of creating multiple parallel flexible strips of calvarium that facilitate remodeling of the skull and initially resemble the stave joints of a barrel (Fig. 6.16). Over time, bone forms between the strips of calvarium, which then acquires a new shape.

6.2.4 Distraction Osteogenesis

Posterior vault expansion using distraction osteogenesis has become a first-line treatment in syndromic craniosynostosis. Indeed, distraction osteogenesis following a monobloc osteotomy has largely superseded traditional grafting and fixation due to the decreased risk of infection and other morbidity. Craniofacial CT with 3D imaging may be obtained during the course of distraction to monitor the progress of the osteogenesis and stability of the distractors (Fig. 6.17).

6.2.5 Periorbital Augmentation

Postoperative depressions in the periorobital region are common following orbital rim advancement and cranial vault remodeling in children. Augmentation of the bony deficiencies can be accomplished using versatile biocompatible materials, such as Medpor and hydroxyapatite. On CT, Medpor appears as low attenuation, while hydroxyapatite appears as high attenuation, similar to cortical bone (Fig. 6.18).

6.2.6 Endoscopic Strip Craniectomy

Endoscopic craniosynostosis surgery is a minimally invasive treatment option mainly available to patients under 5 months of age and is performed in order to prevent or reverse elevation in intracranial pressure and to minimize skull deformity. The technique consists of performing a strip craniectomy, whereby the affected suture is resected (suturectomy). This surgery produces linear defects along the course of the sutures, which are evident on CT during the early (first several months) postoperative period (Fig. 6.19). The calvarium is gradually remodeled through the use of postoperative helmet therapy. Consequently, the skull acquires a more desirable morphology once the craniectomy defects heal.

6.2.7 LeFort III Osteotomy

The LeFort III osteotomy is performed in patients with midfacial retrusion associated with craniofacial dysostoses such as Crouzon, Apert, and Pfeiffer syndromes. The procedure often resolves obstructive sleep apnea syndrome, exorbitism, malocclusions, and esthetic defects. Indeed, a significant increase in orbital volume can be obtained following LeFort III advancement. In particular, the infraorbital rim shifts forward, while the position of the globe remains relatively unaffected. CT with 3D reconstructions can be useful for evaluating the distraction devices and the status of the osteotomy sites – whether these remain open or have healed (Fig. 6.20). Complications include infection, mechanical failure, intraoperative fragment disjunction, velopharyngeal insufficiency, trismus, cerebrospinal fluid leakage, and bony irregularities. Many of the complications can be evaluated using diagnostic imaging.

6.2.8 Frontoethmoidal Encephalocele Repair

Frontoethmoidal encephaloceles, including nasofrontal, nasoethmoidal, and nasooribtal encephaloceles, can result from congenital malformations that may be associated with hypertelorism and proptosis. The aim of the surgical treatment is to restore the position of functional brain

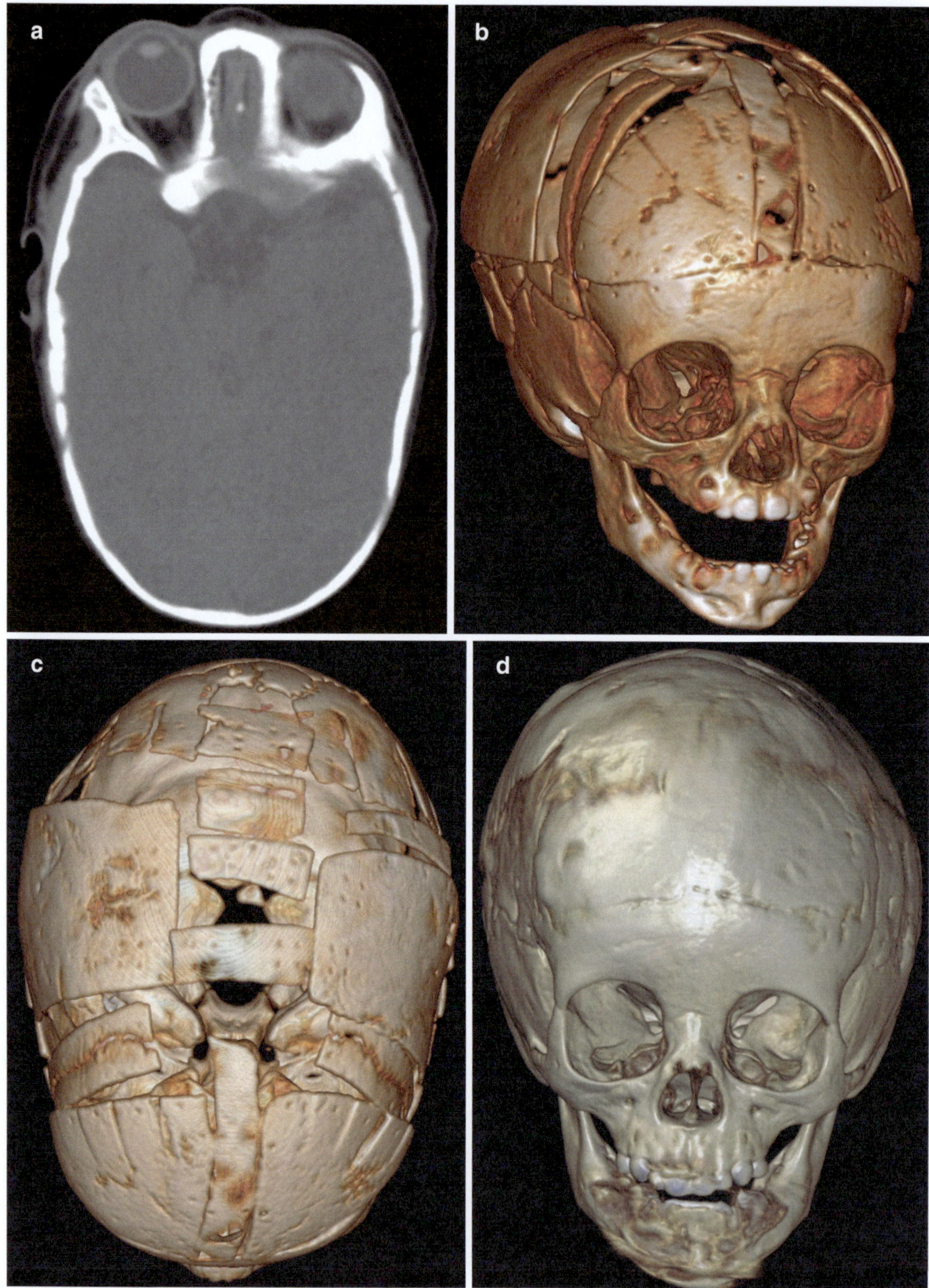

Fig. 6.16 Barrel stave osteotomies. Preoperative axial CT image (**a**) shows scaphocephaly. Oblique frontal and vertex 3D volume rendered CT images (**b**, **c**) show multiple osteotomies and repositioned segments of calvarium. Follow-up frontal 3D volume rendered CT image (**d**) obtained approximately 1 year later shows expected healing of the osteotomies

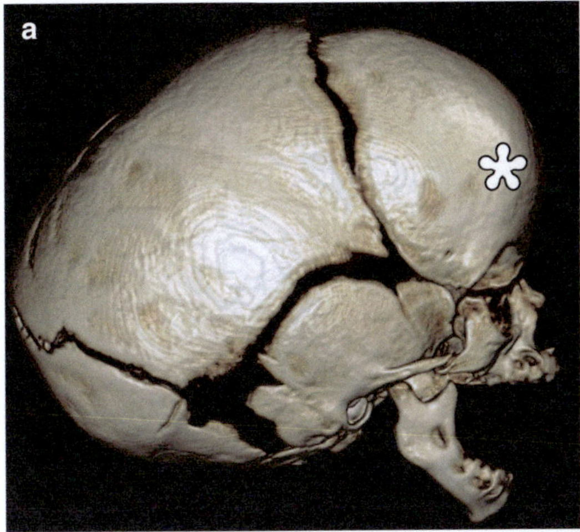

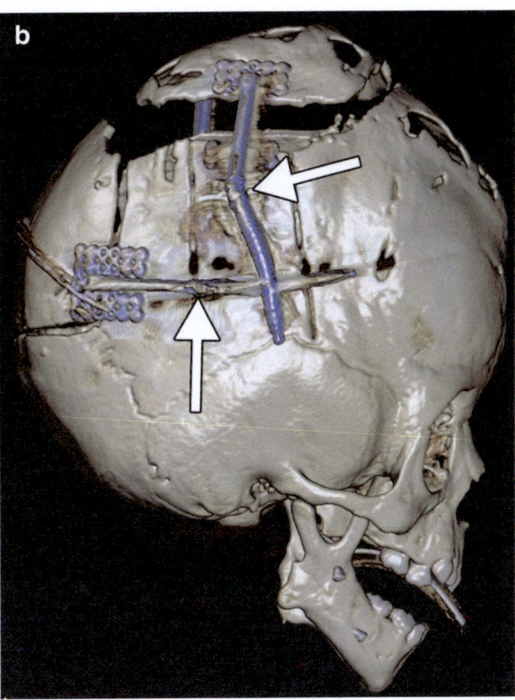

Fig. 6.17 Cranial vault expansion with distraction osteogenesis. Preoperative 3D volume rendered CT (**a**) shows scaphocephaly with frontal bossing (*). Postoperative 3D volume rendered CT (**b**) shows interval osteotomy and application of distraction devices (*arrows*) to the posterior calvarium. There is improvement in the overall shape of the skull

tissue into the cranial cavity, perform dural repair, and close bone defects, and correct associated facial malformations, such as hypertelorism and orbital dystopia. A multidisciplinary approach is required to address the brain herniation and to correct associated skull and maxillofacial malformations. For example a two-stage reconstruction can be implemented whereby the frontoethmoidal encephalocele undergoes neurosurgical repair during the first procedure and craniofacial reconstruction is performed during the second procedure. Calvarial bone graft can be used to close the osseous frontoethmoidal defects. With respect to the craniofacial malformation, a cranial flap with orbital osteotomies can be performed, which enables correction of the hypertelorism and orbital dystopia. In adults, titanium miniplates are often used for fixation, but resorbable devices are used in children in order to accommodate anticipated growth. CSF

leak tends to be the most frequent postoperative complication. High-resolution CT with 3D reconstructions is useful for delineating the altered bony anatomy after surgery (Fig. 6.21). CT can also be used to assess the soft tissues of the orbit and residual or recurrent encephalocele, although MRI may be helpful if CT is indeterminate.

6.2.9 Optic Nerve Decompression for Orbitofrontal Fibrous Dysplasia

Orbitofrontal fibrous dysplasia can lead to optic nerve compression and visual disturbances. Optic nerve decompression can be achieved via coronal transcranial and endonasal approaches. Typically, the roof of the optic canal can be removed using high-speed or ultrasonic drill,

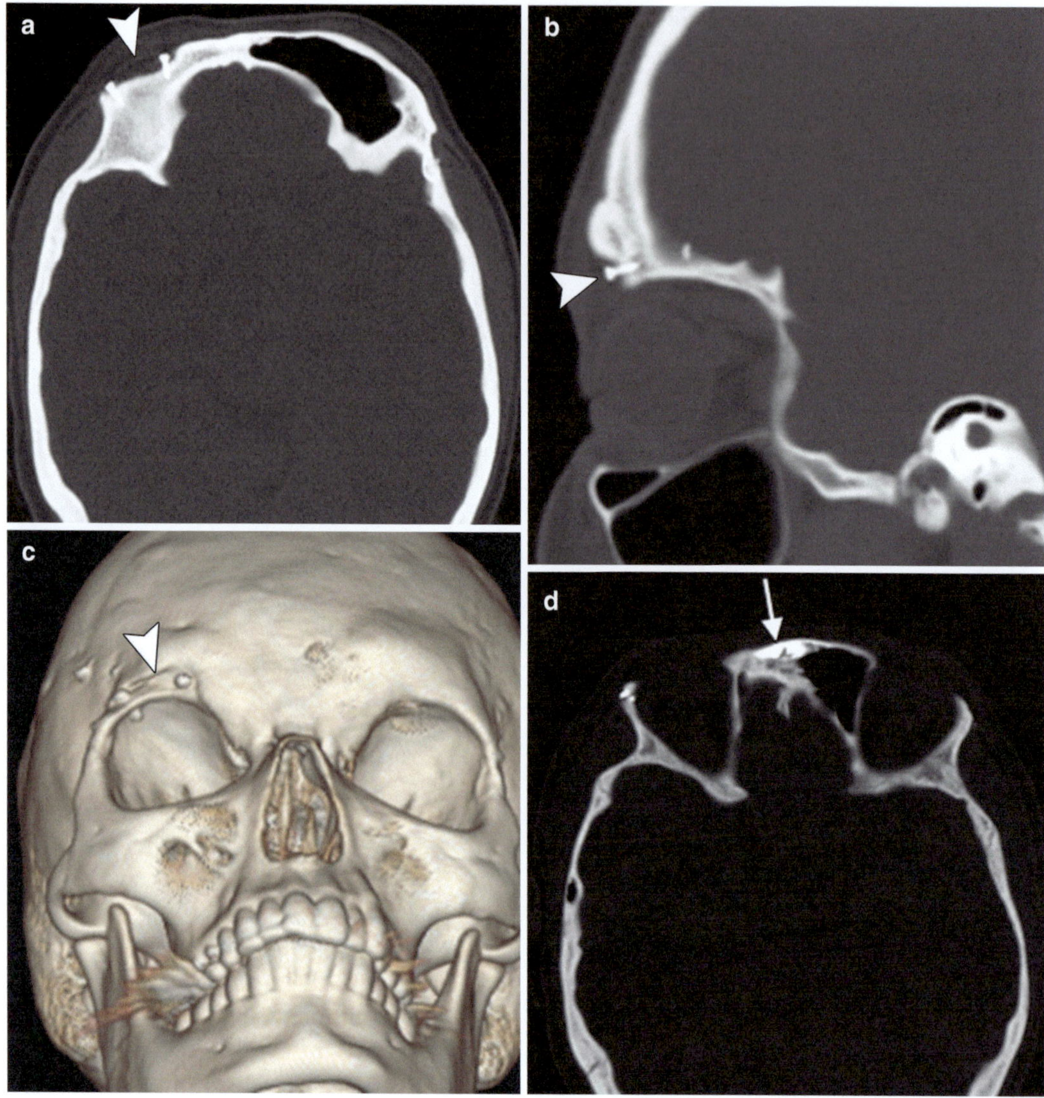

Fig. 6.18 Orbital rim augmentation. This patient with right unilateral coronal synostotic plagiocephaly underwent implantation of carved Medpor right superior lateral orbital rim augmentation and placement of hydroxyapatite cement in the glabellar depression and bilateral frontal temporal depressions. Axial (**a**), sagittal (**b**), and 3D volume rendered (**c**) CT images show the site where the low attenuation Medpor implant has been screwed to the underlying bone (*arrowheads*). Axial CT image (**d**) demonstrates the hyperattenuating hydroxyapatite cement that has been used to fill a depression in the right aspect of the glabella (*arrow*)

curettage, and sphenoid punch. The orbital roof and lateral wall can be reconstructed using bone graft and secured using microplates or titanium wires to ensure structural integrity. Optic nerve decompression can be performed in conjunction with correction of orbital dystopias and craniofacial deformities induced by fibrous dysplasia. Indeed, complementary remodeling resection, dacryocystorhinostomy, and internal optic nerve decompression can be performed. CT can be useful to delineate the optic canal and for planning additional surgery after decompression (Fig. 6.22), particularly if there are progressive or recurrent visual symptoms.

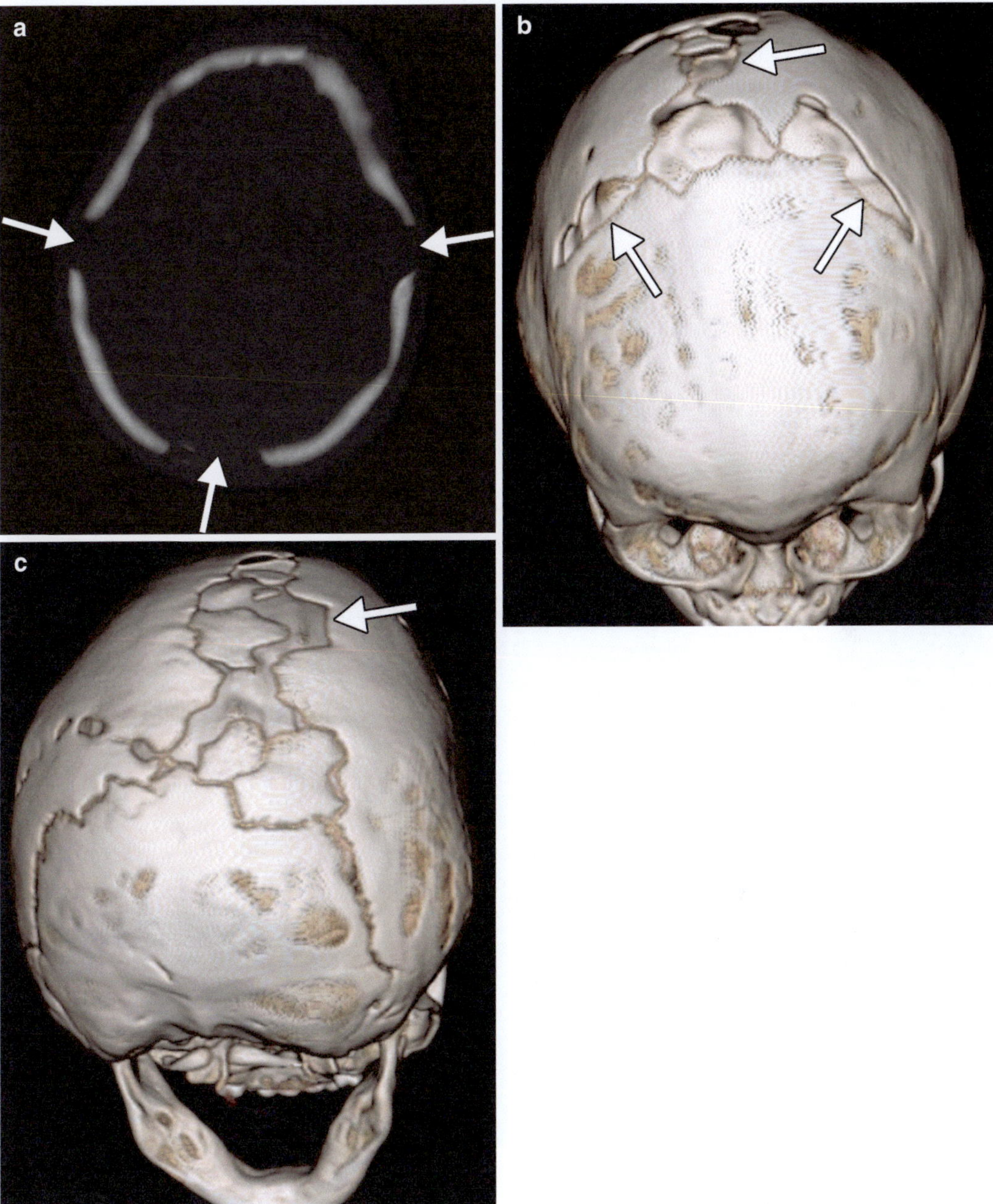

Fig. 6.19 Strip craniectomy. The patient has a history of coronal and sagittal craniosynostosis treated via endoscopic strip craniectomy. Postoperative axial CT (**a**) and 3D surface-rendered CT (**b**, **c**) images show that portions of the calvarium along the expected positions of the coronal and sagittal sutures have been removed (*arrows*)

6.2.10 Complications of Craniofacial Surgery

Imaging with CT during the early postoperative period may be necessary for the evaluation of acute intracranial and orbital hemorrhage (Fig. 6.23), which is an inherent and fairly common risk of cranial and maxillofacial surgery. In addition to such generic complications, there are certain postoperative issues specific to

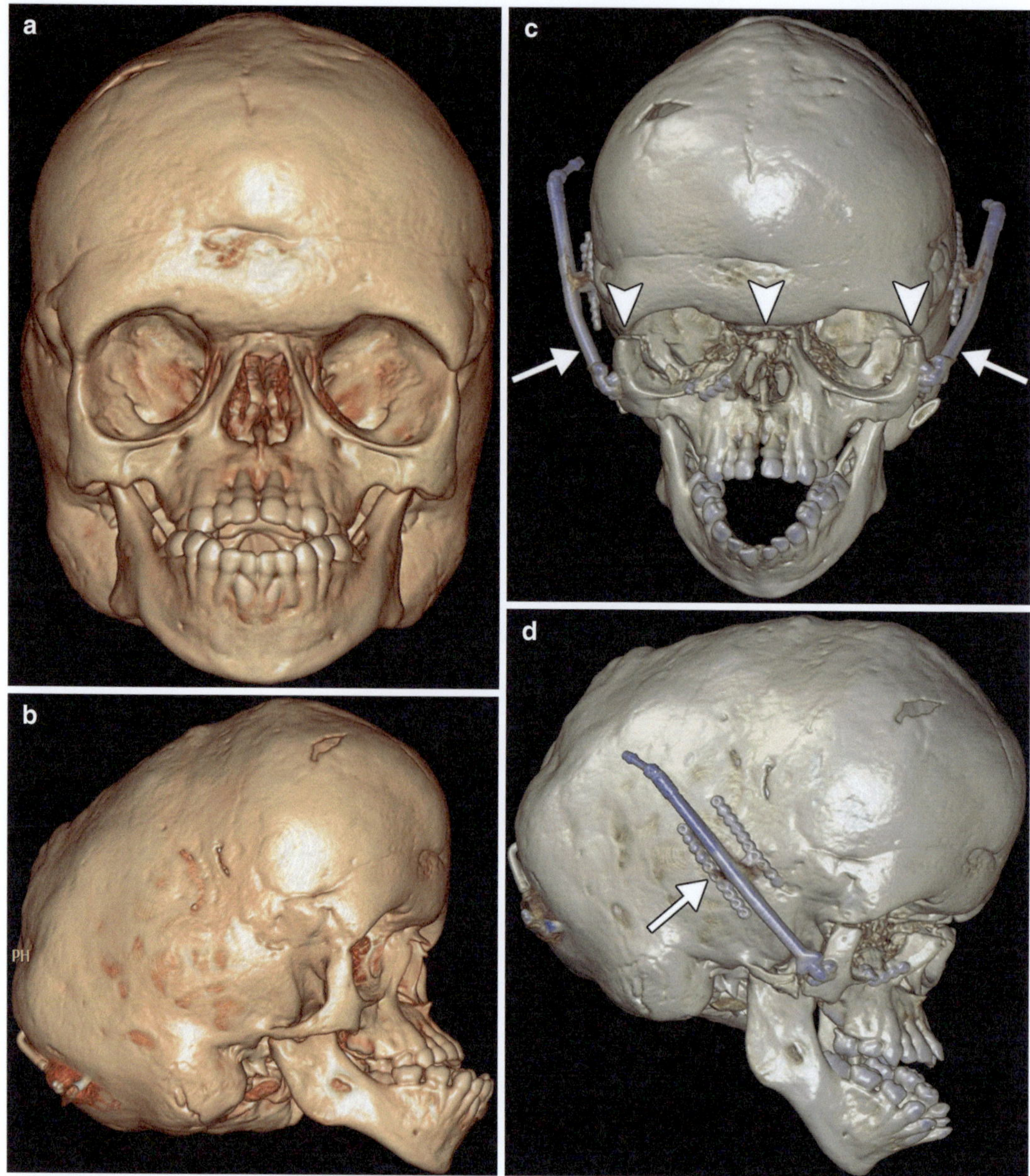

Fig. 6.20 LeFort III osteotomy. Frontal (**a**) and lateral (**b**) 3D volume rendered CT images before LeFort III osteotomy show severe midfacial hypoplasia. There are also the stigmata of prior orbitofrontal advancement. Frontal (**c**) and lateral (**d**) 3D volume rendered CT images after LeFort III osteotomy show bilateral cranio-maxillary distractor devices (*arrows*) in position and a horizontal facial osteotomy that traverses the nasal bridge and orbits (*arrowheads*)

craniosynostosis and midface surgery that can involve the orbits, including persistent strabismus, hardware migration with impingement upon the orbital contents, and nasolacrimal duct obstruction. The strabismus associated with craniosynostosis does not usually resolve with cranial vault or maxillofacial surgery. Orbital MRI may be useful for pre-operative planning of strabismus procedures (Fig. 6.24). Hardware migration can occur months to years after craniofacial surgical repair and typically coincides with growth of the child. New-onset strabismus can result if screws or other hardware project into the globe or extraocular muscles, particularly in a growing child. High-resolution CT can best depict the status of metal hardware and its relationship

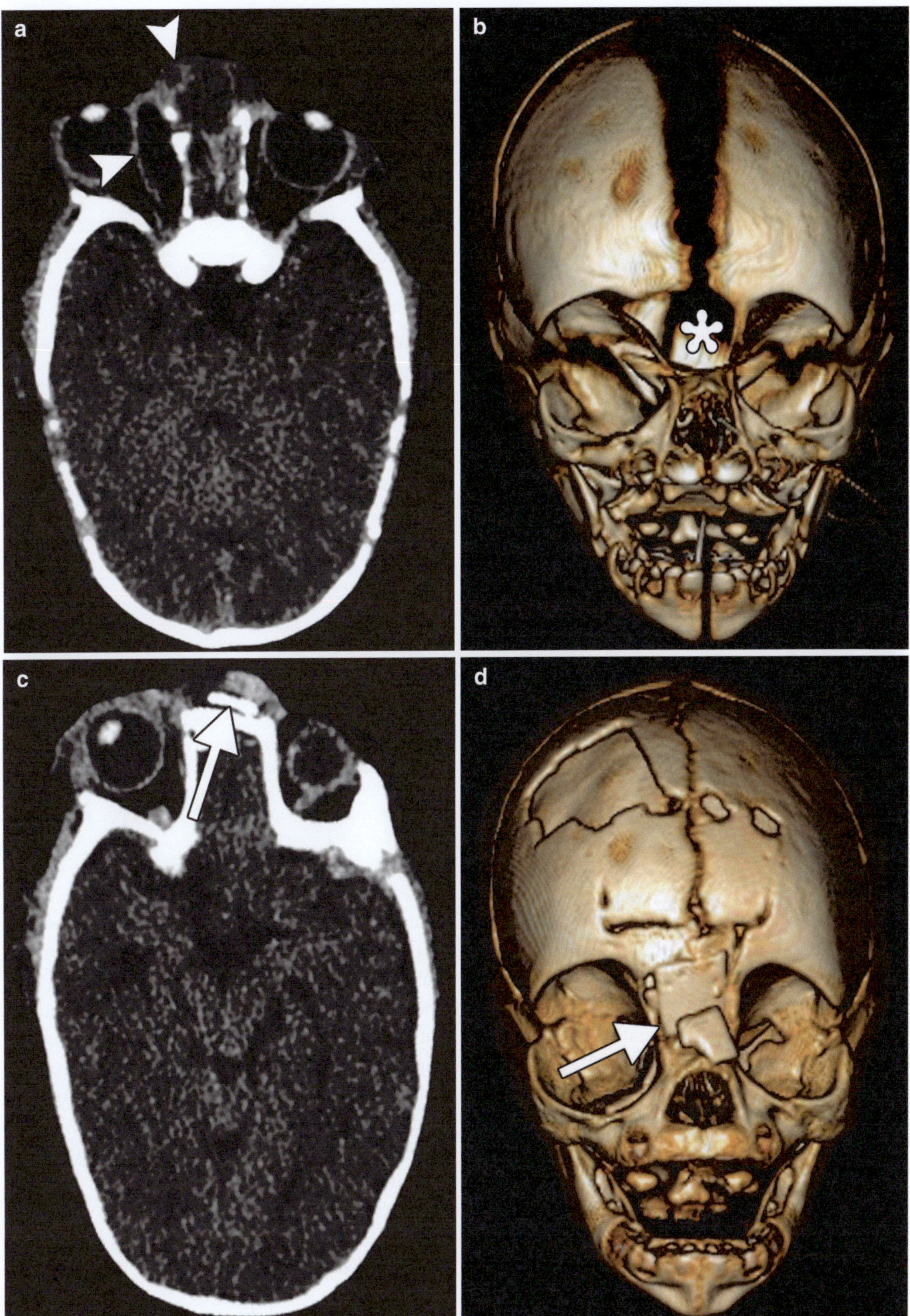

Fig. 6.21 Frontoethmoid encephalocele repair. Preoperative axial (**a**) and 3D volume rendered (**b**) CT images show a frontoethmoidal encephalocele with a defect in the nasal bridge (*) and extension into the right orbit (*arrowheads*), associated with proptosis. There is also hypertelorism. Postoperative axial (**c**) and 3D volume rendered (**d**) CT images show interval excision of the encephalocele, plugging of the defect with calvarial bone graft (*arrows*), decreased hypertelorism, and resolution of the proptosis

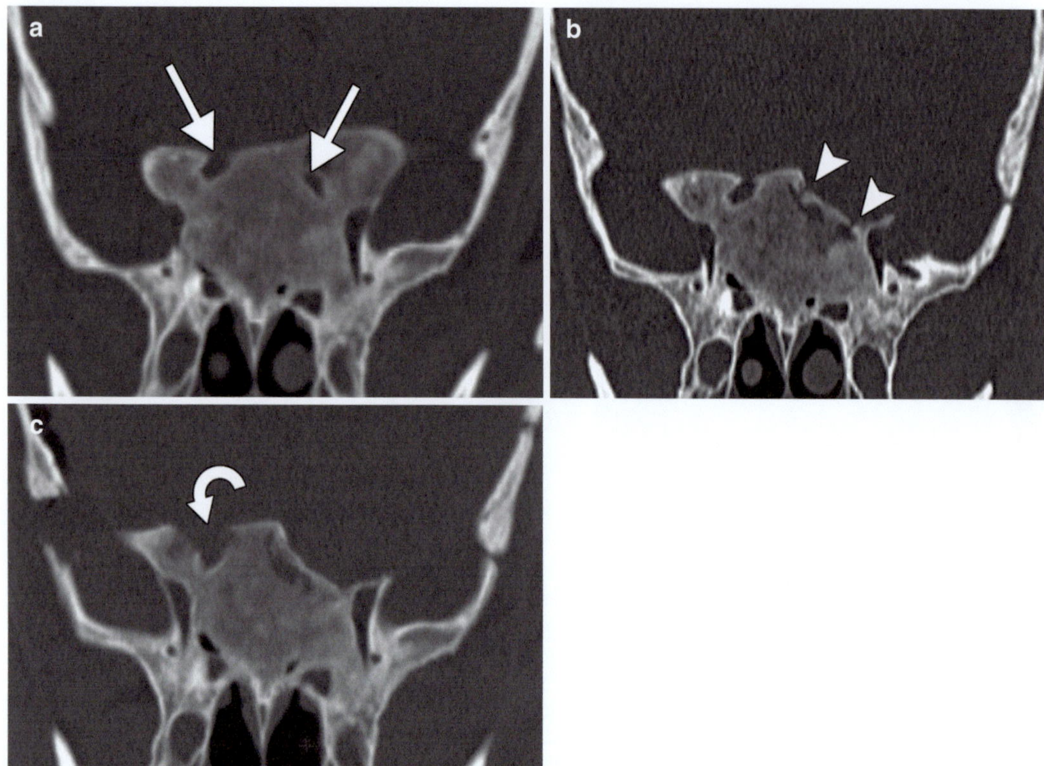

Fig. 6.22 Optic nerve decompression for orbitofrontal fibrous dysplasia. Initial coronal CT image (**a**) shows a diffuse ground glass expansile lesion involving the sphenoid bone with resultant narrowing and deformity of the bilateral optic nerve canals (*arrows*). Follow-up coronal CT image (**b**) obtained after left optic nerve decompression shows resection of the lesser sphenoid wing with uncovering of the superior and lateral walls of the optic canal (*arrowheads*). A subsequent coronal CT image (**c**) shows partial resection of the right lesser sphenoid wing with uncovering of the superior wall of the optic nerve canal (*curved arrow*)

to the soft tissues, although associated streak artifact can undermine image quality (Fig. 6.25). Nasolacrimal duct obstruction can occasionally result from LeFort osteotomy with secondary inflammatory changes associated with indirect injury of the nasolacrimal duct. CT can demonstrate debris within the nasolacrimal duct and mucosal swelling and congestion around the distal nasolacrimal duct opening, which narrows the inferior meatus (Fig. 6.26). This condition can be successfully treated with dacryocystorhinostomy. Finally, the development of intracranial hypertension, both before, and even after cranial vault expansion can lead to neurological and visual deterioration. This may be attributable to persistent inadequate intracranial space, which can often be apparent with CT (Fig. 6.27). Radiological imaging, particularly via CT with 3D volume renderings, is also useful for planning revision surgery, which consists of reexpanding and recontouring of the calvarium. Likewise, maxillofacial CT with 3D volume renderings is useful for quantifying orbital deformities that persist or progress after initial craniosynostosis surgery and planning subsequent reconstructive operations that specifically address the orbital region (Fig. 6.28).

6.3 Summary

- Surgery for strabismus and craniofacial malformations often results in complex findings on diagnostic neuroimaging. Thus, familiarity

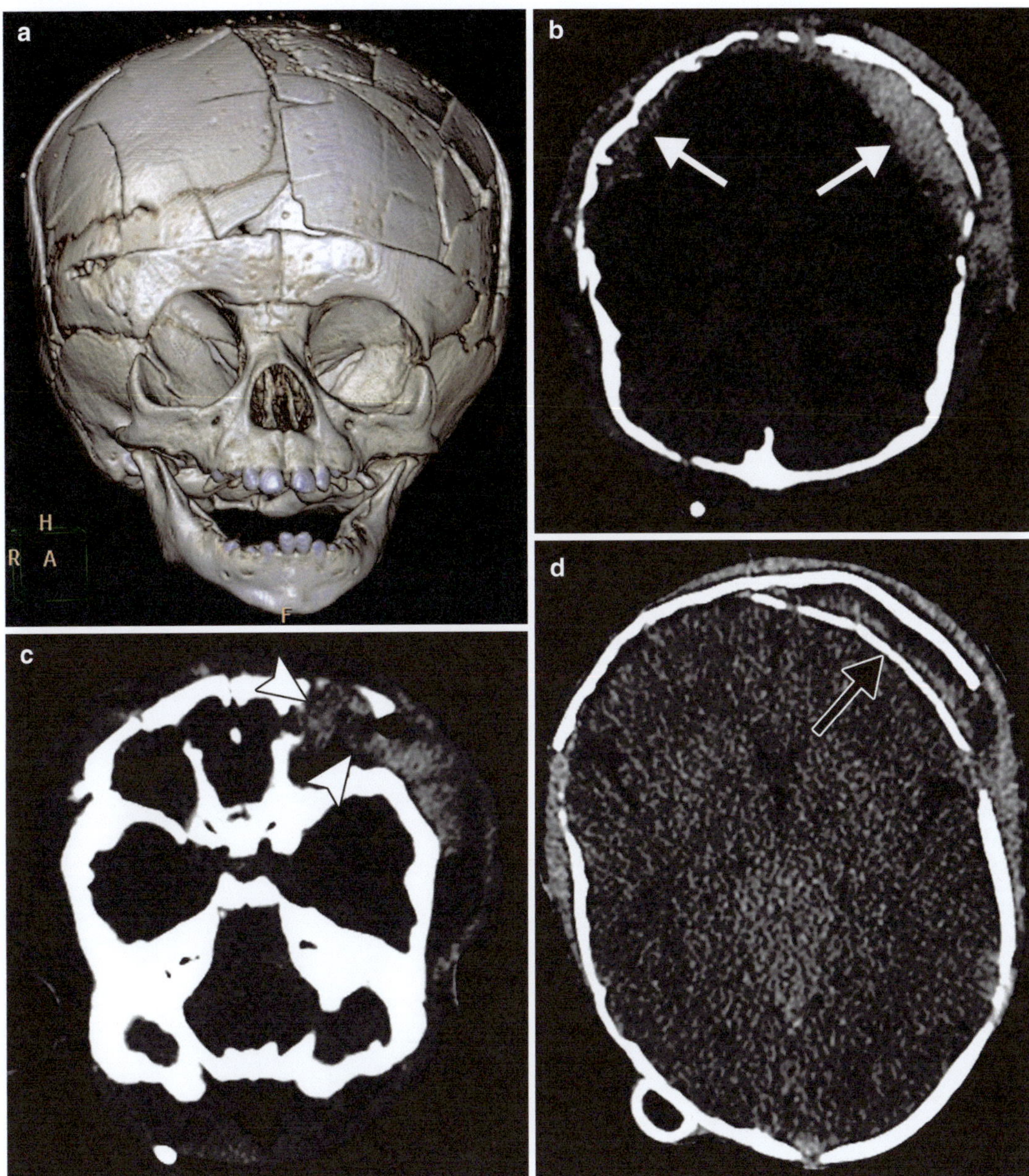

Fig. 6.23 Postoperative hemorrhage. The patient underwent recent orbitofrontal advancement, as shown on the 3D volume rendered CT image (**a**). The corresponding axial CT images (**b**, **c**) show acute hyperattenuating extra-axial hemorrhage in the bilateral frontal convexities, left greater than right (*arrows*), and left orbit (*arrowheads*). Follow-up axial CT image (**d**) demonstrates resolution of the right frontal convexity hematoma and decrease in size of the left frontal convexity hematoma with development of calcification of the dura (*black arrow*)

with the spectrum of procedures can facilitate interpretation of postoperative imaging.

- High spatial resolution MRI of the orbit is the modality of choice for evaluating the configuration of the extraocular muscles after strabismus surgery and planning of subsequent revision surgery, although postoperative changes can be very subtle.

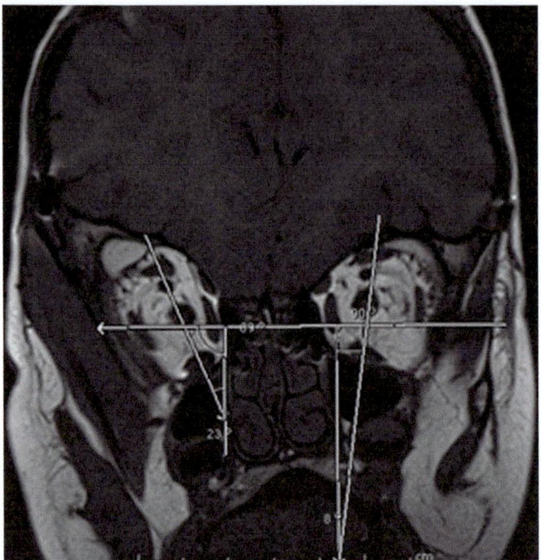

Fig. 6.24 Persistent strabismus after craniosynostosis surgery. Coronal T1-weighted MRI shows asymmetry in the alignment of the left and right extra-ocular muscles with significant excyclorotation on the right in a child with unilateral coronal synostosis

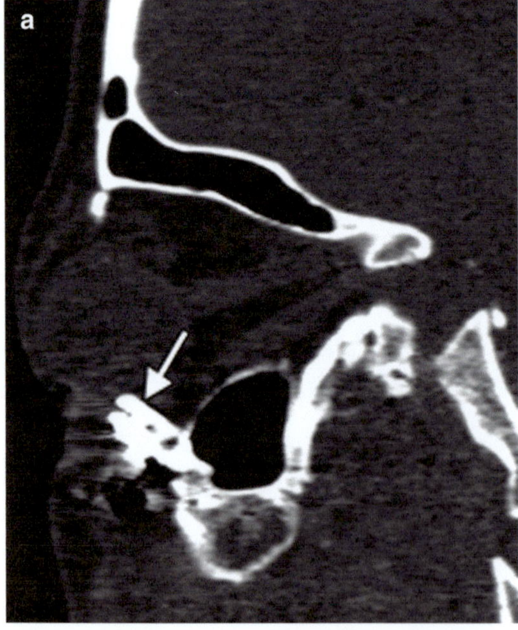

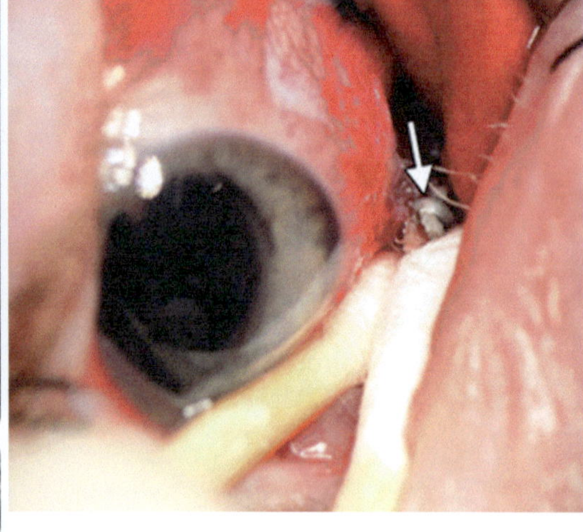

Fig. 6.25 Hardware impingement due to orbital growth. The patient underwent craniofacial surgery several years before and now presents with strabismus. Coronal CT image (**a**) shows metal screws (*arrow*) that project into the orbit, indenting the inferior rectus muscle and globe. The corresponding intraoperative photograph (**b**) shows that tip of the screws (*arrow*) indent the globe, where there is conjunctival injection (Adapted with permission from Sadiq et al. (2013))

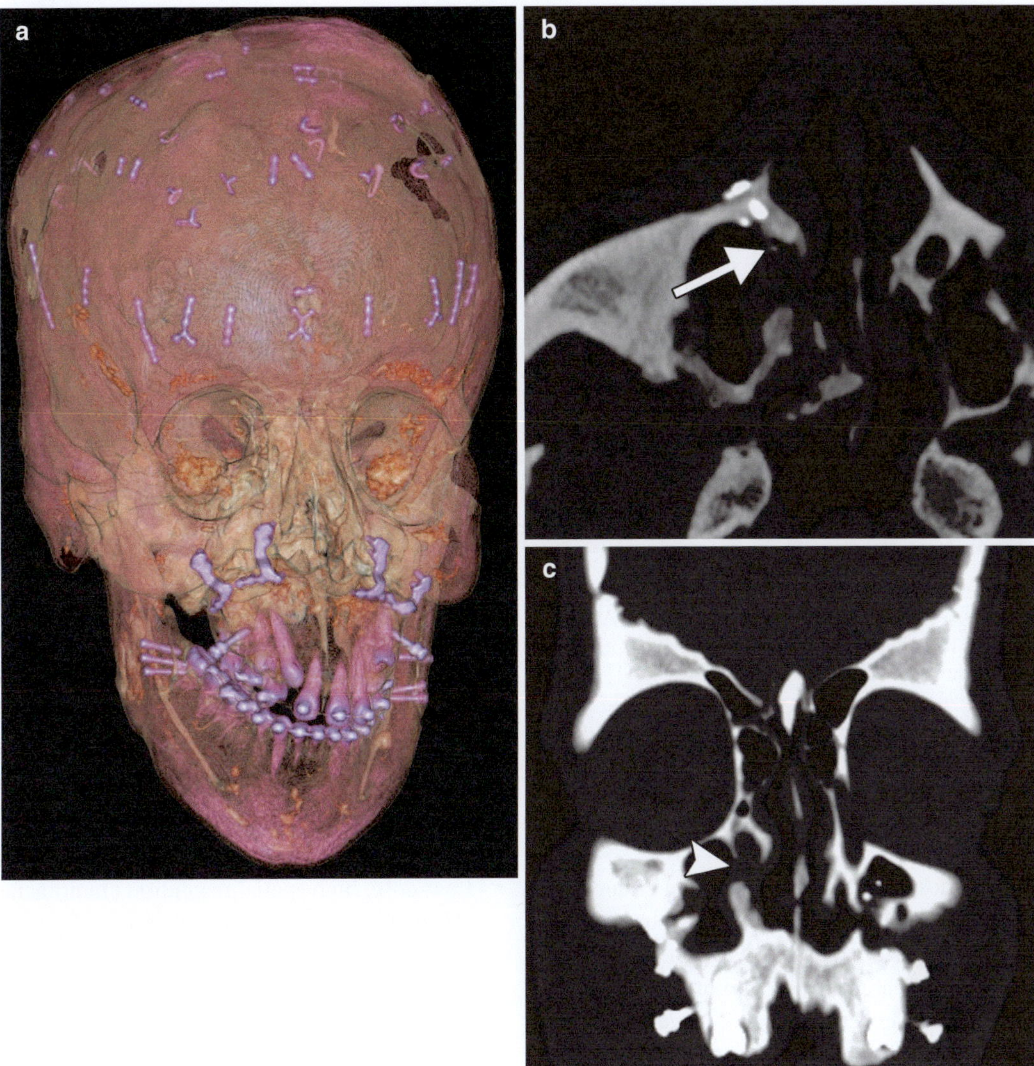

Fig. 6.26 Nasolacrimal duct obstruction. The patient presented with right nasolacrimal duct obstruction status post-craniofacial surgery for craniosynostosis. The 3D surface-rendered CT image (**a**) show extensive postoperative findings related to orbitofrontal advancement and LeFort osteotomy. Axial (**b**) and coronal (**c**) CT images show opacification of the right nasolacrimal duct with hyperattenuating debris (*arrow*) and opacification at the inferior meatus adjacent to the expected location of the nasolacrimal duct opening (*arrowhead*)

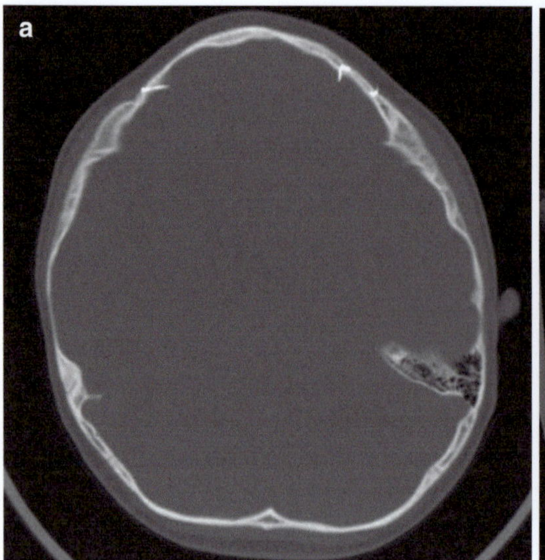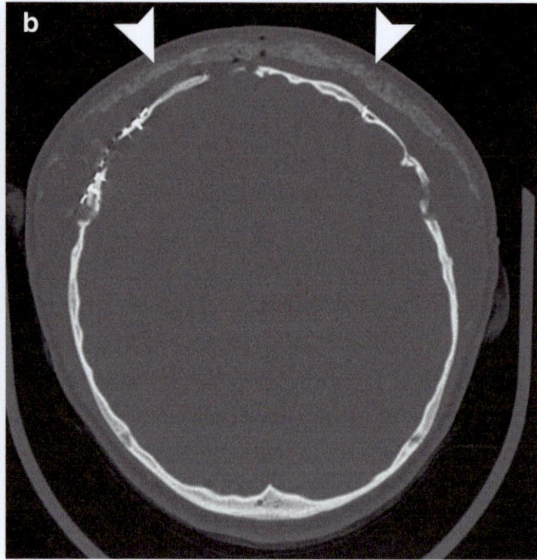

Fig. 6.27 Persistent cranial deformity after craniosynostosis surgery. The patient has a history of bicoronal synostosis and had orbitofrontal advancement but presents with sign of elevated intracranial pressure with visual blurring, progressive headaches, and imaging findings suggestive of inadequate intracranial space. Axial CT image after initial orbitofrontal advancement (**a**) shows a relatively small capacity cranial vault, particularly in the frontal region, where there is mild beaking. Axial CT image obtained after revision surgery (**b**) shows interval frontal osteotomies with a more capacious frontal region and a more regular contour of the skull. Only hydroxyapatite, which appears hyperattenuating (*arrowheads*), has been applied to the outer table of the frontal calvarium for cosmetic purposes. There is still extensive scalp edema from recent surgery

- Low-dose, high spatial resolution craniofacial CT with 3D volume rendered imaging is useful for the postoperative assessment of the orbit after surgical reconstruction of cranial malformations. This enables quantitative assessment of orbital volumes and osseous morphology, aiding the planning of further surgery.
- Low-dose, high spatial resolution craniofacial CT is also useful for the evaluation of potential hardware and osseous complications.
- Minimizing radiation exposure is particularly important in young patients who may undergo repeated CT imaging before and after treatment of the craniofacial anomalies.

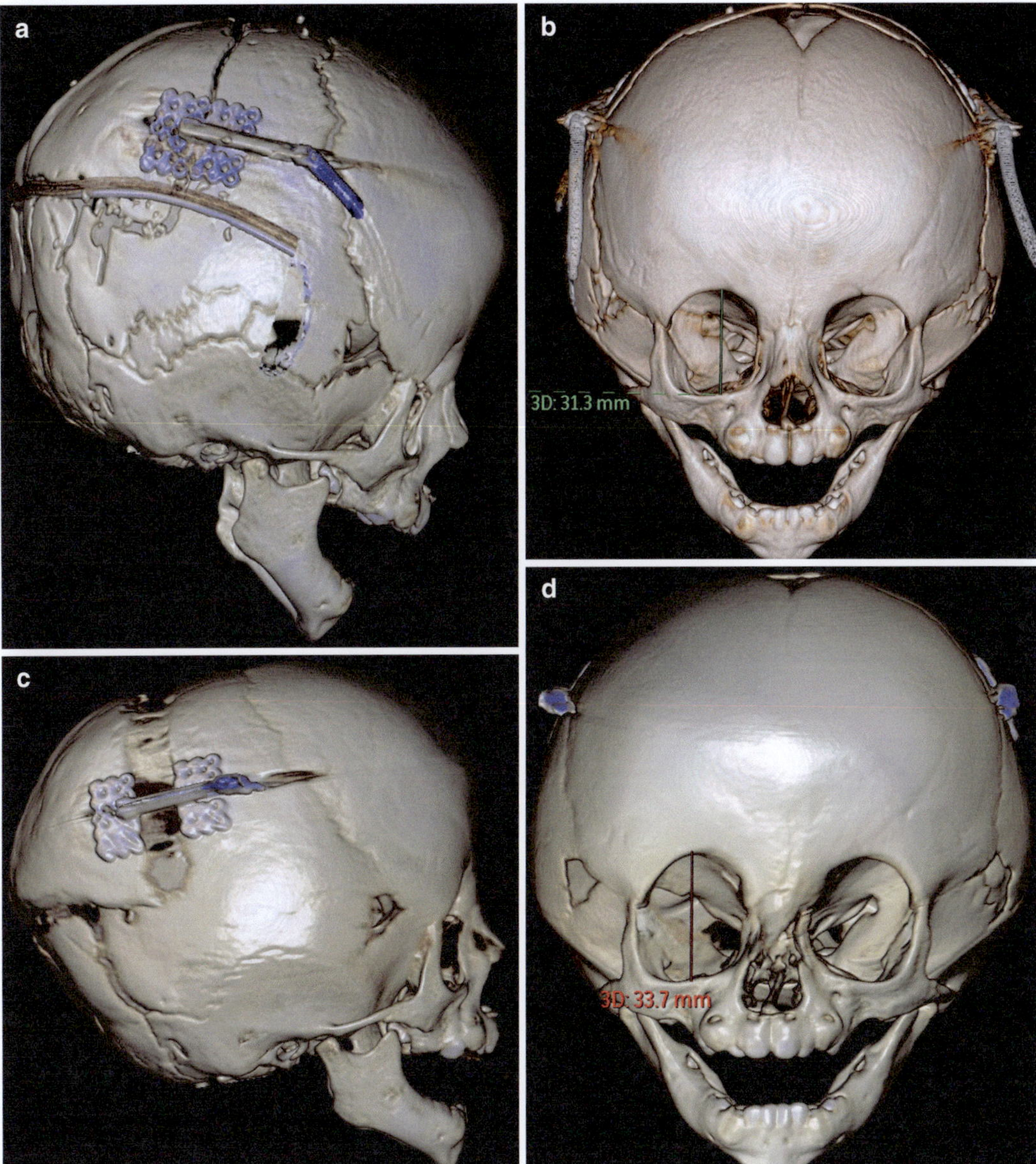

Fig. 6.28 Increased orbital deformity after craniosynostosis surgery. The patient has a history of multiple prematurely fused sutures. Initial 3D volume rendered CT images (**a, b**) obtained after posterior cranial vault expansion show bilateral parietal distraction devices and trigonocephaly. Follow-up 3D volume rendered CT images (**c, d**) obtained nearly 1 year later show increase in size of the cranial vault, but increased deformity of the orbits, with a "quizzical" appearance

Further Reading

Abe T, Satoh K, Wada A. Optic nerve decompression for orbitofrontal fibrous dysplasia: recent development of surgical technique and equipment. Skull Base. 2006; 16(3):145–55.

Anantheswar YN, Venkataramana NK. Pediatric craniofacial surgery for craniosynostosis: our experience and current concepts: Parts -2. J Pediatr Neurosci. 2009a; 4(2):100–7.

Anantheswar YN, Venkataramana NK. Pediatric craniofacial surgery for craniosynostosis: our experience and current concepts: Part -1. J Pediatr Neurosci. 2009b;4(2):86–99.

Andrews BT, Meara JG. Reconstruction of frontoethmoidalencephalocele defects. Atlas Oral Maxillofac Surg Clin North Am. 2010;18(2):129–38.

Baker RS, Conklin JD. Acquired Brown syndrome from blunt orbital trauma. J Pediatr Ophthalmol Surg. 1987; 18:893.

Barley GB, Dyer JA. Strengthening the superior oblique muscle. Ophthalmic Surg. 1987;18:893.

Bentley RP, Sgouros S, Natarajan K, Dover MS, Hockley AD. Changes in orbital volume during childhood in cases of craniosynostosis. J Neurosurg. 2002;96(4): 747–54.

Béquignon E, Cardinne C, Lachiver X, Wagner I, Chabolle F, Baujat B. Craniofacial fibrous dysplasia surgery: A functional approach. Eur Ann Otorhinolaryngol Head Neck Dis. 2013 Jul 18. pii: S1879–7296(12) 00141-X.

Binning M, Ragel B, Brockmeyer DL, Walker ML, Kestle JR. Evaluation of the necessity of postoperative imaging after craniosynostosis surgery. J Neurosurg. 2007; 107(1 Suppl):43–5.

Campbell JW, Albright AL, Losken HW, Biglan AW. Intracranial hypertension after cranial vault decompression for craniosynostosis. Pediatr Neurosurg. 1995;22(5):270–3.

Clark RA, Demer JL. Magnetic resonance imaging of the effects of horizontal rectus extraocular muscle surgery on pulley and globe positions and stability. Invest Ophthalmol Vis Sci. 2006;47(1):188–94.

Clark RA, Rosenbaum AL, Demer JL. Magnetic resonance imaging after surgical transposition defines the anteroposterior location of the rectus muscle pulleys. J AAPOS. 1999;3(1):9–14.

Crouch ER. Use of botulinum toxin in strabismus. Curr Opin Ophthalmol. 2006;17(5):435–40.

Curtis TH, Stout AU, Drack AV, Durairaj VD. Giant orbital cysts after strabismus surgery. Am J Ophthalmol. 2006;142(4):697–9.

David L, Argenta L, Fisher D. Hydroxyapatite cement in pediatric craniofacial reconstruction. J Craniofac Surg. 2005;16(1):129–33.

De Ponte FS, Pascali M, Perugini M, Lattanzi A, Gennaro P, Brunelli A. Surgical treatment of frontoethmoidal encephalocele: a case report. J Craniofac Surg. 2000; 11(4):342–5.

Derderian CA, Bastidas N, Bartlett SP. Posterior cranial vault expansion using distraction osteogenesis. Childs Nerv Syst. 2012;28(9):1551–6.

Edelman PM. Functional benefits of adult strabismus surgery. Am Orthopt J. 2010;60:43–7.

Eley KA, Witherow H, Hayward R, Evans R, Young K, Clark A, Dunaway D. The evaluation of bony union after frontofacial distraction. J Craniofac Surg. 2009;20(2): 275–8.

Festa F, Pagnoni M, Valerio R, Rodolfino D, Saccucci M, d'Attilio M, Caputi S, Iannetti G. Orbital volume and surface after Le Fort III advancement in syndromiccraniosynostosis. J Craniofac Surg. 2012;23(3):789–92.

Francis CS, Shetty A, Frank R, Meltzer HS, Cohen SR. In situ fronto-orbital advancement with medial orbital

osteotomies for trigonocephaly-associated hypotelorism. J Craniofac Surg. 2011;22(1):281–4.

Ginat DT, Gupta R. Advances in computed tomography imaging technology. Annu Rev Biomed Eng. 2014;16: 431–53.

Gosain AK. Hydroxyapatite cement paste cranioplasty for the treatment of temporal hollowing after cranial vault remodeling in a growing child. J Craniofac Surg. 1997;8(6):506–11.

Holmes AD, Wright GW, Meara JG, Heggie AA, Probert TC. LeFort III internal distraction in syndromiccraniosynostosis. J Craniofac Surg. 2002;13(2):262–72.

Hopper RA. New trends in cranio-orbital and midface distraction for craniofacial dysostosis. Curr Opin Otolaryngol Head Neck Surg. 2012;20(4):298–303.

Hunter DG, Lam GC, Guyton DL. Inferior oblique muscle injury from local anesthesia for cataract surgery. Ophthalmology. 1995;102:501.

Iannetti G, Fadda T, Agrillo A, Poladas G, Iannetti G, Filiaci F. LeFort III advancement with and without osteogenesis distraction. J Craniofac Surg. 2006;17(3): 536–43.

Imai K, Fujimoto T, Takahashi M, Maruyama Y, Yamaguchi K. Preoperative and postoperative orbital volume in patients with Crouzon and Apert syndrome. J Craniofac Surg. 2013;24(1):191–4.

Jang SY, Kim MK, Choi SM, Jang JW. Nasolacrimal duct obstruction after maxillary orthognathic surgery. J Oral Maxillofac Surg. 2013;71(6):1085–98.

Kowal L, Wong E, Yahalom C. Botulinum toxin in the treatment of strabismus. A review of its use and effects. DisabilRehabil. 2007;29(23):1823–31.

Kushner BJ. The efficacy of strabismus surgery in adults: a review for primary care physicians. Postgrad Med J. 2011a;87(1026):269–73.

Kushner BJ. Insertion slanting strabismus surgical procedures. Arch Ophthalmol. 2011b;129(12):1620–5.

Lee DW, Kim JY, Lew DH. Use of rapidly hardening hydroxyapatite cement for facial contouring surgery. J Craniofac Surg. 2010;21(4):1084–8.

Lenart TD, Lambert SR. Slipped and lost extraocular muscles. Ophthalmol Clin North Am. 2001;14(3): 433–42.

Mahapatra AK, Suri A. Anterior encephaloceles: a study of 92 cases. Pediatr Neurosurg. 2002;36(3):113–8.

Mehendale RA, Dagi LR, Wu C, Ledoux D, Johnston S, Hunter DG. Superior rectus transposition and medial rectus recession for Duane syndrome and sixth nerve palsy. Arch Ophthalmol. 2012;130(2):195–201.

Mehendale RA, Stemmer-Rachimamov AO, Dagi LR. A 50 year old man with a long-standing large angle exotropia and limitation of adduction in the left eye. Digital J Ophthalmol. 2012;19:64–7.

Metz HS, Searl S, Rosenberg P, Sterns G. Giant orbital cyst after strabismus surgery. J AAPOS. 1999;3(3):185–7.

Miller JM, Demer JL, Rosenbaum AL. Effect of transposition surgery on rectus muscle paths by magnetic resonance imaging. Ophthalmology. 1993;100(4):475–87.

Mills MD, Coats DK, Donahue SP, Wheeler DT, American Academy of Ophthalmology. Strabismus surgery for adults: a report by the American Academy of Ophthalmology. Ophthalmology. 2004;111(6):1255–62.

Nasu W, Kobayashi S, Kashiwa K, Honda T. Secondary craniofacial reconstruction of huge frontoethmoidalencephalomeningocele after primary neurosurgical repair. J Craniofac Surg. 2008;19(1):171–4.

Neely KA, Ernest JT, Mottier M. Combined superior oblique paresis and Brown syndrome after blepharoplasty. Am J Ophthalmol Strabismus. 1987;24:309.

Negishi T, Hikoya A, Isoda H, Tsuchiya Y, Sawada M, Hotta Y, Sato M. Magnetic resonance imaging of the medial rectus muscle of patients with consecutive exotropia after medial rectus muscle recession. Ophthalmology. 2010;117(10):1876–82.

Nout E, van Bezooijen JS, Koudstaal MJ, Veenland JF, Hop WC, Wolvius EB, van der Wal KG. Orbital change following Le Fort III advancement in syndromiccraniosynostosis: quantitative evaluation of orbital volume, infra-orbital rim and globe position. J Craniomaxillofac Surg. 2012;40(3):223–8.

Ohba M, Ohtsuka K, Hosaka Y, Ogawa K, Osanai H. A case of a slipped medial rectus muscle after strabismus surgery. Binocul Vis Strabismus Q. 2004;19(3): 165–8.

Panchal J, Uttchin V. Management of craniosynostosis. Plast Reconstr Surg. 2003;111(6):2032–48; quiz 2049.

Papay FA, Morales Jr L, Flaharty P, Smith SJ, Anderson R, WAlker JM, WAlker RS, WAlker S. Optic nerve decompression in cranial base fibrous dysplasia. J Craniofac Surg. 1995;6(1):5–10; discussion 11-4.

Pelo S, Gasparini G, Di Petrillo A, Tamburrini G, Di Rocco C. Distraction osteogenesis in the surgical treatment of craniostenosis: a comparison of internal and external craniofacial distractor devices. Childs Nerv Syst. 2007;23(12):1447–53. Epub 2007 Sep 18.

Pollack IF, Losken HW, Biglan AW. Incidence of increased intracranial pressure after early surgical treatment of syndromiccraniosynostosis. Pediatr Neurosurg. 1996;24(4):202–9.

Posnick JC, Armstrong D, Bite U. Metopic and sagittal synostosis: intracranial volume measurements prior to and after cranio-orbital reshaping in childhood. Plast Reconstr Surg. 1995;96(2):299–309; discussion 310–5.

Prata JA, Minckler DS, Green RL. Pseudo-Brown syndrome as a complication of glaucoma drainage implant surgery. Ophthalmic Surg. 1993;24:608.

Purdy EP. Oculoplastic and orbital applications of porous high-density polyethylene implants. Curr Opin Ophthalmol. 1997;8(5):57–63.

Sadiq MA, Prabhu SP, Fearon JA, Taghinia AH, Dagi LR. Screw implantation in the globe: the risk of delayed hardware migration from craniofacial repair. J Craniofac Surg. 2013;24(5):1650–2.

Schatz CJ, Ginat DT. Imaging of cosmetic facial implants and grafts. AJNR Am J Neuroradiol. 2013;34(9):1674–81.

Shah AS, Prabu SP, Sadiq MA, Mantagos IS, Hunter DG, Dagi LR. Adjustable nasal transposition of split lateral rectus muscle. JAMA Ophthalmol. 2014;10:1–7.

Simon JW. Complications of strabismus surgery. Curr Opin Ophthalmol. 2010;21(5):361–6.

Singh KA, Burstein FD, Williams JK. Use of hydroxyapatite cement in pediatric craniofacial reconstructive surgery: strategies for avoiding complications. J Craniofac Surg. 2010;21(4):1130–5.

Song JJ, Finger PT, Kurli M, Wisnicki HJ, Iacob CE. Giant secondary conjunctival inclusion cysts: a late complication of strabismus surgery. Ophthalmology. 2006;113(6): 1049.e1–2.

Songür E, Mutluer S, Gürler T, Bilkay U, Görken C, Güner U, Celik N. Management of frontoethmoidal (sincipital) encephalocele. J Craniofac Surg. 1999; 10(2):135–9.

Steinbach MJ, Kirshner EL, Arstikaitis MJ. Recession vs marginal myotomy surgery for strabismus: effects on spatial localization. Invest Ophthalmol Vis Sci. 1987; 28(11):1870–2.

Imaging After Vitreoretinal Surgery

Justin Kanoff, Daniel Thomas Ginat, Arun Singh, and Ivana Kim

7.1 Overview

The retina is the neurosensory tissue in the posterior aspect of the globe, which converts light to electrical signals that are transmitted via the optic nerves. The retina comprises several layers, including Bruch's membrane, retinal pigment epithelium, photoreceptor layer, external limiting membrane, outer nuclear layer, outer plexiform layer, inner plexiform layer, ganglion cell layer, nerve fiber layer, and inner limiting membrane at the vitreoretinal interface. Retinal detachment consists of a separation of the neurosensory retina from the retinal pigment epithelium. There are three types of retinal detachment: rhegmatogenous, tractional, and exudative. Treatment for retinal detachment depends on the particular type of detachment. Exudative detachments involve fluid collections under the retina from neoplastic or inflammatory conditions and are not associated with a retinal break. These are generally managed nonsurgically. Tractional retinal detachment occurs when a fibrous or fibrovascular membrane from trauma or neovascularization mechanically pulls the retina away from the retinal pigment epithelium. Rhegmatogenous detachments occur when there is a full thickness break in the retina and fluid enters the subretinal space from the vitreous cavity. Both rhegmatogenous and tractional retinal detachments may be treated surgically. The main options for retinal detachment repair include scleral buckling, vitrectomy with gas or silicone oil injection, or a combination of these. These procedures have a common goal, which is to reappose the neurosensory retina to the retinal pigment epithelium. The imaging findings after the treatment of retinal detachment and other procedures pertaining to the retina and vitreous are described and depicted in the following sections.

J. Kanoff, MD • I. Kim, MD
Department of Ophthalmology, Massachusetts Eye and Ear Infirmary, Boston, MA, USA

D.T. Ginat, MD, MS (✉)
Director of Head and Neck Imaging,
Department of Radiology, University of Chicago,
5841 S Maryland Avenue, Chicago, IL 60637, USA
e-mail: ginatd01@gmail.com

A. Singh, MD
Department of Ophthalmology, Cole Eye Institute,
Cleveland Clinic, Cleveland, OH, USA

7.2 Scleral Buckling

Scleral buckling is a surgical technique in which an encircling band or segmental element is sutured onto the scleral surface for reattaching the retina in cases of rhegmatogenous retinal detachment. The scleral buckle indents the globe, thereby relieving the vitreous traction and bringing the retinal break in closer apposition to the retinal pigment epithelium. This prevents more fluid from passing through the break and

D.T. Ginat, S.K. Freitag (eds.), *Post-treatment Imaging of the Orbit*,
DOI 10.1007/978-3-662-44023-0_7, © Springer-Verlag Berlin Heidelberg 2015

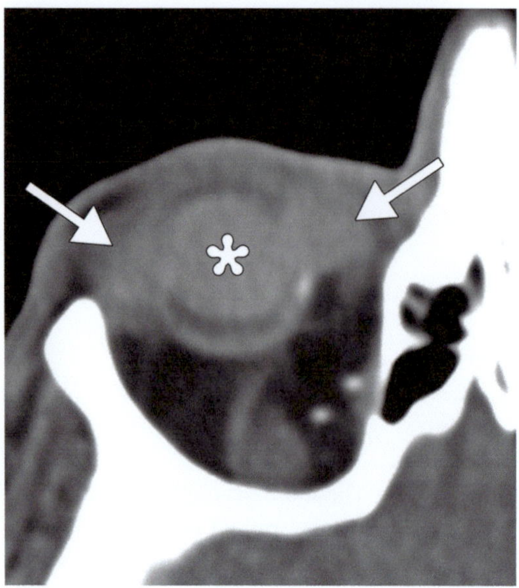

Fig. 7.1 Hydrogel scleral buckle. Axial CT image shows a bulky soft tissue attenuation structure encircling the right globe (*arrows*). There is a punctate calcification associated within the buckle medially. Silicone oil is present within the globe (*)

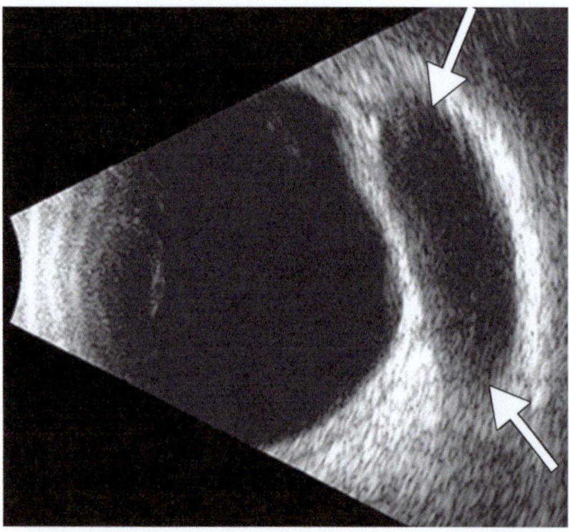

Fig. 7.2 Hydrogel scleral buckle on ultrasound. B-mode ultrasound image shows a nearly anechoic structure adjacent to and slightly indenting the posterior globe (*arrows*)

underneath the retina which allows the retinal pigment epithelium to pump out the remaining subretinal fluid. Scleral buckling is a surgical technique that was introduced in 1951 by Schepens et al. and has been perfected to yield a very high surgical success rate. Several materials have been used as scleral buckles, including hydrogel, silicon rubber, and silicon sponge. In the past, these materials were implanted underneath a partial-thickness flap of sclera, but modern scleral buckling utilizes exoplants almost exclusively. Each of these materials has characteristic imaging findings.

Hydrogel scleral exoplants, such as MIRAgel (MIRA, Waltham, MA), are composed of hydrophilic polymers, for which the key ingredient is copoly(methyl acrylate-2-hydroxyethyl acrylate) cross-linked with ethylene diacrylate in 15 % water. These scleral buckles were designed to be pliable and flexible during implantation and subsequently hydrate and expand. Perceived benefits included a lower chance of infection due to the solid rather than porous structure and a lower chance of extrusion. However, many patients had complications from these exoplants including buckle extrusion and hydrolytic degradation leading to their removal from the market. Nevertheless, many patients still have these exoplants in place and are at continued risk of complications. Patients with hydrogel scleral buckles may present for orbital imaging because of complaints of diplopia, proptosis, or palpable orbital mass. These exoplants should not be mistaken for neoplasm or abscess. On CT, the attenuation is intermediate between soft tissue and fluid, although rim calcifications may also be present (Fig. 7.1). On B-mode ultrasound, the exoplants appear hypoechoic to nearly anechoic (Fig. 7.2). On MRI, the hydrogel demonstrates slightly higher T1 and T2 signal with respect to the vitreous or aqueous fluid (Fig. 7.3). Swollen hydrogel scleral buckles can potentially mimic cystic orbital tumors or fluid collections, although the circular or semicircular morphology of the buckle suggests otherwise (Fig. 7.4). However, fragmentation and migration of the exoplants within the orbit can pose more of a diagnostic dilemma without the relevant clinical history (Fig. 7.5).

Currently, silicone exoplants are almost exclusively used for scleral buckling. These are available as either solid silicone rubber or porous sponges. The solid silicone elements are non-

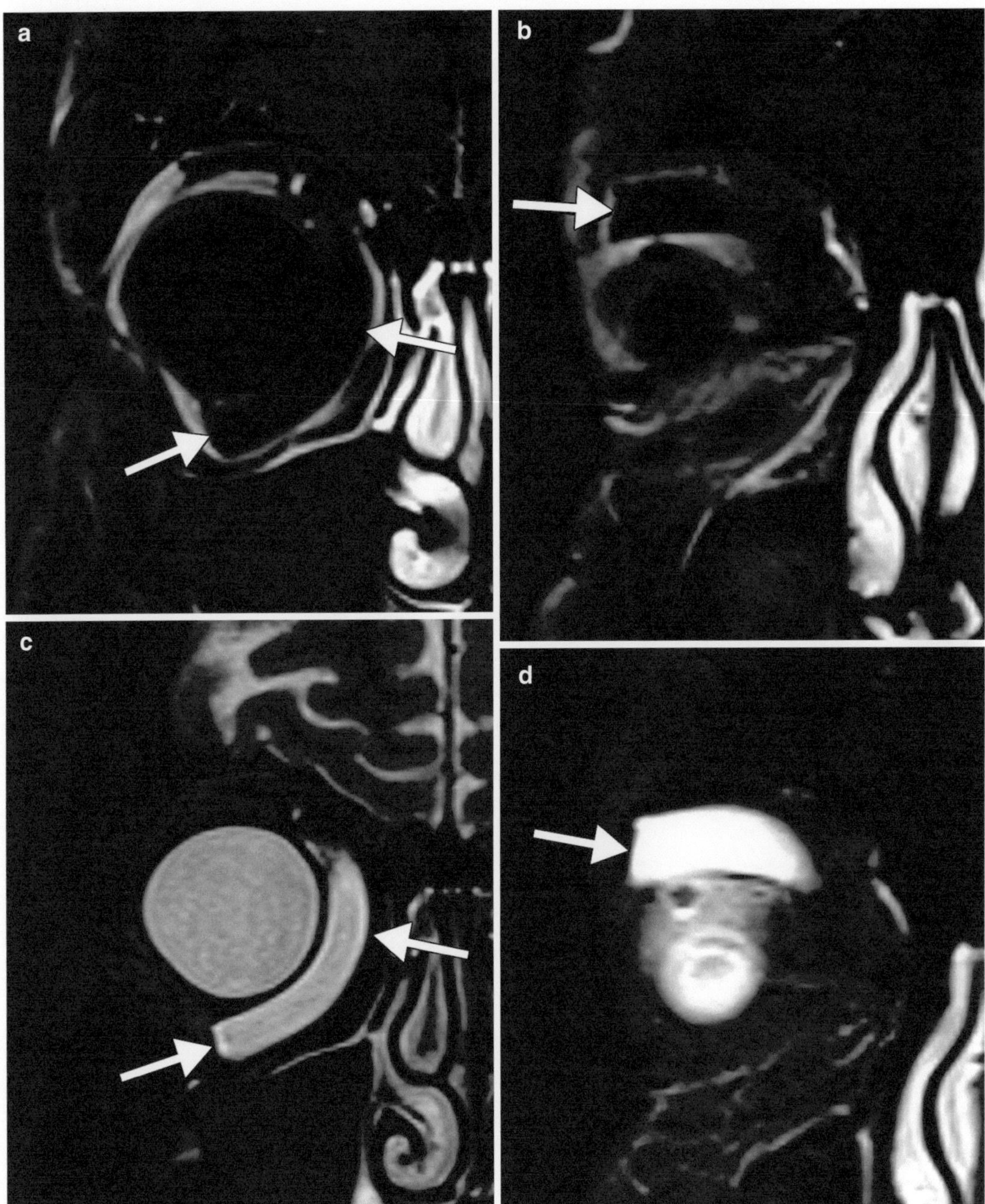

Fig. 7.3 Segmental hydrogel scleral buckle. Coronal fat-suppressed post-contrast T1-weighted (**a**, **b**) and fat-suppressed T2-weighted (**c**, **d**) MR images show a semicircular right scleral buckle in the medial orbit (*arrows*). The device has similar signal characteristics as fluid

compressible compared to the silicone sponges which, because of the multiple air cells, deform when under pressure. On B-scan ultrasound, silicone scleral buckles are hyperechoic (Fig. 7.6).

On CT, the solid rubber silicone scleral buckle appears hyperattenuating (Fig. 7.7), while the silicone sponge scleral buckles are hypoattenuating, similar to air (Fig. 7.8). Solid silicone bands are

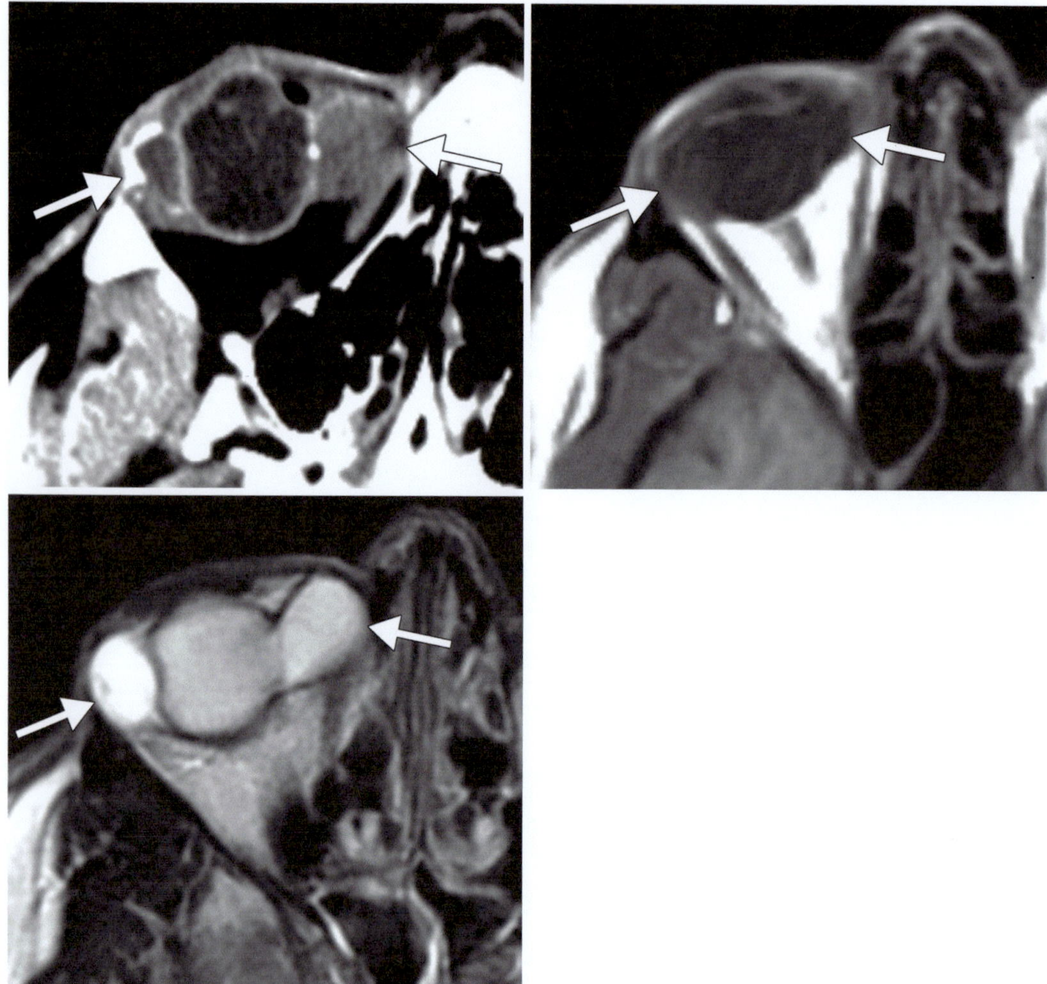

Fig. 7.4 Hydrated hydrogel scleral buckle with mass effect. Axial CT image (**a**) shows a markedly expanded buckle with associated rim calcifications. Axial T1-weighted (**b**) and axial T2 (**c**) images show that the expanded scleral buckle has signal characteristics similar to that of fluid

occasionally used in combination with the silicone sponge elements (Fig. 7.9). Silicone scleral buckles are MRI compatible and appear hypointense on all sequences (Fig. 7.10).

An uncommon but serious complication of scleral buckling is infection. Acute infections associated with silicone scleral buckles may show diffuse scleral thickening and preseptal soft tissue swelling with enhancement on imaging (Fig. 7.11). Scleral thickening may decrease as infection improves in response to appropriate antibiotic therapy. On imaging, silicone sponge has low attenuation when not infected and high attenuation in the presence of infection. In cases of chronically infected scleral buckles, the sclera may be thickened around the buckle, but with scleral melting under the buckle. Salient findings on MRI include increased T2 signal intensity and corresponding enhancement in the preseptal and postseptal tissues of the orbit and thickening of the sclera (Fig. 7.12). Most often the infected scleral buckle needs to be surgically removed to adequately treat the infection.

Imaging, particularly with ultrasound, is useful for characterizing the position of the scleral buckle and associated complications.

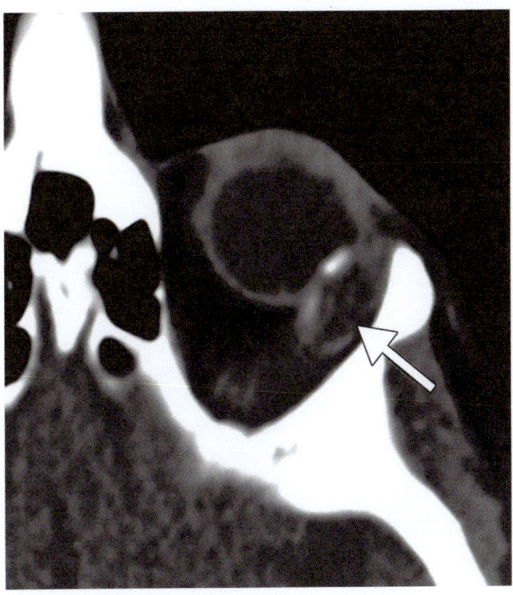

Fig. 7.5 Fragmented and migrated hydrogel scleral buckle. Axial CT image shows posterolateral displacement of a portion of the swollen scleral buckle with rim calcifications (*arrow*)

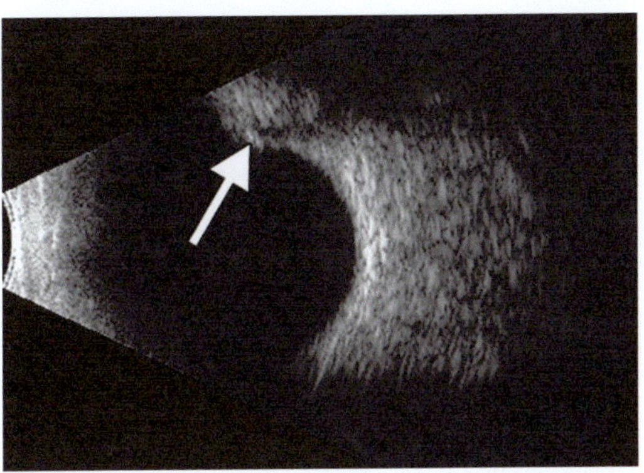

Fig. 7.6 Silicone scleral buckle depicted on ultrasound. B-mode ultrasound image shows a hyperechoic scleral buckle mildly indenting the globe (*arrow*), as intended (Courtesy of Karen Capaccioli and Lois Hart)

7.3   Vitrectomy

Vitrectomy is another option for surgical repair of retinal detachment. During a vitrectomy, the vitreous gel is removed from the posterior segment of the eye using an instrument which provides high-speed cutting and aspiration. Removal of the vitreous gel eliminates the tractional forces on the retinal break and the retina as a whole. After removal of the vitreous, the fluid in the eye is exchanged for air; at the same time, the subretinal fluid is removed by aspiration, thereby reattaching the retina. In complicated retinal detachments, it is not always possible to remove the subretinal fluid with suction alone. Laser or cryopexy is applied around the retinal breaks to seal them. At the conclusion of the case, the eye is filled with an agent to tamponade the retinal breaks, preventing further passage of fluid through the breaks into the subretinal space until the chorioretinal scar from laser or cryopexy fully develops. Either gas (perfluoropropane, C_3F_8, or sulfur hexafluoride, SF_6) or silicone oil may be chosen for tamponade. The intraocular gas is slowly reabsorbed into the bloodstream and replaced with fluid produced by the ciliary body while the silicone oil remains in the eye until surgically removed at a later date.

During the postoperative period, the intraocular gas is readily depicted on CT by the presence of an air-fluid level within the globe (Fig. 7.13). On MRI, there is corresponding low signal intensity on T1- and T2-weighted sequences (Fig. 7.14). On ultrasound, the gas appears as echogenic foci with associated ring-down artifact (Fig. 7.15). The intraocular gas is gradually reabsorbed into the bloodstream and the space it occupied becomes fluid-filled.

7.4   Intraocular Silicone Oil

The presence of silicone oil can impede sonographic evaluation. Therefore, CT or MRI may be required to evaluate the orbital contents in such cases. Alternatively, intraocular silicone oil may be encountered incidentally on imaging of the orbits or brain performed for unrelated reasons.

Intraocular silicone oil has unique imaging characteristics. On CT, the substance demonstrates high attenuation, typically 80–130 HU, depending upon the preparation (Fig. 7.16). On MRI, the appearance of silicone oil is

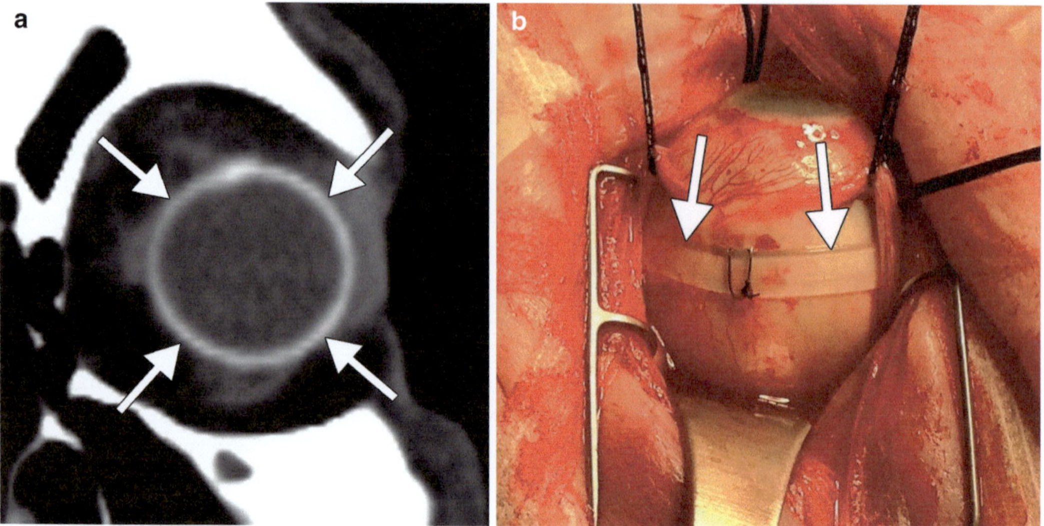

Fig. 7.7 Silicone rubber scleral buckle depicted on CT and intraoperatively. Coronal (**a**) CT image shows the hyperattenuating implant encircling the globe (*arrows*). Intraoperative photograph (**b**) shows a scleral buckle in situ (*arrows*)

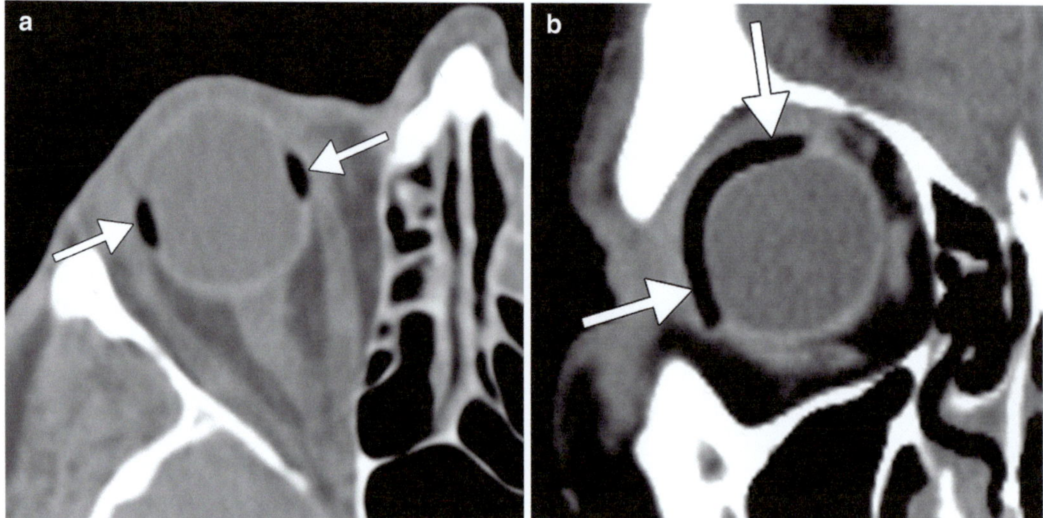

Fig. 7.8 Encircling and segmental silicone sponge scleral buckles depicted on CT. Axial CT image (**a**) shows the low attenuation device encircling the scleral buckle that mildly indents the right globe (*arrows*). Axial CT image in a different patient (**b**) shows the low-attenuation segmental device partially encircles the temporal aspect of the right globe (*arrows*)

variable, usually appearing as intermediate signal on T1-weighted sequences and as high signal on T2-weighted sequences, with no internal enhancement (Fig. 7.17). Consequently, the imaging features can mimic hemorrhage. However, the presence of chemical shift artifact, which manifests as bright and dark bands at the margins of the silicone oil, is helpful for differentiating silicone oil from hemorrhage. Elimination of the chemical shift artifact on MRI can be

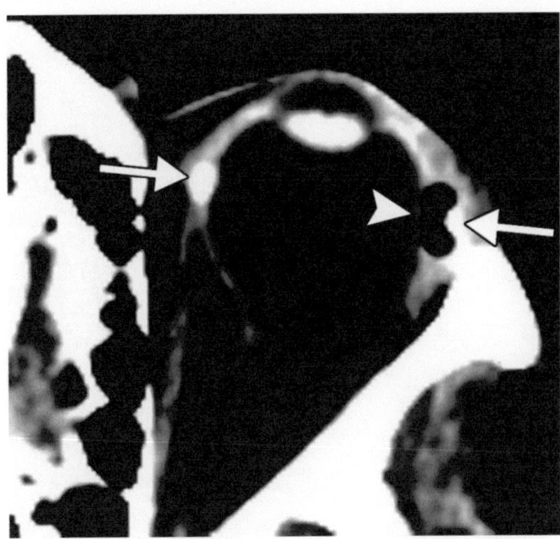

Fig. 7.9 Combined encircling silicone rubber and segmental silicone sponge scleral buckles depicted on CT. Axial CT image shows a thin high attenuation band that encircles the right globe (*arrow*) and a thicker high-attenuation buckle along the superomedial quadrant of the right globe (*arrowhead*)

achieved with selective saturation of the silicone resonance, which can otherwise improve evaluation of the globe.

There are several complications related to instillation of intraocular silicone oil, including emulsification and migration. Emulsification consists of droplets that form between the oil and the intraocular fluids or at the surface of the ocular tissues. On ultrasound, the vitreous body can appear "dirty" with scattered foci of echogenicity and acoustic shadowing (Fig. 7.18). On cross-sectional imaging, larger fragmented droplets can be discerned (Fig. 7.19), and knowledge of this occurrence is important for complete removal of the oil. Droplets of silicone oil can migrate into the angle and may induce secondary glaucoma, particularly if emulsified, by obstruction of the trabecular meshwork. The responsible silicone oil droplets are best delineated using high-resolution imaging, such as optical coherence tomography (OCT) (Fig. 7.20). Chronic intraocular pressure elevation occurs in approximately 10 % of cases treated with intraocular silicone oil. The presence of silicone oil in the anterior chamber can also result in corneal

edema and opacification if there is prolonged contact with the corneal endothelium. Rarely, silicone oil can also track into the optic nerve sheath and even extend into the ventricular system (Fig. 7.21).

7.5 Perfluoro-N-Octane

Perfluoro-N-octane (PFO) is a perfluorocarbon liquid that is used in many cases of complex retinal detachment repair. Since PFO is a dense, heavy liquid, it is useful to stabilize the retina and "push out" subretinal fluid. The PFO is removed before the end of the procedure since long term it has ocular toxicity. However, it is not uncommon that some small amount of PFO remains after the procedure and may be encountered on imaging. On CT, PFO appears hyperattenuating (approximately 500 HU) and may have a corrugated or bubbly surface. On MRI, PFO appears as low signal intensity on both T1- and T2-weighted sequences (Fig. 7.22). The PFO layers dependently in the globe upon which other materials, such as silicone oil, may float.

7.6 Intraocular Implants

In the past, a ganciclovir implant was used to treat CMV retinitis in HIV-positive patients. Currently, the two most common implants are Ozurdex (dexamethasone intravitreal implant, Allergan) and Retisert (fluocinolone acetonide intravitreal implant, Bausch and Lomb). Ozurdex is approved to treat macular edema from central retinal vein occlusions and branch retinal vein occlusions as well as noninfectious uveitis. It is injected into the vitreous cavity in an office procedure using an insertion device. Retisert is approved to treat chronic noninfectious uveitis. It is implanted into the eye in the operating room and sutured to the inside wall of the eye through the pars plana. Complications of both implants include steroid-associated glaucoma, development of cataract in phakic patients, and migration of the implant (Fig. 7.23).

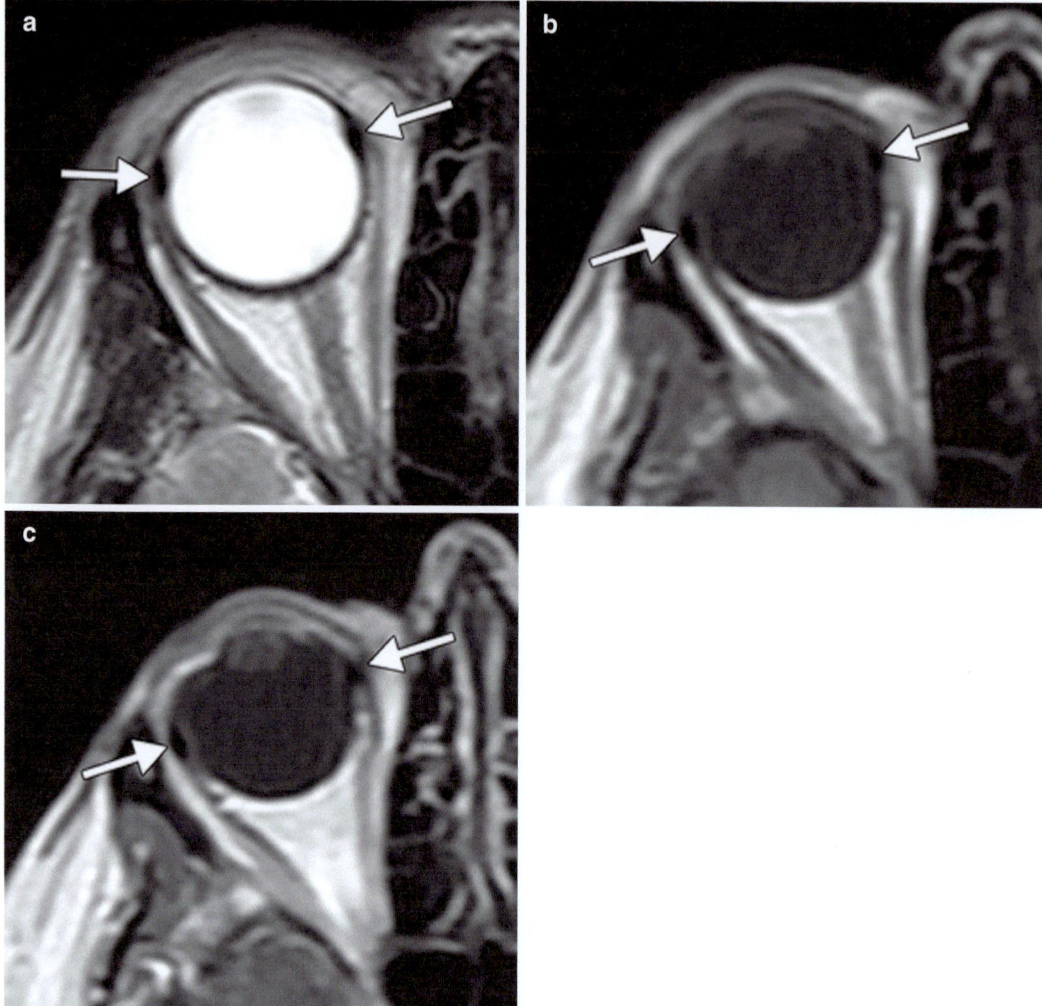

Fig. 7.10 Encircling silicone scleral buckle depicted on MRI. Axial T2-weighted (**a**), T1-weighted (**b**), and post-contrast T1-weighted (**c**) MR images show the non-enhancing hypointense scleral buckle encircling the right globe (*arrows*)

7.7 Globe Rupture Repair

Traumatic globe rupture is an ophthalmological emergency. The goals of primary repair are to repair the wound in a watertight manner to restore globe integrity, remove contaminated and nonviable tissue, remove foreign bodies, and prevent an infection from developing. Initial surgery for globe rupture essentially consists of exploring the globe to determine the location and extent of the lacerations, repositioning prolapsed intraocular tissue, removing foreign bodies, and suturing the wounds. It is essential to obtain a preoperative CT scan to evaluate for the presence of an intraocular foreign body in all cases of globe rupture. A plain film is not sufficient to definitively exclude the presence of a foreign body. CT may be acquired after globe repair to document adequate removal of foreign bodies and to evaluate for post-traumatic or postoperative complications. Otherwise, restoration of the globe volume and contours may be incidentally appreciated (Fig. 7.24). The lens may be unapparent due to traumatic expulsion. Although B-scan ultrasound is rarely used preoperatively in the setting of an open-globe injury (due to the risk of expulsion of intraocular

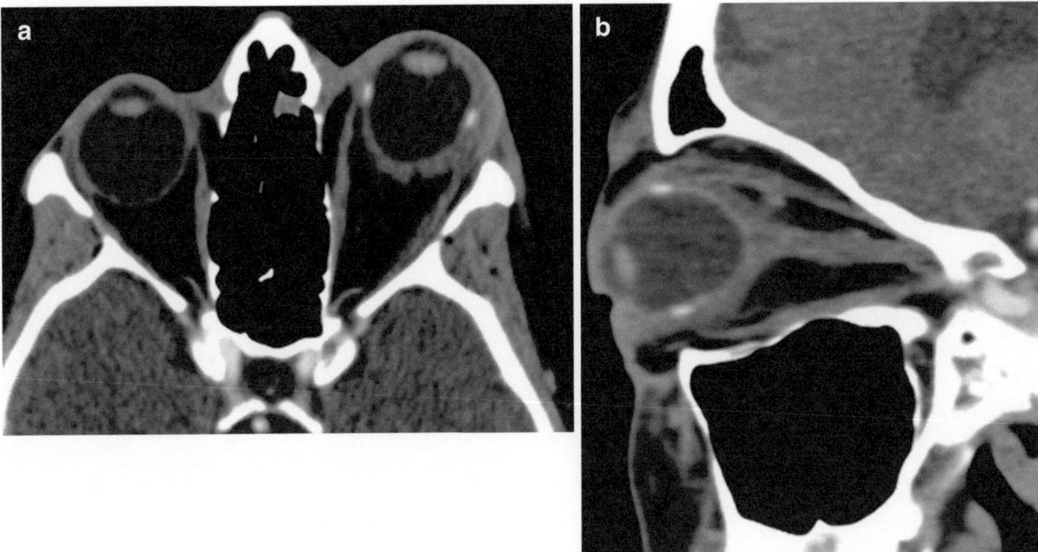

Fig. 7.11 Infected scleral buckle depicted on CT. Axial (**a**) and sagittal (**b**) CT images show proptosis of the left globe with preseptal edema and scleral thickening associated with a hyperattenuating left silicone scleral buckle

contents), it is a routine diagnostic tool after globe repair, particularly for evaluating potential complications, such as vitreous hemorrhage and retinal or choroidal detachment (Fig. 7.25).

7.8   Summary

- Diagnostic imaging is particularly useful in cases of media opacity when direct visualization of the ocular fundus is otherwise obscured.
- Multiple modalities, including CT, MRI, and ultrasound can be exploited, each with its advantages and disadvantages.
- It is important to be familiar with the variety of devices used to treat retinal diseases that can be identified on diagnostic imaging and their potential complications in order to optimize patient management.

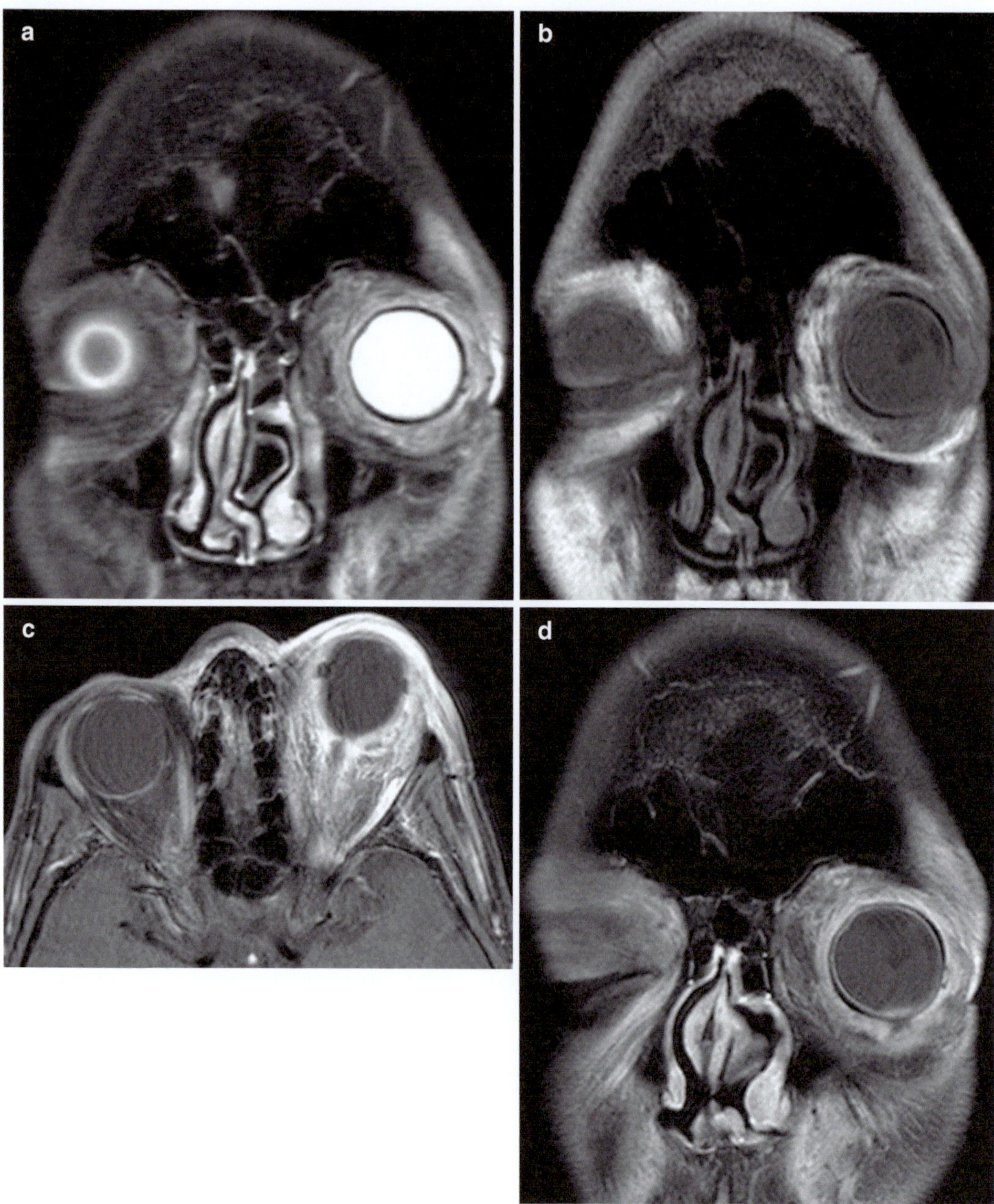

Fig. 7.12 Infected scleral buckle depicted on MRI. Coronal T2-weighted (**a**), coronal T1-weighted (**b**), and axial (**c**) and coronal (**d**) fat-suppressed T1-weighted MR images show proptosis with preseptal and postseptal inflammatory changes in the left orbit, particularly surrounding the scleral implant, which is hypointense on all sequences

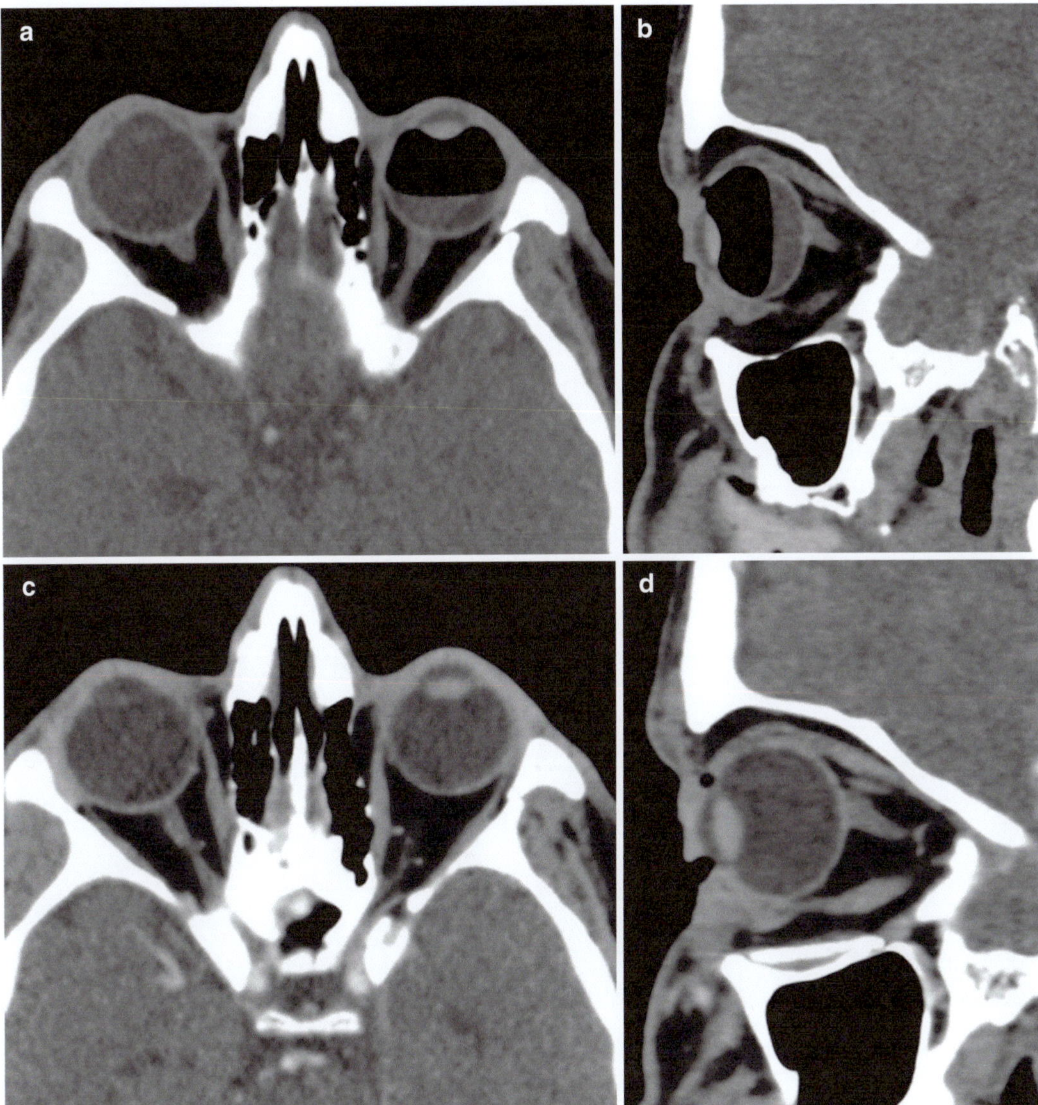

Fig. 7.13 Intraocular gas depicted on CT. Initial postoperative axial (**a**) and sagittal (**b**) CT images show a gas-fluid level within the left globe. Follow-up axial (**c**) and sagittal (**d**) CT images show the globe is now filled with fluid

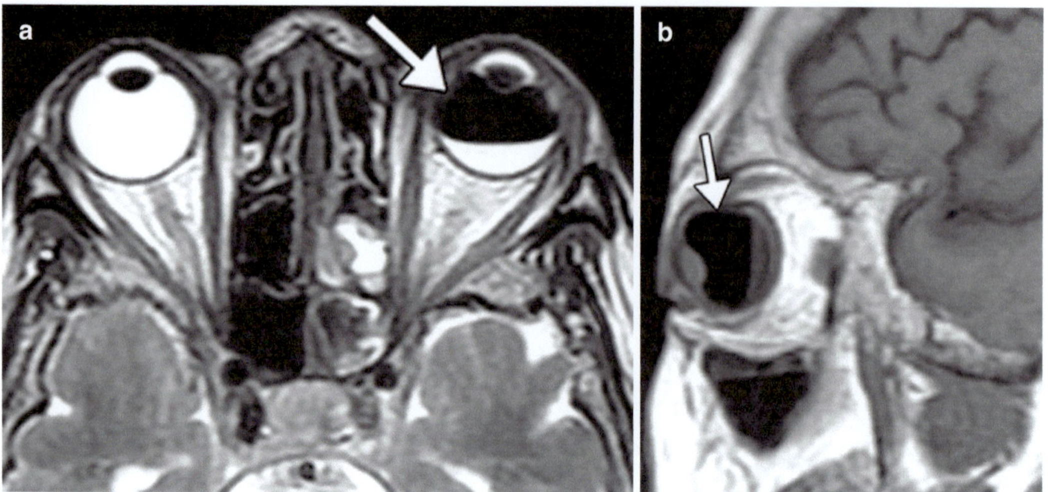

Fig. 7.14 Intraocular gas depicted on MRI. Axial T2-weighted (**a**) and sagittal T1-weighted (**b**) MR images show an anti-dependent signal void within the left globe (*arrows*), which represents the gas

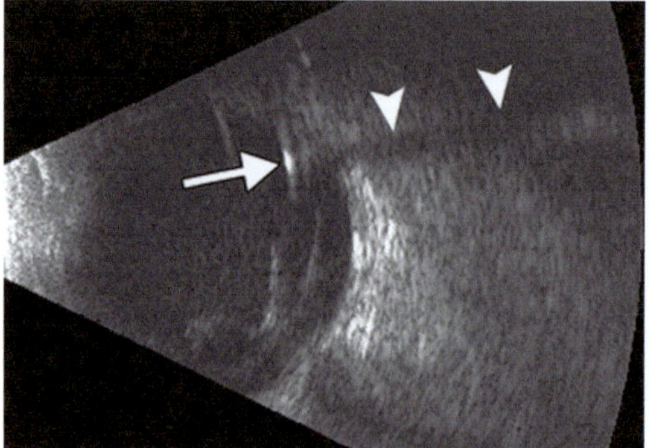

Fig. 7.15 Residual intraocular gas tamponade depicted on ultrasound. B-mode ultrasound image shows a hyper-echoic focus (*arrow*) with associated ring-down artifact and acoustic shadowing (*arrowheads*), resulting from a residual bubble of gas (Courtesy of Karen Capaccioli and Lois Hart)

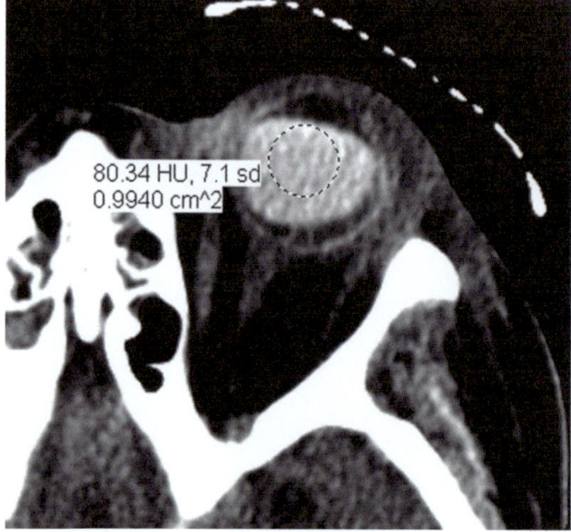

Fig. 7.16 Intraocular silicone oil depicted on CT. Axial CT image shows globular hyperattenuating material within the posterior left globe (ROI with 80 HU), which floats upon the residual vitreous humor. The intraocular lens is absent and the silicone oil is not present within the anterior chamber due to the residual capsular bag, which prevents migration of the silicone oil

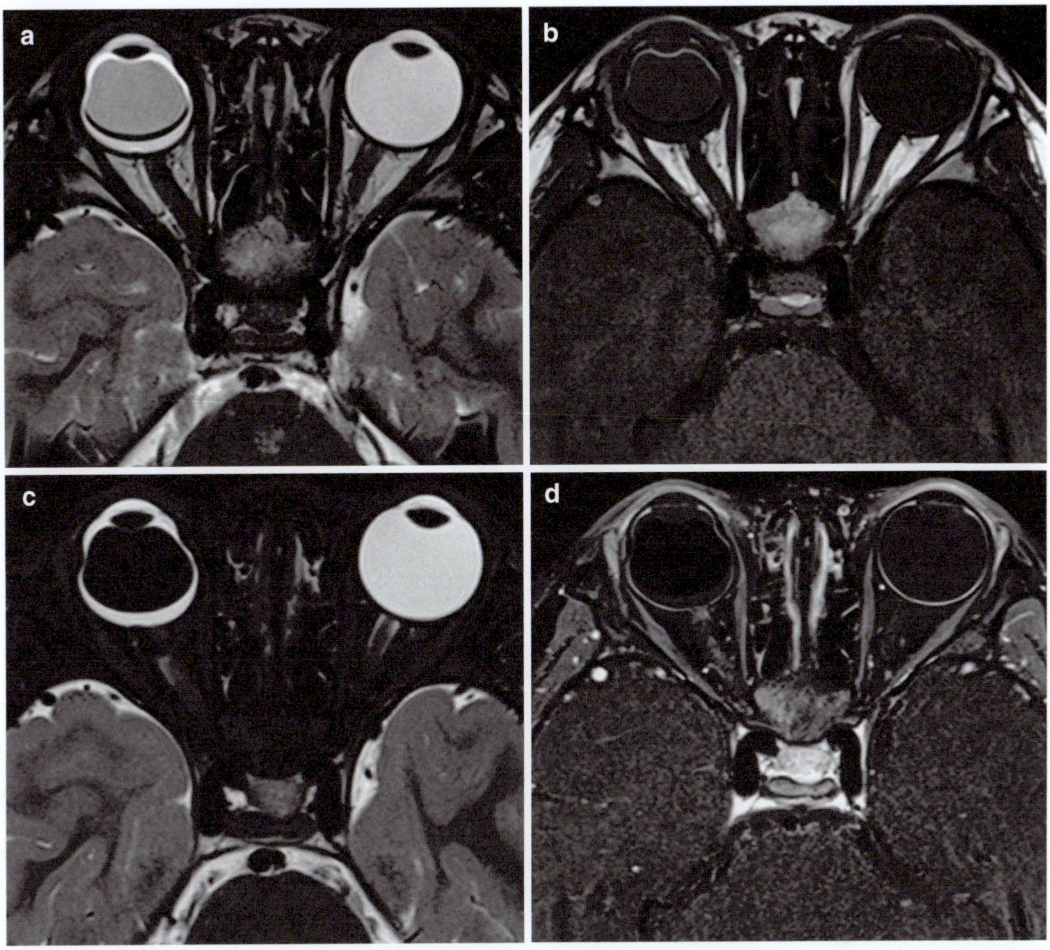

Fig. 7.17 Intraocular silicone oil depicted on MRI. Axial T2-weighted (**a**), axial T1-weighted (**b**), axial fat-suppressed T2-weighted (**c**), and axial post-contrast fat-suppressed T1-weighted (**d**) MR images show that the silicone oil within the vitreous chamber of the right globe displays high T2 signal, intermediate T1 signal, and chemical shift artifact and signal dropout with fat suppression. A scleral buckle is also present on the right eye (Courtesy of Sanjay Prabhu MD)

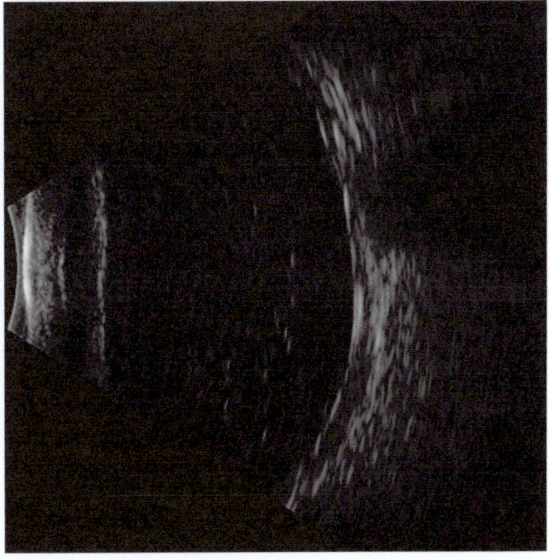

Fig. 7.18 Emulsified silicone oil depicted on sonography. B-scan ultrasound image of the globe shows numerous scattered foci of hyperechogenicity with acoustic shadowing (Courtesy of Karen Capaccioli and Lois Hart)

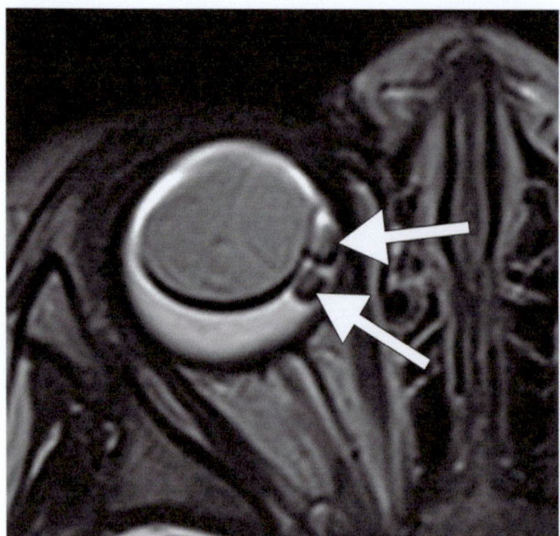

Fig. 7.19 Fragmented silicone oil droplets depicted on MRI. Axial T2 MRI shows droplets of silicone oil (*arrows*) that have separated from the main collection

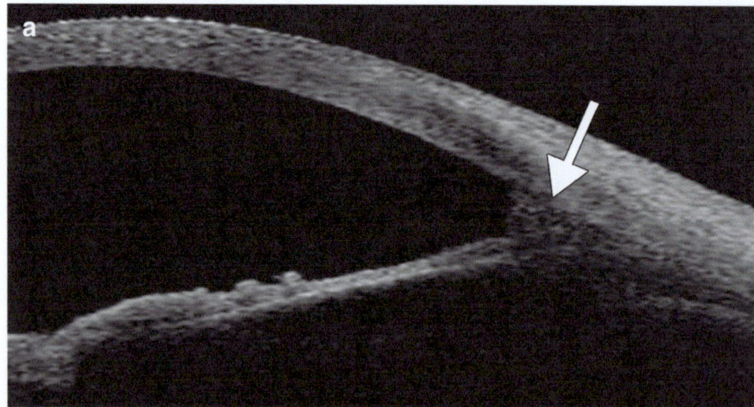

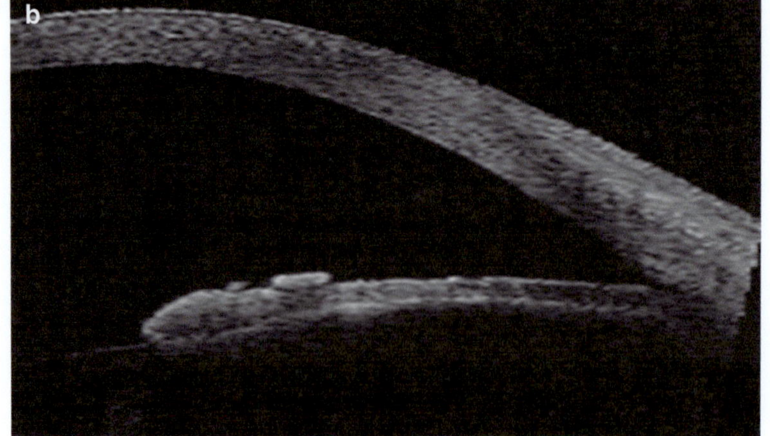

Fig. 7.20 Silicone oil migration into the anterior chamber with secondary glaucoma. The patient has a history of pars plana vitrectomy with silicone oil injection and developed secondary open-angle glaucoma due to silicone oil clogging the trabecular meshwork. Anterior segment OCT (**a**) shows silicone oil in the superior angle (*arrow*). Normal anterior segment OCT (**b**) for comparison (Courtesy of Lili Farrokh-Siar MD and Fatoumata Yanoga MD)

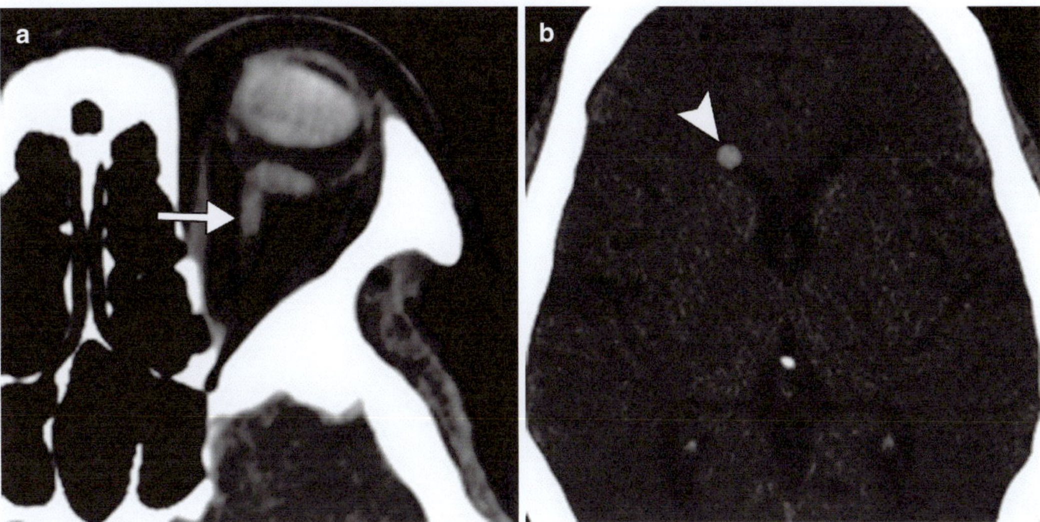

Fig. 7.21 Silicone oil migration into the optic nerve sheath and ventricular system. Axial CT images (**a**, **b**) show silicone in the left eye with extension along the optic nerve (*arrow*) and in the nondependent portion of the lateral ventricle (*arrowhead*) (Adapted with permission from Chang et al. (2013))

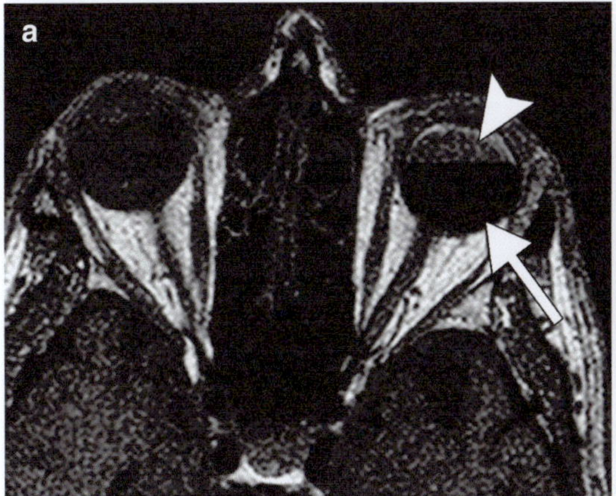
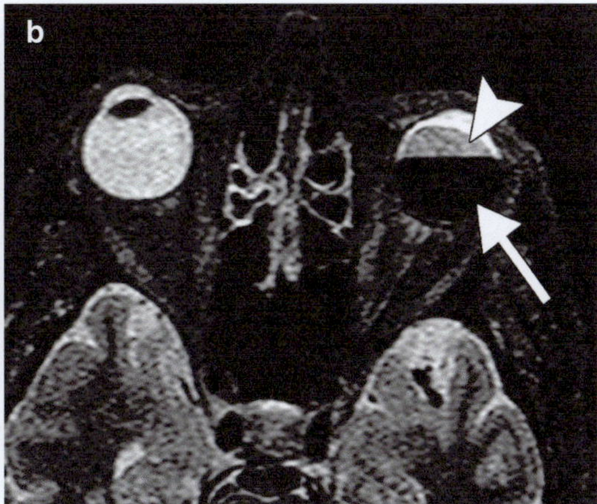

Fig. 7.22 Intraocular PFO depicted on MRI. Axial T1 (**a**) and fat-suppressed T2 (**b**) MR images show the hypointense PFO layering dependently within the left globe (*arrows*). Silicone oil is also present in the left globe, which floats upon the PFO (*arrowheads*) (Courtesy of John Christoforidis MD)

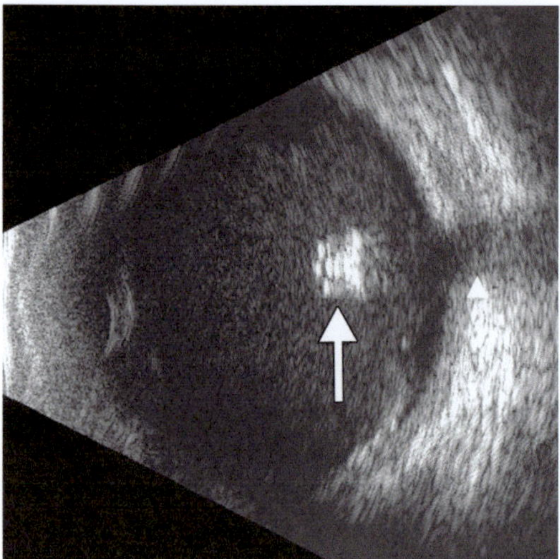

Fig. 7.23 Dislocated Retisert. B-mode ultrasound shows a dislocated Retisert pellet (*arrow*) in the vitreous chamber

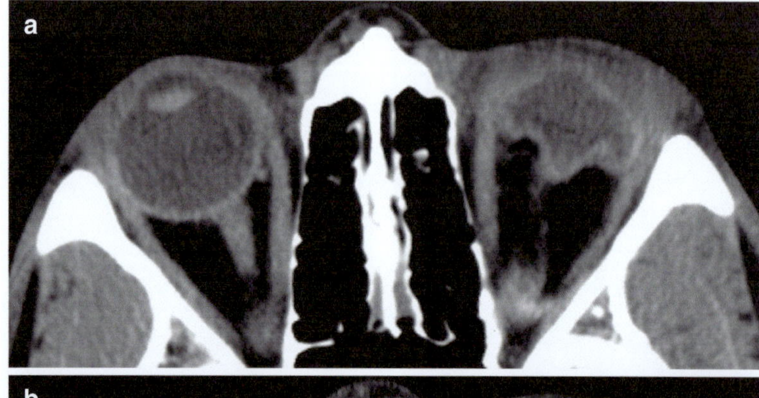

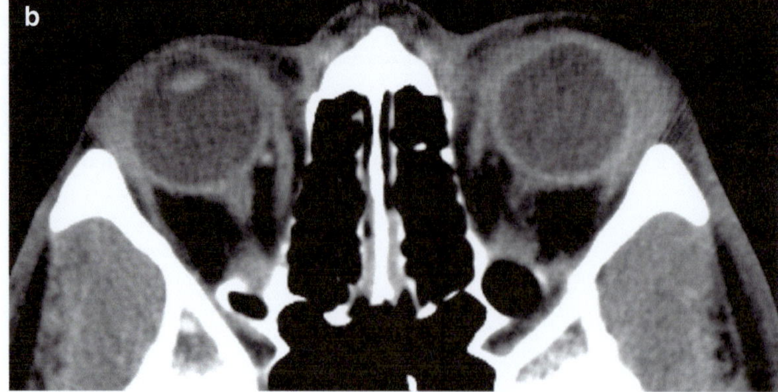

Fig. 7.24 Ruptured globe repair. The patient sustained a globe laceration from blunt trauma to the left eye. Preoperative axial CT image (**a**) shows severe contour deformity of the left globe with a "flat tire" sign and no discernable lens, presumably due to a lens expulsion. Postoperative axial CT image (**b**) obtained a few days later for suspected orbital cellulitis shows normalization of the left globe contour

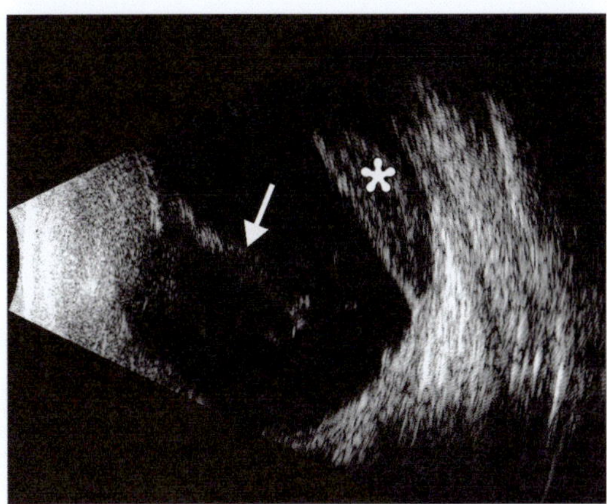

Fig. 7.25 Vitreous hemorrhage and hemorrhagic choroidal detachment after traumatic ruptured globe repair. B-mode ultrasound demonstrates linear hyperechogenicity with in the globe (*arrow*) corresponding to vitreous hemorrhage and echogenic material posterior to the displaced choroid (*) corresponding to hemorrhagic choroidal detachment

Further Reading

Acar N, Unver YB, Altan T, Kapran Z. Acute endophthalmitis after 25-gauge sutureless vitrectomy. Int Ophthalmol. 2007;27(6):361–3. Epub 2007 May 11.

Adelman RA, Parnes AJ, Sipperley JO, Ducournau D, European Vitreo-Retinal Society (EVRS) Retinal Detachment Study Group. Strategy for the management of complex retinal detachments: the European vitreo-retinal society retinal detachment study report 2. Ophthalmology. 2013;120(9):1809–13.

Akduman L, Cetin EN, Levy J, Becker MD, Mackensen F, Lim LL. Spontaneous dissociation and dislocation of Retisert pellet. Ocul Immunol Inflamm. 2013;21(1):87–9.

Al-Jazzaf AM, Netland PA, Charles S. Incidence and management of elevated intraocular pressure after silicone oil injection. J Glaucoma. 2005;14(1):40–6.

Andreoli MT, Yiu G, Hart L, Andreoli CM. B-scan ultrasonography following open globe repair. Eye (Lond). 2014;28(4):381–5.

Bernardino CR, Mihora LD, Fay AM, Rubin PA. Orbital complications of hydrogel scleral buckles. Ophthal Plast Reconstr Surg. 2006;22(3):206–8.

Budenz DL, Taba KE, Feuer WJ, Eliezer R, Cousins S, Henderer J, Flynn Jr HW. Surgical management of secondary glaucoma after pars plana vitrectomy and silicone oil injection for complex retinal detachment. Ophthalmology. 2001;108(9):1628–32.

Chan CK, Lin SG, Nuthi AS, Salib DM. Pneumatic retinopexy for the repair of retinal detachments: a comprehensive review (1986–2007). Surv Ophthalmol. 2008;53(5):443–78.

Chang CC, Chang HS, Toh CH. Intraventricular silicone oil. J Neurosurg. 2013;118(5):1127–9.

Ginat DT, Singh AD, Moonis G. Multimodality imaging of hydrogel scleral buckles. Retina. 2012;32(8):1449–52.

Herrick RC, Hayman LA, Maturi RK, Diaz-Marchan PJ, Tang RA, Lambert HM. Optimal imaging protocol after intraocular silicone oil tamponade. AJNR Am J Neuroradiol. 1998;19(1):101–8.

Honavar SG, Goyal M, Majji AB, Sen PK, Naduvilath T, Dandona L. Glaucoma after pars plana vitrectomy and silicone oil injection for complicated retinal detachments. Ophthalmology. 1999;106(1):169–76; discussion 177.

Kiilgaard JF, Milea D, Løgager V, la Cour M. Cerebral migration of intraocular silicone oil: an MRI study. Acta Ophthalmol. 2011;89(6):522–5.

Lambiase A, Abdolrahimzadeh S, Recupero SM. An update on intravitreal implants in use for eye disorders. Drugs Today (Barc). 2014;50(3):239–49.

Lane JI, Watson Jr RE, Witte RJ, McCannel CA. Retinal detachment: imaging of surgical treatments and complications. Radiographics. 2003;23(4):983–94.

Mansour AM, Han DP, Kim JE, Uwaydat SH, Sibai A, Medawar WA, Li HK, Rjeily JA, Salti HI, Bashshur Z, Hourani M. Radiologic findings in infected and noninfected scleral buckles. Eur J Ophthalmol. 2007;17(5):804–11.

Mathews VP, Elster AD, Barker PB, Buff BL, Haller JA, Greven CM. Intraocular silicone oil: in vitro and in vivo MR and CT characteristics. AJNR Am J Neuroradiol. 1994;15(2):343–7.

Nazemi PP, Chong LP, Varma R, Burnstine MA. Migration of intraocular silicone oil into the subconjunctival space and orbit through an Ahmed glaucoma valve. Am J Ophthalmol. 2001;132(6):929–31.

Nemet AY, Ferencz JR, Segal O, Meshi A. Orbital cellulitis following silicone-sponge scleral buckles. Clin Ophthalmol. 2013;7:2147–52.

Nguyen QD, Lashkari K, Hirose T, Pruett RC, McMeel JW, Schepens CL. Erosion and intrusion of silicone rubber scleral buckle. Presentation and management. Retina. 2001;21(3):214–20.

Oshitari K, Hida T, Okada AA, Hirakata A. Long-term complications of hydrogel buckles. Retina. 2003;23(2):257–61.

Sallam A, Taylor SR, Lightman S. Review and update of intraocular therapy in noninfectious uveitis. Curr Opin Ophthalmol. 2011;22(6):517–22.

Shields CL, Demirci H, Marr BP, Mashayekhi A, Materin MA, Shields JA. Expanding MIRAgel scleral buckle simulating an orbital tumor in four cases. Ophthal Plast Reconstr Surg. 2005;21(1):32–8.

Uji A. Suprachoroidal gas injection as a complication of pars plana vitrectomy confirmed by computed tomography. Clin Ophthalmol. 2012;6:533–6.

Wirostko WJ, Han DP, Perkins SL. Complications of pneumatic retinopexy. Curr Opin Ophthalmol. 2000;11(3):195–200.

Yonekawa Y, Chodosh J, Eliott D. Surgical techniques in the management of perforating injuries of the globe. Int Ophthalmol Clin. 2013;53(4):127–37.

Zaidi AA, Alvarado R, Irvine A. Pneumatic retinopexy: success rate and complications. Br J Ophthalmol. 2006;90(4):427–8.

Imaging After Orbital and Intraocular Oncology Therapies

8

Jeffrey Bonham, Daniel Thomas Ginat, and Suzanne K. Freitag

8.1 Overview

A wide variety of benign and malignant neoplasms can affect the orbit, either primarily or secondarily, such as via extension of a tumor from a neighboring structure or as a metastasis. Likewise, there are a multitude of orbital oncological therapeutic modalities available, including surgery, chemotherapy, radiation, cryotherapy, and laser therapy. Diagnostic imaging plays an important role not only in the pretreatment evaluation of orbital region tumors but also for follow-up after treatment in order to monitor tumor response or recurrence. CT and MRI are generally suitable modalities for posttreatment surveillance of the orbit. Positron emission tomography (PET) using [18 F]-2-deoxy-D-glucose (18FDG) serves a role as a staging tool in ophthalmic oncology, particularly for detecting distant metastatic lesions that conventional imaging studies may otherwise miss. Besides the initial workup of orbital tumors, 18FDG-PET can be useful for the assessment of treatment response. Ultrasound with color and spectral Doppler is useful for evaluating small intraocular tumors that are otherwise inconspicuous on CT and MRI. The interpretation of posttreatment imaging can be particularly challenging due to the altered anatomy and tissue properties caused by many forms of treatment. Furthermore, many oncological treatments can cause complications that warrant investigation via diagnostic imaging. Some of these complications have particularly characteristic and interesting imaging findings. In order to optimally approach an imaging study of the orbit after treatment, it is important to know what the original tumor was like, the type and timing of the therapy that was administered, and the clinical status of the patient at the time of the scan. The various types of orbital oncologic treatments and their corresponding expected and complicated imaging features are reviewed in the following sections.

J. Bonham, MD
Department of Radiology, University of Chicago,
5841 S Maryland Avenue, Chicago, IL 60637, USA

D.T. Ginat, MD, MS (✉)
Director of Head and Neck Imaging,
Department of Radiology, University of Chicago,
5841 S Maryland Avenue, Chicago, IL 60637, USA

S.K. Freitag, MD
Director, Ophthalmic Plastic Surgery Service,
Department of Ophthalmology, Massachusetts Eye
and Ear Infirmary, Harvard Medical School,
Boston, MA, USA

8.2 Intraocular Biopsy

Biopsy is often performed for the diagnosis of orbital masses. Incisional biopsy, which involves sampling a small portion of a lesion, may be useful when a tissue diagnosis is desired, but the lesion is infiltrative and cannot be separated from surrounding structures. Excisional biopsy consists of removing the tumor in its entirety and

D.T. Ginat, S.K. Freitag (eds.), *Post-treatment Imaging of the Orbit*,
DOI 10.1007/978-3-662-44023-0_8, © Springer-Verlag Berlin Heidelberg 2015

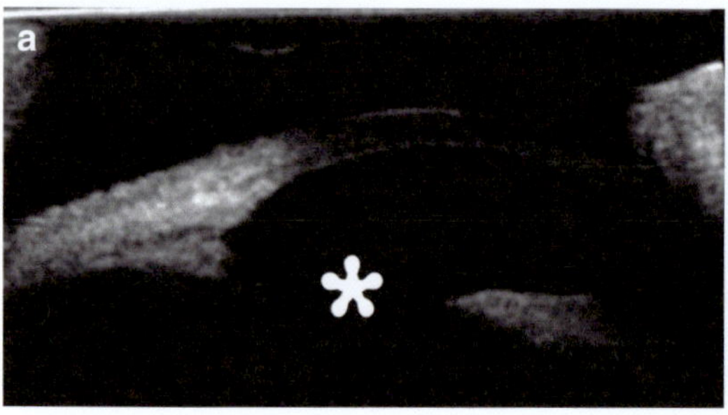
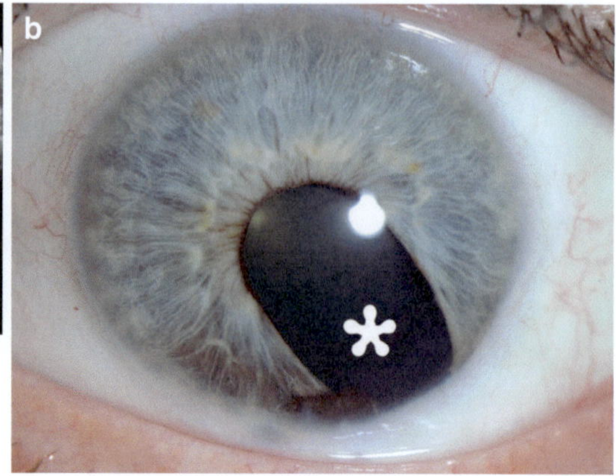

Fig. 8.1 Excisional biopsy of an anterior segment tumor. The patient has a history of iris melanoma excised many years earlier. UBM (**a**) and corresponding clinical photo-graph (**b**) show a defect in the iris and ciliary body (*) (Courtesy of Ivana Kim MD)

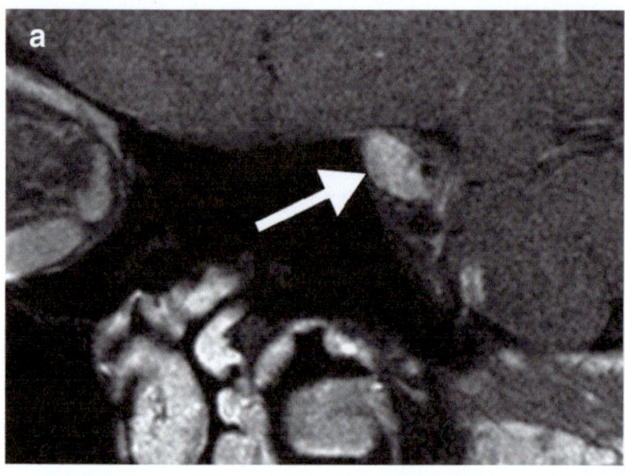
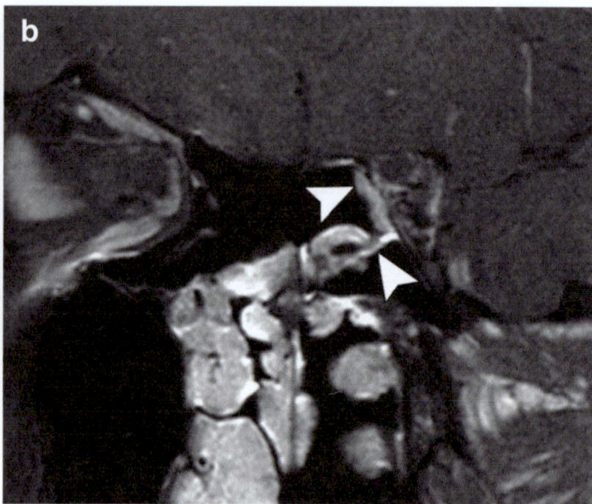

Fig. 8.2 Nasoseptal flap. The patient presented with left optic neuropathy due to a cavernous hemangioma in the orbital apex and underwent excisional biopsy via a transnasal endoscopic technique with access through the medial wall of the orbit. Due to the risk of postoperative enophthalmos, the medial wall of the orbit has been reconstructed with a vascularized pedicle flap from the mucosa of the nasal septum. Preoperative coronal post-contrast, fat-suppressed T1-weighted MRI (**a**) shows a well-defined enhancing lesion in the left orbital apex (*arrow*). Postoperative coronal post-contrast, fat-suppressed T1-weighted MRI (**b**) shows linear enhancement along the medial wall of the orbital apex extending from the nasal septum, which corresponds to the transposed mucosal flap (*arrowheads*). The mucosal flap enhances avidly similar to the preoperative appearance of the tumor. However, there was no evidence of residual tumor (postoperative imaging was obtained to confirm complete tumor resection)

is both diagnostic and therapeutic. Aside from absence of the lesion, complete excisional biopsy may leave no changes on postoperative imaging. However, there may be perceptible defects in normal anatomic structures that were removed along with the tumor (Fig. 8.1). In addition, there may be alterations in the structures remaining in the region of the excision due to reconstructive efforts. For example, a vascularized nasoseptal mucosal flap used to reconstruct a medial orbital wall defect created during endoscopic transnasal orbitotomy can demonstrate avid enhancement on MRI (Fig. 8.2), potentially mimicking residual tumor. However, the flap has a distinctive linear configuration with a connection to the nasal septum.

Complications related to orbital biopsy that may lead to imaging evaluation are uncommon and include infection, hemorrhage, visual loss, diplopia, and CSF leak. CT and MRI are both

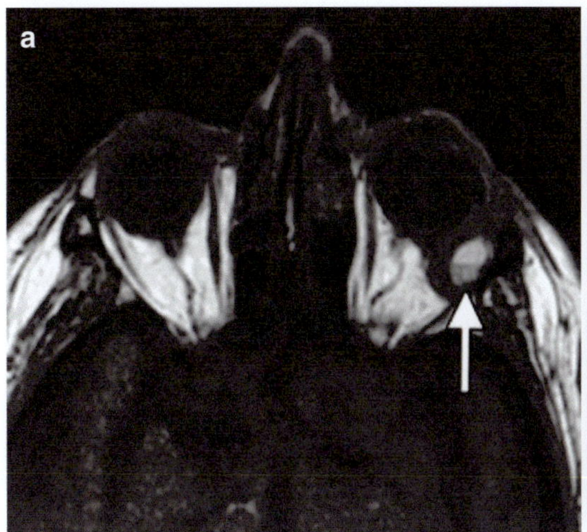
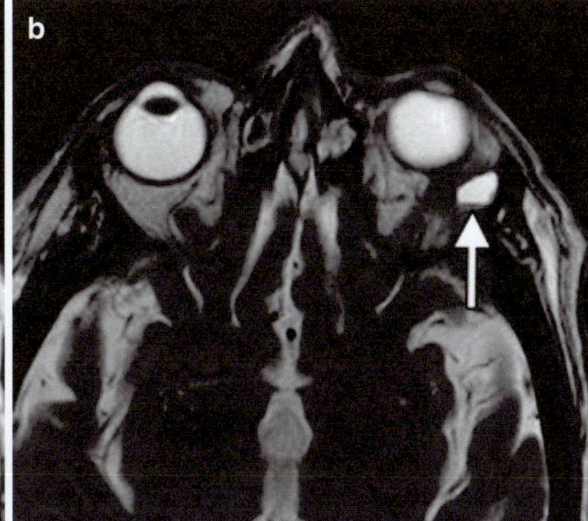

Fig. 8.3 Post-biopsy hemorrhage. The patient underwent recent left anterolateral orbitotomy for biopsy of a left orbital tumor. Axial T1-weighted (**a**) and T2-weighted (**b**) MR images show a fluid-fluid level within the left orbital mass (*arrows*)

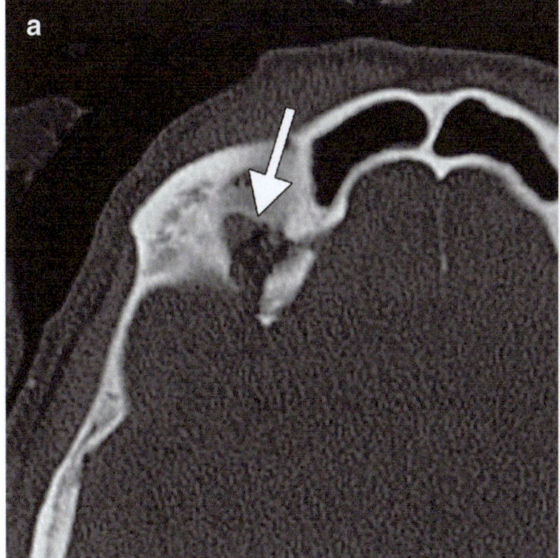
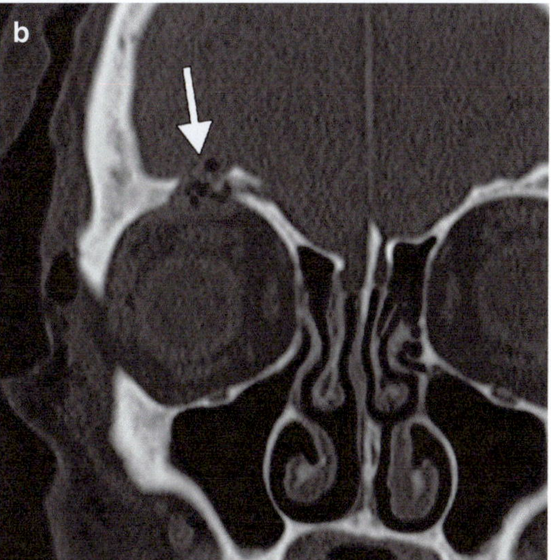

Fig. 8.4 Post-biopsy CSF leak. The patient underwent recent orbital tumor biopsy. Axial (**a**) and coronal (**b**) CT images show a defect in the right orbital roof and a small amount of pneumocephalus (*arrows*). The biopsy was performed to evaluate for perineural tumor spread involving the supraorbital nerve

appropriate modalities for evaluating postoperative infection, which can manifest as preseptal and/or postseptal cellulitis, with or without abscess. Hemorrhage can occur anywhere along the path of the biopsy, including within or adjacent to the remaining portions of the biopsied tumor, which can result in transient expansion of the mass. Noncontrast CT and MRI are suitable for the evaluation of post-biopsy hemorrhage, in order to characterize the extent and site of hemorrhage. There can be an acute change in the appearance of the tumor if it has hemorrhaged, which can manifest with fluid-fluid levels on CT or MRI (Fig. 8.3). Disruption of the orbital roof during a biopsy can lead to a CSF leak, which can manifest as an accumulation of fluid within the orbit and pneumocephalus. Thin-section, multiplanar CT without contrast is useful for delineating the defect and planning surgical repair, if necessary (Fig. 8.4). Alternatively, an encephalocele can form through the iatrogenic defect and MRI is useful for characterizing this entity prior to surgical repair.

8.3   Enucleation

Enucleation refers to removal of the eye. The main oncological indications for enucleation include uveal melanoma, retinoblastoma, or other less common intraocular tumors that are large, recurrent, or poorly responsive to treatment. The extraocular muscles are disinserted from the globe prior to its removal from the socket. The muscles may be reattached to the orbital implant in a variety of ways, including suturing muscle to muscle in front of the implant, suturing the muscle directly to the implant, or suturing the muscle to the material used to wrap the implant. The void created by removing the globe is typically filled with an orbital implant (Fig. 8.5). The most commonly used implants are composed of silicone, hydroxyapatite, and porous polyethylene (Medpor). The imaging features of the various implant materials are discussed and depicted in extensive detail in Chap. 5. However, notably, certain implants, such as Medpor, can demonstrate internal enhancement due to fibrovascular ingrowth, which should not be mistaken for tumor involvement (Fig. 8.6). Furthermore, in the early postoperative period,

enhancement and T2 hyperintensity of the orbital tissues are expected findings (Fig. 8.7) and may represent granulation tissue or a transient inflammation. Although this is a characteristically diffuse process, it can be difficult to discern an underlying tumor, and follow-up imaging is recommended if there is any doubt. Despite the potential artifacts, MRI with contrast is generally the best modality for surveillance imaging after enucleation for retinoblastoma in order to delineate local and regional tumor recurrence, trilateral retinoblastoma, as well as distant metastases to the spine. In addition, intraocular melanoma has a particular propensity to metastasize to the liver (95 % of metastases) and occasionally to the brain (Fig. 8.8). Contrast-enhanced CT and 18FDG-PET are also appropriate imaging modalities for metastatic workup in the bones, chest, and abdomen, depending upon the type of primary tumor and location of the suspected metastasis. For example, melanoma and squamous cell carcinoma tend to be markedly hypermetabolic on 18FDG-PET, unless there is considerable necrosis, while adenoid cystic carcinoma tends to not be so conspicuous. A potential pitfall on 18FDG-PET

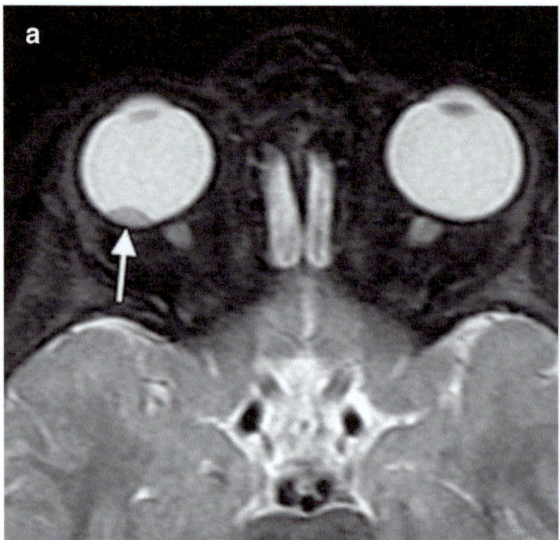
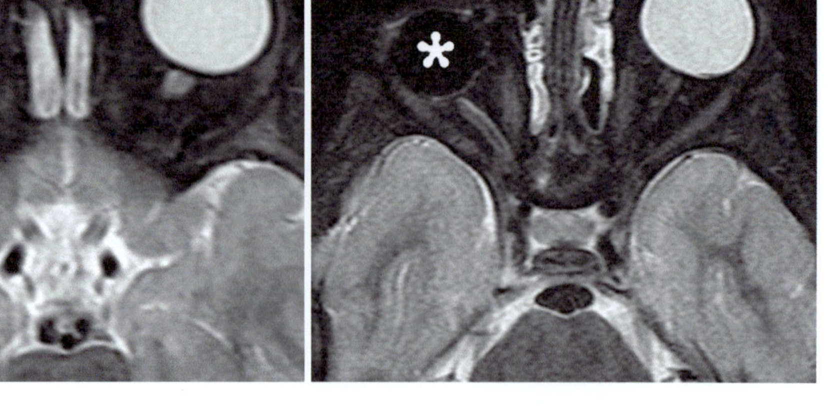

Fig. 8.5 Enucleation. Preoperative axial fat-suppressed T2-weighted MRI (**a**) shows a right intraocular mass, consistent with retinoblastoma (*arrow*). Postoperative axial fat-suppressed T2-weighted MRI (**b**) shows interval removal of the right globe and insertion of a silicone implant (*). Much of the right optic nerve remains

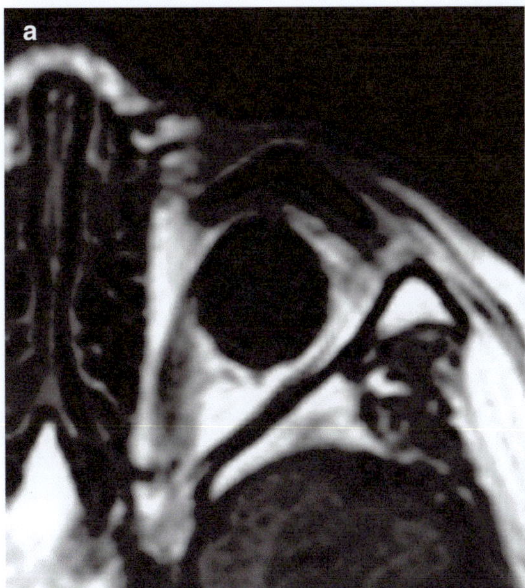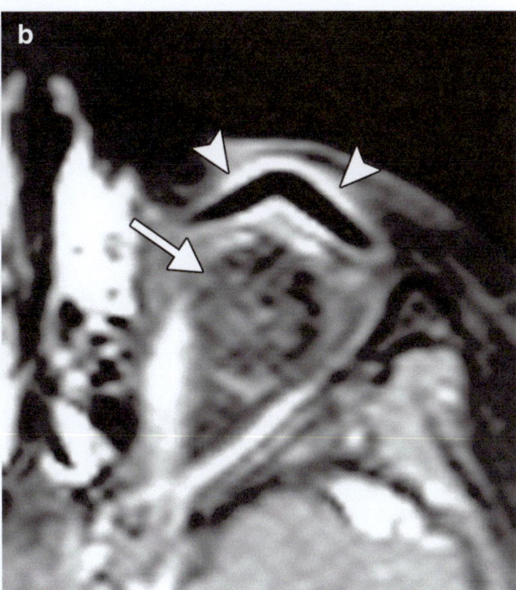

Fig. 8.6 Porous polyethylene (Medpor) implant fibrovascular ingrowth and ocular prosthesis artifact. Axial T1-weighted (**a**) and axial post-contrast fat-suppressed T1-weighted (**b**) MR images show expected diffuse enhancement of the Medpor implant (*arrow*). There is also linear enhancement of the conjunctiva surrounding the ocular prosthesis (*arrowheads*)

is the presence of orbital implants. While silicone implants do not appear hypermetabolic on 18FDG-PET (Fig. 8.9), Medpor and hydroxyapatite implants with fibrovascular ingrowth can appear diffusely hypermetabolic (Fig. 8.10) due to physiologic activity. This should not be mistaken for neoplasm or infection, which tends to display a greater degree of hyperpigmentation in components beyond the implant itself.

Besides surveillance of tumor recurrence and metastases, diagnostic imaging is also useful for evaluating complications related to enucleation, which are depicted in Chap. 5. However, enucleation during infancy due to retinoblastoma or other causes can lead to the development of microorbitalism due to the decreased growth stimulation from the globe and surrounding soft tissues (orbital arrest syndrome). The ipsilateral maxillary sinus is frequently hypoplastic as well. High-resolution multiplanar facial bone CT imaging (Fig. 8.11) is useful for characterizing the abnormalities and for corrective surgical planning, which may consist of osteotomy and expansion of the orbital vault.

8.4 Exenteration

Exenteration involves removal of the orbital contents, including the globe and varying amounts of periorbital tissue. Exenteration is a radically disfiguring procedure that is most often reserved for the treatment of life-threatening malignancies arising from the orbit, paranasal sinuses, or periocular skin. The most common diagnoses requiring orbital exenteration include basal cell carcinoma, sebaceous carcinoma, squamous cell carcinoma, melanoma, and lacrimal gland malignancies. There are various classifications of exenteration surgery based on which tissues are removed. For example, Meyer and Zaoli's classification describes four types of exenteration. In type I, the palpebral skin and conjunctiva are spared. In type II, only the palpebral skin is spared and the globe and its appendages are removed with the conjunctiva. In type III, the eyelid is removed with the orbital contents. In type IV, the globe, eyelids, and appendages of the eye are removed with the involved bony

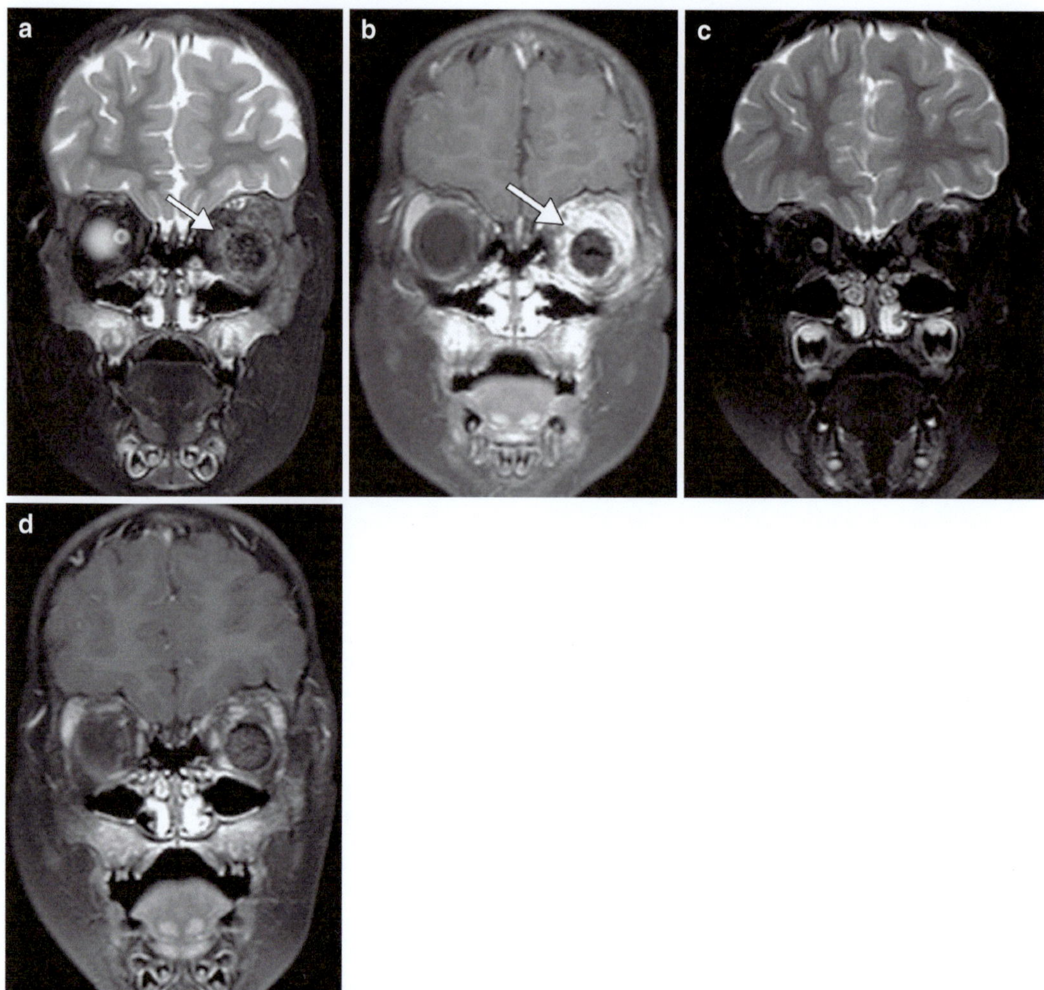

Fig. 8.7 Expected early postoperative findings related to enucleation. Initial postoperative coronal fat-suppressed T2-weighted (**a**) and post-contrast fat-suppressed T1-weighted (**b**) MR images show diffuse T2 hyperintensity and enhancement of the orbit surrounding the implant (*arrows*). The corresponding follow-up MR images obtained 6 months later (**c**, **d**) show near interval resolution of these findings, although there is persistent mild enhancement and swelling of the extraocular muscles. A Medpor implant is present

structures. Various methods for reconstruction of the exenteration cavity can be implemented, including partial- or full-thickness skin graft, dermis fat grafts, free or pedicled musculocutaneous flaps, and artificial implants (Figs. 8.12, 8.13, and 8.14). Of note, on postoperative MRI or CT imaging, the viable muscular portion of myocutaneous flaps normally displays enhancement, which should not be mistaken for tumor recurrence. Patients may wear an eye patch following surgery or have an ectoprosthesis that features the globe and eyelids, which are custom fit for cosmetic purposes. The prostheses can be made from a variety of materials, such as polymethyl methacrylate and silicone. These prostheses are retained with adhesives, tissue undercuts, or magnets once the socket has healed. The prosthesis is not always removed during diagnostic imaging exams of the region, which usually does not pose an issue with regard to artifacts since the

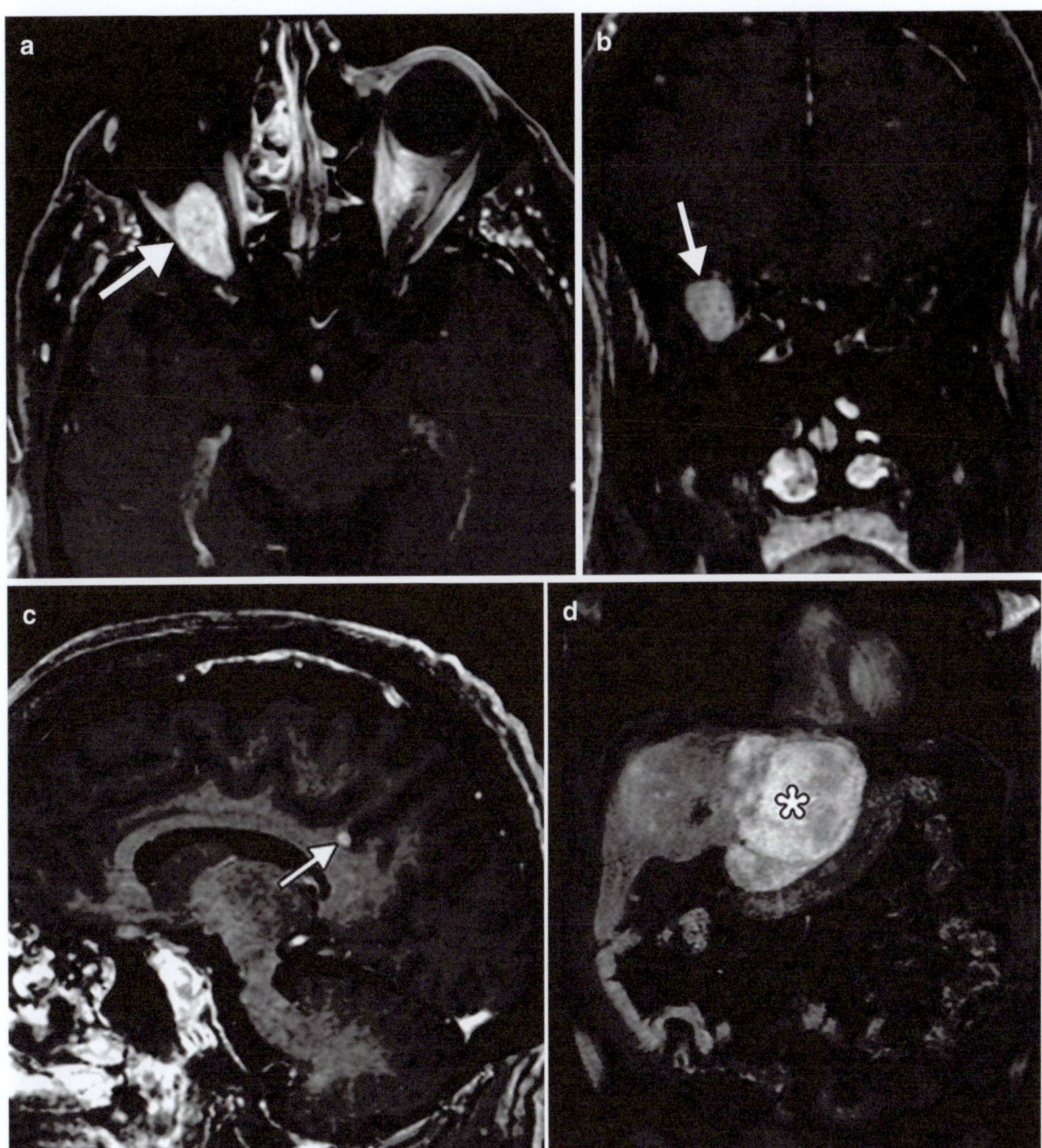

Fig. 8.8 Recurrent choroidal melanoma with metastases. Post-contrast fat-suppressed axial (**a**) and coronal (**b**) T1-weighted MR images show an enhancing mass in the right orbit, posterior to the ocular implant. Sagittal post-contrast T1-weighted MRI (**c**) shows an enhancing metastasis in the brain (*arrow*). Coronal post-contrast T1-weighted MRI (**d**) of the abdomen shows a large enhancing metastasis within the liver (*)

majority of these do not contain metallic components and the underlying exenteration cavity can be readily delineated (Fig. 8.15).

Complications have been reported in over 20 % of exenterations in the setting of orbital oncology and include fistula formation, infec-tion, flap necrosis, CSF leak, and tumor recur-rence. Fistulas most commonly occur from the orbit to the ethmoid sinuses but can extend to other sites. On imaging, fistulas may appear as air-filled channels, which are best depicted on CT (Fig. 8.16). Fistulas are sometimes associated

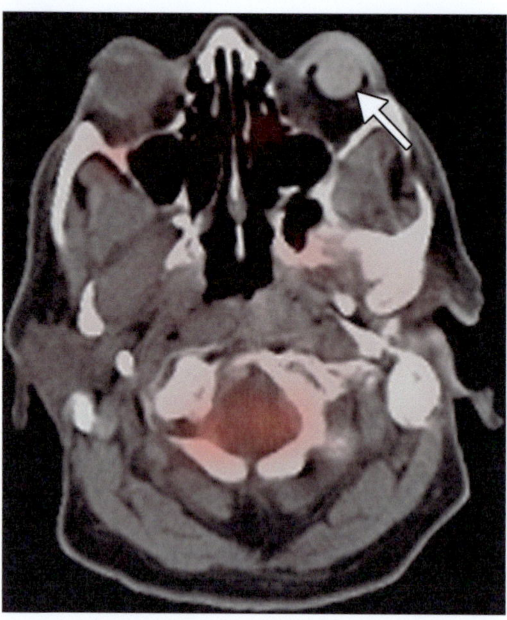

Fig. 8.9 Silicone orbital implant on positron emission tomography/CT imaging. The 18FDG-PET/CT fusion image shows absence of hypermetabolism in the left orbital prosthesis (*arrow*)

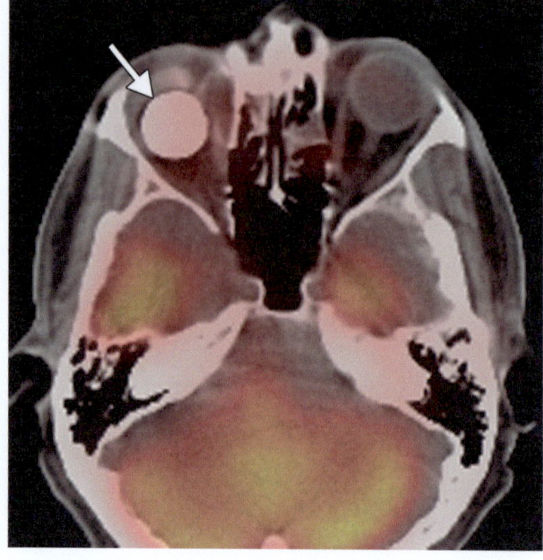

Fig. 8.10 Hydroxyapatite implant on positron emission tomography/CT. The 18FDG-PET/CT fusion image shows mild diffuse hypermetabolism within the right orbital hydroxyapatite prosthesis (*arrow*). There were no symptoms related to the implant and there was no evidence of tumor in the orbits

with infection. Otherwise, infections appear as nonspecific fluid collections that can be difficult to distinguish from seromas or CSF leaks based on imaging alone. Tumor recurrence most commonly occurs at the margins of the reconstruction flap (Fig. 8.17). It is also important to be vigilant for lymph node metastases, intracranial metastases, and perineural tumor spread, all of which can manifest after exenteration. CT with contrast is typically adequate for delineating lymph nodes, while MRI with contrast is more sensitive for depicting intracranial metastases. MRI with contrast is also particularly useful for depicting the presence of perineural tumor spread, which appears as excess thickening and enhancement of the involved nerve segments (Fig. 8.18). The incidence and form of tumor recurrence are highly dependent on the tumor histology and staging. For example, squamous cell carcinomas and adenoid cystic carcinomas have a relative propensity for perineural spread. In addition, adenoid cystic carcinomas can metastasize to the dura and mimic meningiomas (Fig. 8.19).

8.5 Optic Nerve Resection

Resection of the optic nerve along with optic nerve sheath meningiomas was first described by Cushing and Eisenhardt in 1938. En bloc resection of the tumor and involved optic nerve is sometimes performed for patients who have progressive growth of the tumor posteriorly that threatens to involve the optic chiasm or intracranial structures. The globe is typically left intact if it is not involved by the tumor, for cosmetic purposes and to avoid the difficulties associated with orbital implants. MRI is the modality of choice for the postoperative assessment of residual or recurrent optic nerve meningioma. In particular, it is important to evaluate for the presence of intracranial optic nerve meningioma, which can potentially spread to the contralateral side. Nevertheless, the surgery itself can produce a striking appearance on imaging, in which the globe is present, while both the optic nerve sheath and optic nerve are absent along variable lengths, and if the canalicular

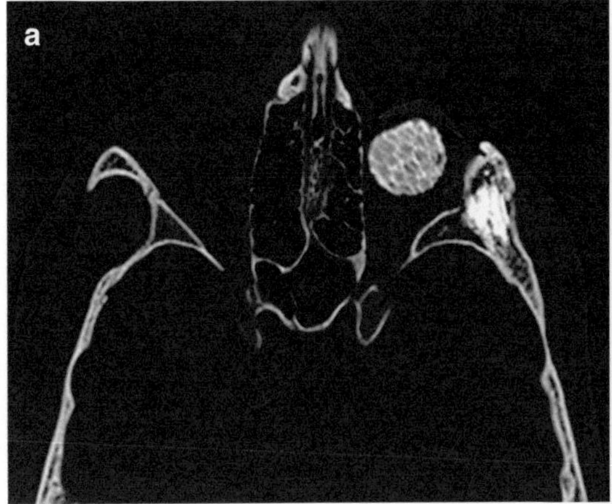
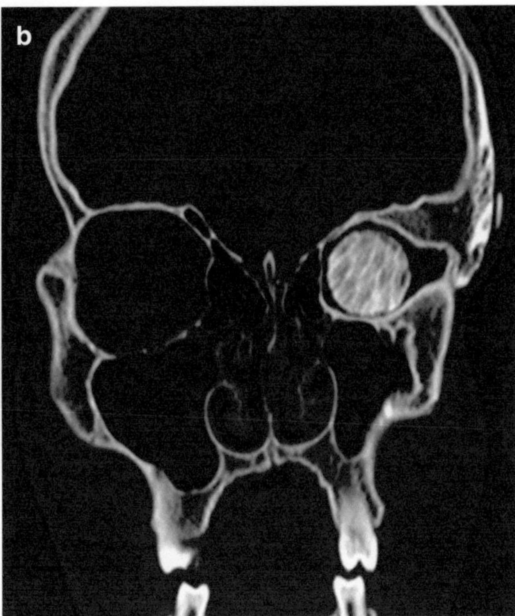

Fig. 8.11 Orbital arrest syndrome (microorbitalism). Axial (**a**) and coronal (**b**) CT images show a relatively small left orbital cavity, which contains a hydroxyapatite implant. In particular, there is sclerosis and thickening of portions of the left orbital walls. There is also hypoplasia of the left maxillary sinus, which is depicted on the coronal image

segment is removed, the optic canal fills with CSF (Fig. 8.20).

8.6 Radiation Therapy

External beam radiation therapy (EBRT) is widely used for the treatment of a variety of orbital tumors. EBRT is delivered using photons or particles such as protons or neutrons via a linear accelerator. Stereotactic radiosurgery (SRS) typically involves a single fraction of radiation and has different subtypes including the gamma knife and proton irradiation. The gamma knife uses over 200 converging gamma-ray beams and is ideal for treatment of small- to medium-sized lesions. Proton beam therapy involves the delivery of high energy protons to the tumor. A dose of 50–70 Gy is typically given in 4–5 fractions. If the site of treatment is the globe, such as in the case of choroidal melanoma, small rings made of tantalum are first surgically sutured to the eye for localization of the tumor during the treatment (Fig. 8.21).

These rings are MRI compatible. Brachytherapy involves the surgical placement of a radioactive material onto the sclera directly adjacent to the tumor. Tumors of the bulbar conjunctiva, squamous carcinoma, and malignant melanoma can be treated with a radioactive plaque: strontium-90, ruthenium-106 (Ru-106), or iodine-125 (I-125), after excision. Alternatively, an I-125 interstitial implant can be used with shielding of the cornea and lens. Brachytherapy implants are usually left in place transiently and therefore are uncommonly encountered on imaging. However, if perioperative ultrasound is performed to evaluate for potential complications, the implants appear as linear hyperechogenicity along the surface of the globe (Fig. 8.22).

Many side effects from radiation therapy delivered for treatment of orbital region tumor can be encountered on imaging, both in the early and late posttreatment periods and within or beyond the confines of the orbit. These include orbital fat atrophy, vasculopathy, optic neuropathy, osteoradionecrosis, and secondary neoplasms.

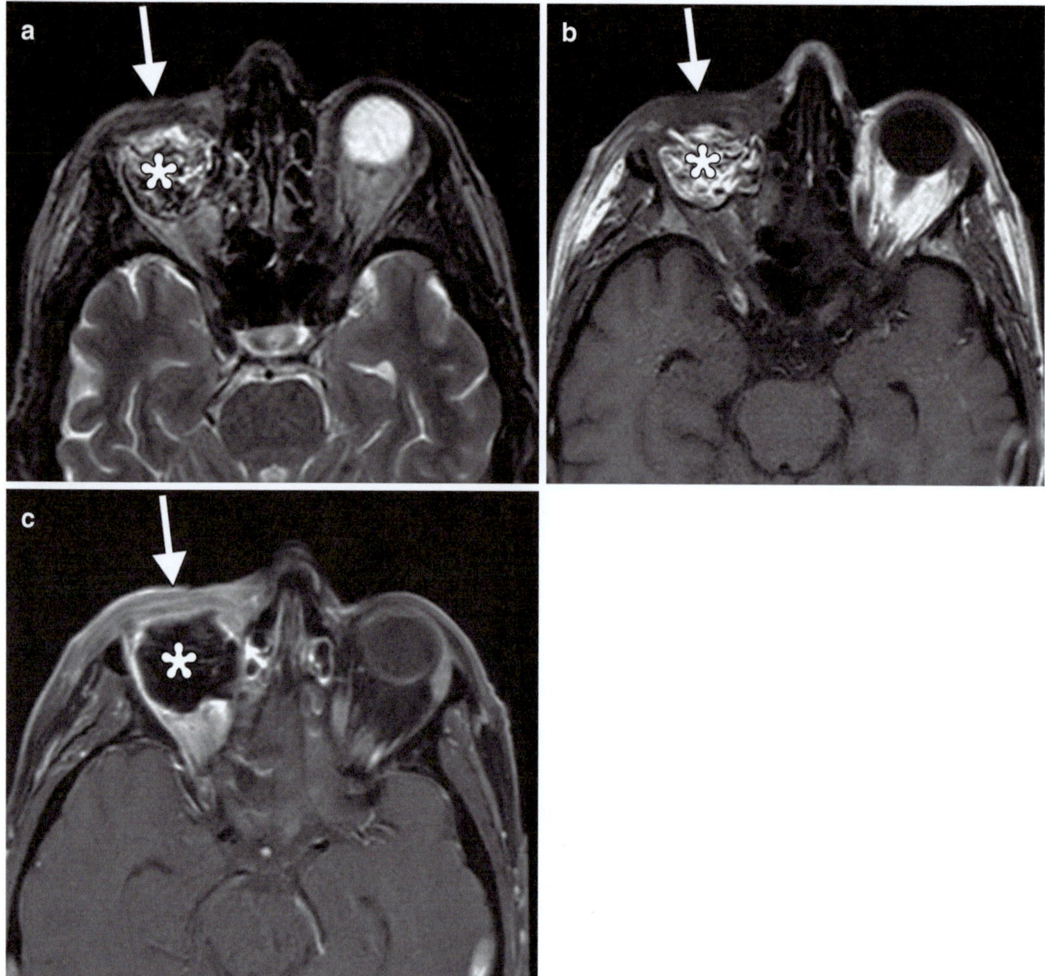

Fig. 8.12 Eyelid-sparing exenteration with fat graft reconstruction. The patient had a history of recurrent choroidal melanoma after enucleation. Axial T2-weighted (**a**), T1-weighted (**b**), and post-contrast fat-suppressed T1-weighted (**c**) images show preservation of the eyelids (*arrows*), which are mildly swollen and enhancing due to recent surgery. Fat graft (*) is present within the exenteration cavity

Radiation-induced orbital fat atrophy can result in enophthalmos and reduced ocular motility. There can also be contractile fibrosis of the orbital connective tissues and extraocular muscles, which contributes to the symptoms. Diagnostic imaging can be used to assess the reduction in orbital volume (Fig. 8.23).

Radiation-induced vasculopathy can present many years after radiation to the orbit and can manifest as transient ischemic attacks or strokes. CTA or MRA are useful for the evaluation of the associated cerebrovascular steno-occlusive disease. This complication can affect small vessels as well as large vessels, such as the internal carotid artery (Fig. 8.24).

Radiation necrosis of the brain is not an uncommon phenomenon in patients with orbital region malignancies treated with external beam radiation. The anterior temporal pole and inferior frontal lobes are the most commonly affected sites. On CT, brain radiation necrosis appears as confluent areas of hypoattenuation, while on MRI there is confluent T2 hyperintensity that corresponds to vasogenic edema and areas of enhancement that may display a "Swiss cheese," "cut pepper," or "spreading

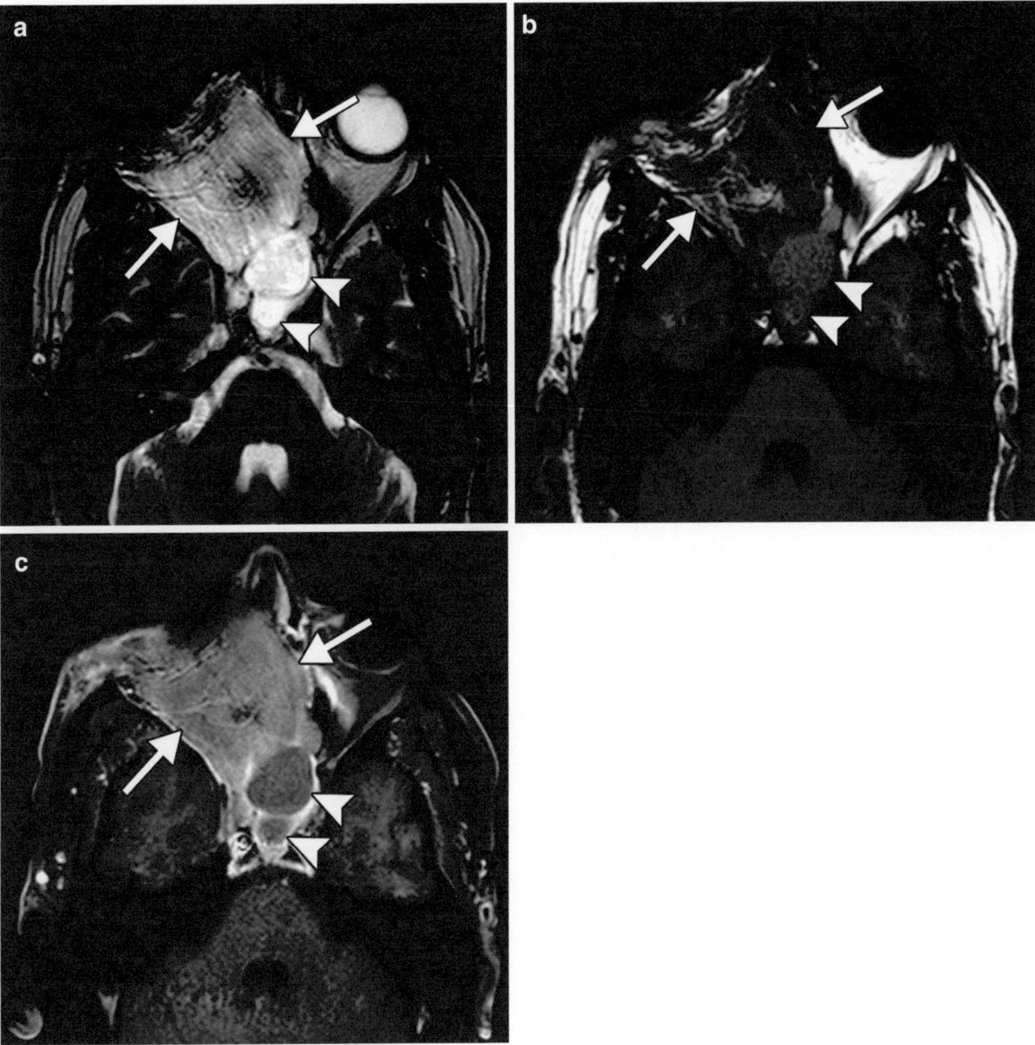

Fig. 8.13 Orbital exenteration and maxillectomy with myocutaneous graft reconstruction. The patient has a history of a salivary gland malignancy involving the right orbit. Axial T2-weighted (**a**), T1-weighted (**b**), and fat-suppressed, post-contrast T1-weighted (**c**) MR images show striations and enhancement of the muscular component of the flap (*arrow*) and trapped secretions in the sphenoid sinuses (*arrowheads*)

wave front" pattern (Fig. 8.25). However, the appearance of radiation necrosis can sometimes mimic brain metastases, and advanced imaging techniques can help differentiate tumor and radiation necrosis, such as MRI perfusion. For example, elevated perfusion suggests metastases over radiation necrosis. 18FDG-PET can also be useful, whereby radiation necrosis appears as hypometabolism, while metastases tend to display hypermetabolism, although this modality is limited by the underlying normal high cortical metabolism and low spatial resolution.

Radiation-induced optic neuropathy is a devastating late complication of radiotherapy to the anterior visual pathway that can result in acute and potentially irreversible visual loss. This complication may result from radiation necrosis of the anterior visual pathway and occurs on an average of 18 months after treatment, but the onset may range from 3 months to 9 years. Cumulative doses of radiation that exceed 50 Gy or single

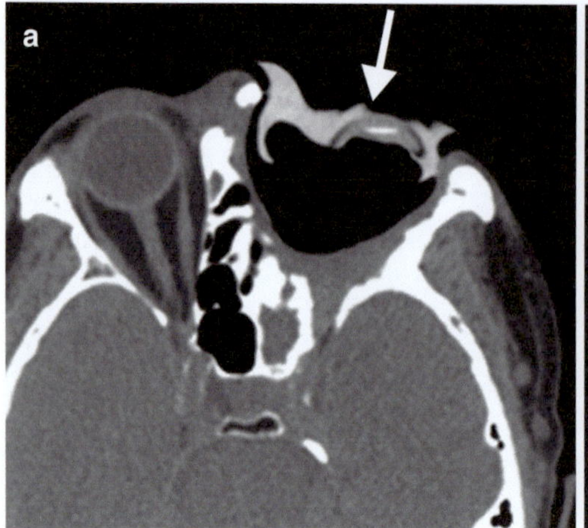 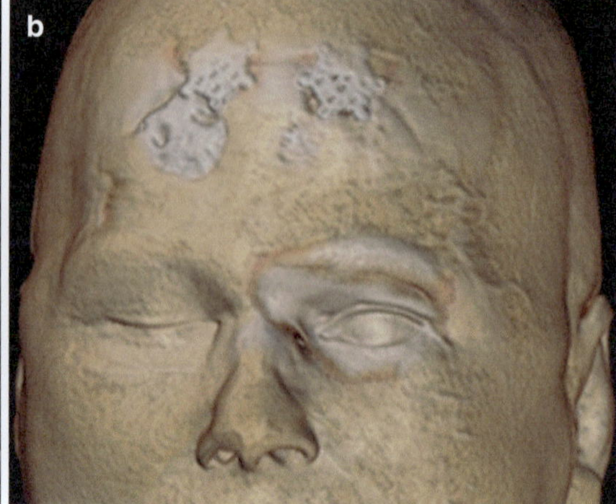

Fig. 8.14 Orbital exenteration with cosmetic ectoprosthesis. The patient has a history of basal cell carcinoma involving the left face with orbital invasion and is status post orbital exenteration. Axial (**a**) CT image shows a custom-fit hyperattenuating prosthesis (*arrow*) that covers the left orbital exenteration cavity, which is lined by a skin graft. The 3D volume-rendered CT image (**b**) shows a satisfactory cosmetic result, although the artificial eyelids do not blink

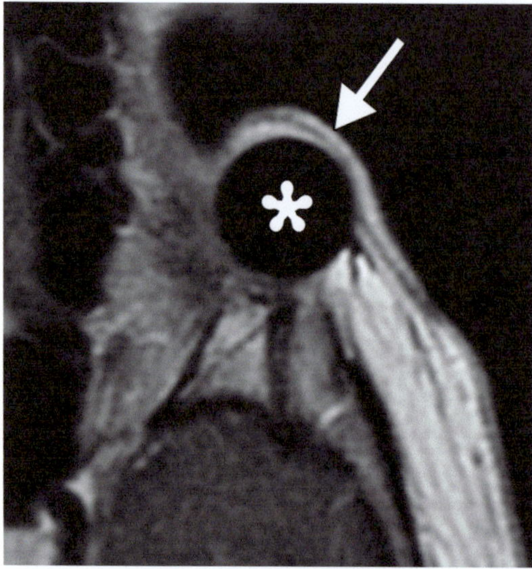

Fig. 8.15 Exenteration with implant. The patient has a history of left choroidal melanoma with extrascleral extension, status post left orbital exenteration with augmentation of the cavity with a spherical silicone implant affixed to the lateral orbital rim, as shown on the axial T1-weighted MRI, in which the hypointense implant (*) is covered by skin graft (*arrow*)

doses to the anterior visual pathway greater than 10 Gy usually precede radiation-induced optic neuropathy. MRI is the best modality for depicting radiation-induced optic neuropathy. On MRI, the affected optic nerve can display diffuse T2 hyperintensity, mild enhancement, and swelling (Fig. 8.26).

Osteoradionecrosis is relatively uncommon in the region of the orbit compared to other sites in the head and neck. Nevertheless, this is an important complication that is difficult to treat and can be responsible for delayed socket healing. Osteoradionecrosis is defined as an area of exposed devitalized irradiated bone, with failure to heal during a period of at least 3 months, in the absence of local neoplastic disease. It is important to differentiate osteoradionecrosis from local recurrence of malignancy, bone metastasis, radiation-induced sarcoma, and infection. Both CT and MRI are effective and often complementary diagnostic modalities for the evaluation of osteoradionecrosis, which can appear as areas of irregular bone destruction and sclerosis (Fig. 8.27). There may also be associated enhancement of the involved bone and surrounding soft tissues.

A variety of secondary tumors can arise from radiation therapy to the orbit, including meningiomas, leiomyosarcomas, fibrosarcomas, chondrosarcomas, and osteosarcomas. Osteosarcoma is the most common secondary malignant neoplasm in survivors of retinoblastoma treated with radiation

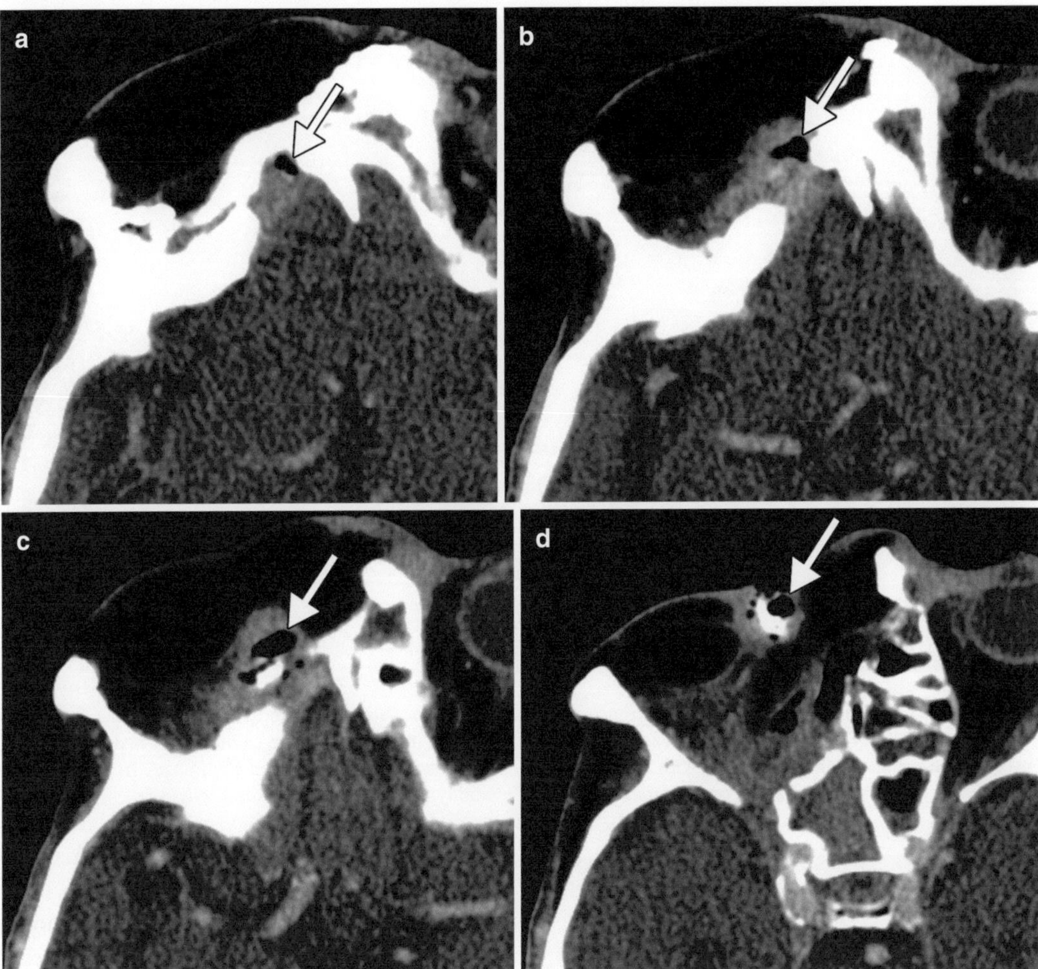

Fig. 8.16 Fistula. The patient underwent orbital exenteration with removal of a portion of the orbital roof and paranasal sinuses. Axial CT images (**a–d**) show an air-filled tract (*arrows*) that extends from the epidural space adjacent to an area of bony dehiscence to a skin defect along margins of the myocutaneous flap

and typically develops after a latency period of 5–10 years after doses in excess of 3,000 Gy. These tumors characteristically occur at the edge of the radiation field because the administered radiation in this location does not cause cell death but is sufficient to induce malignant transformation. CT is superior for depicting the presence of matrix mineralization, periosteal reaction, and cortical destruction, whereas MRI is better for delineating soft tissue and intracranial extension and for differentiating enhancing tumor from non-enhancing sinus secretions (Fig. 8.28). Tumor matrix mineralization and aggressive bone destruction are strongly suggestive of osteosarcoma. Matrix mineralization and periosteal new bone formation favor a diagnosis of osteosarcoma over metastatic carcinoma, lymphoma, and myeloma; a destructive mass is generally not found in radiation osteitis. A less aggressive osteosarcoma may be radiologically indistinguishable from chondrosarcoma.

8.7　Chemotherapy

Primary chemotherapy is indicated for selected cases of intraocular retinoblastoma, optic glioma, rhabdomyosarcoma and other malignant mesenchymal tumors, and metastases. Induction

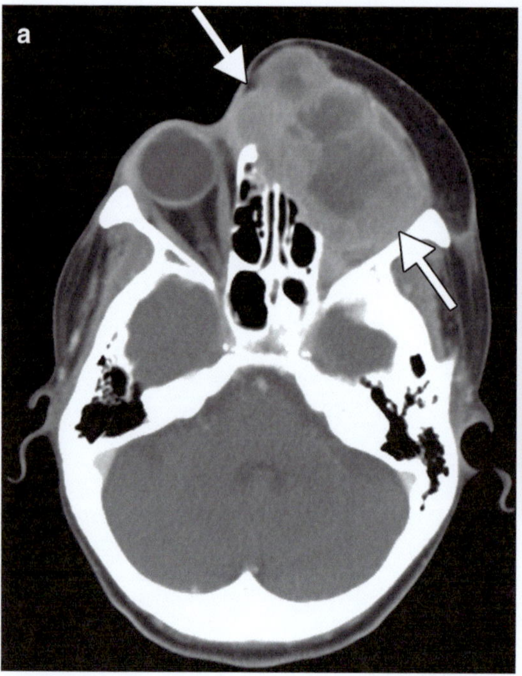

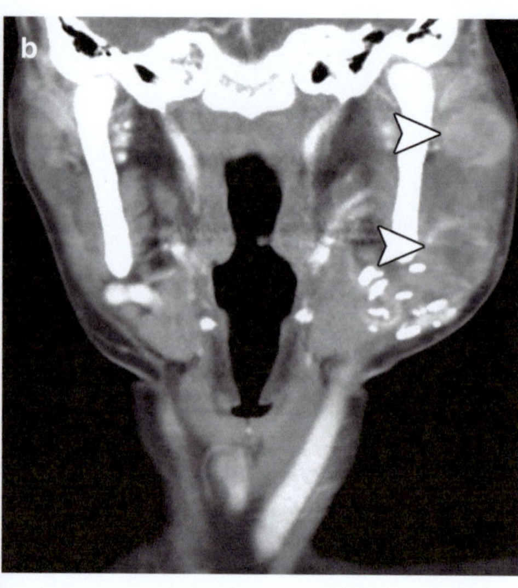

Fig. 8.17 Local and regional tumor recurrence. The patient has a history of squamous cell carcinoma that involved the orbit, which was treated with orbital exenteration and myocutaneous flap reconstruction. Axial CT image (**a**) shows a heterogeneously enhancing mass (*arrows*) that occupies the exenteration bed, deep to the flap. In addition, the coronal CT image (**b**) shows metastatic lymphadenopathy (*arrowheads*)

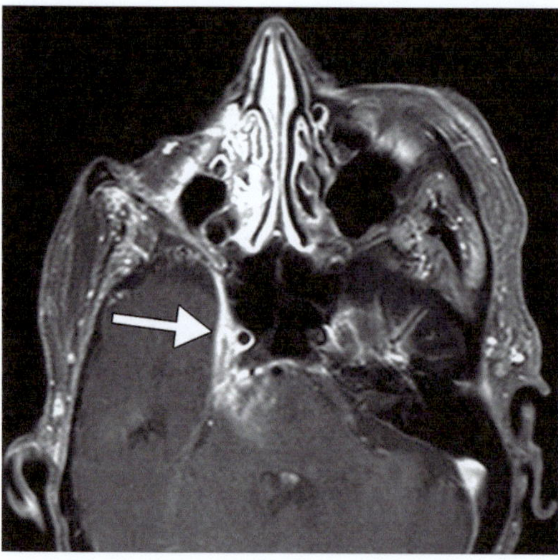

Fig. 8.18 Perineural tumor spread. The patient has a history of facial squamous cell carcinoma with invasion of the right orbit and is status post orbital exenteration. Axial post-contrast fat-suppressed T1-weighted MRI shows diffuse thickening and enhancement of the right trigeminal nerve with extension into the pons (*arrow*)

chemotherapy is also frequently administered to reduce the size of the tumor to facilitate other treatments, such as cryotherapy, laser photocoagulation, resection, and radiation. Finally, chemotherapy may be administered as an adjunct to radiation and surgery. There are many chemotherapy agents and regimens used in clinical practice and they are in constant evolution.

The main role of imaging in patients receiving primary chemotherapy for orbital tumors is for evaluation of treatment response. Furthermore, treated lesions can show changes in signal characteristic on MRI. For example, regressing tumors may show decreased enhancement and increased diffusivity in echo-planar diffusion-weighted imaging (Fig. 8.29). The increased diffusivity often observed in treated tumors is attributable to cell death and an increased proportion of water content. Potential pitfalls of diffusion-weighted imaging include the presence of calcifications and hemorrhage, which can affect ADC values.

In addition, the orbital region is often affected by distortion from susceptibility effects at the air-tissue interfaces, and measurements made on very small lesions may be subject to the effects of partial volume averaging.

There are potential limitations of orbital imaging in these patients. For example, although visual deterioration may prompt an MRI of the orbits in the case of optic gliomas, the change in clinical status is not always accompanied by a discernable change in the MRI appearance of the optic glioma. Furthermore, some chemotherapy agents, such as ipilimumab, can induce a flare response that appears as a spurious increase in hypermetabolism on 18FDG-PET that can be misinterpreted as tumor progression. In addition to the possibility of local and regional tumor recurrence, it is important to monitor distant involvement. In the case of retinoblastoma, follow-up with brain MRI is routinely performed to assess for involvement of the suprasellar and/or pineal regions (Fig. 8.30). Furthermore, these tumors can rarely have spine leptomeningeal drop metastases. MRI with contrast is the modality of choice for evaluating this phenomenon, since the lesions tend to avidly enhance.

8.8 Management of the Orbit in Malignant Sinonasal Disease

Malignant ethmoid and maxillary sinus tumors may involve the orbit. The periorbita, which surrounds the orbital contents, generally provides a barrier against invading tumors from coming into direct contact with or infiltrating the orbital structures. In these cases, tumor resections often spare the orbital contents. The pressure exerted by such tumors may, however, result in globe distortion and compressive optic neuropathy. Tumors may occasionally penetrate the periorbita and invade the orbital soft tissues. Cross-sectional imaging plays a major role in posttreatment follow-up for identifying and characterizing residual or recurrent tumor in the orbit and its surroundings (Fig. 8.31). Another postsurgical complication specific to the orbit that can be evaluated via CT and/or MRI is malposition of the globe, which can result from inadequate reconstruction of the orbital walls, extraorbital fluid collections, or hemorrhage (Figs. 8.32 and 8.33).

8.9 Summary

- Diagnostic neuroimaging plays a key role in the posttreatment management of orbital region neoplasms.
- The main modalities used for posttreatment surveillance and metastatic workup are CT and MRI, with the exception of small intraocular tumors, which are best depicted on ultrasound. In some cases, 18FDG-PET can be useful for screening distant metastases.
- Diagnostic neuroimaging is also useful for evaluating many posttreatment complications, including hemorrhage, infection, radiation necrosis, secondary malignancies, vasculopathy, and graft and implant failures.
- Ultimately interpretation of posttreatment orbit imaging studies benefits from a thorough familiarity with the various types of treatment modalities and complications, availability of relevant clinical history, and a systematic approach towards reviewing the images.

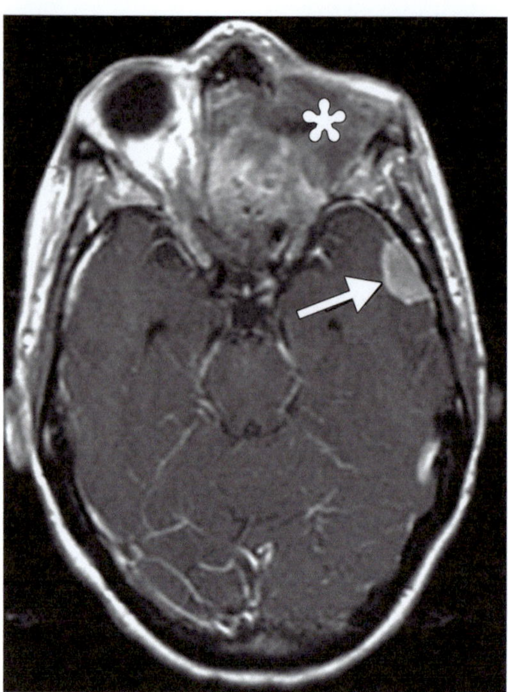

Fig. 8.19 Intracranial metastases mimicking meningioma after orbital exenteration. The patient has a history of adenoid cystic carcinoma of the lacrimal gland. Axial post-contrast T1-weighted MRI shows a dural metastasis along the left temporal convexity (*arrow*). There is a myocutaneous flap within the left orbital exenteration cavity (*)

Fig. 8.20 Optic nerve resection. The patient has a history of right optic nerve meningioma with complete loss of vision and intracranial extension. Preoperative axial (**a**) and coronal (**b**) post-contrast T1-weighted MR images show an enhancing, diffuse, plaque-like mass along the right optic nerve sheath (*arrows*). Postoperative coronal T2-weighted MR images (**c–f**) show that the right globe remains intact, but the right optic nerve and nerve sheath are absent. There was no evidence of recurrent tumor

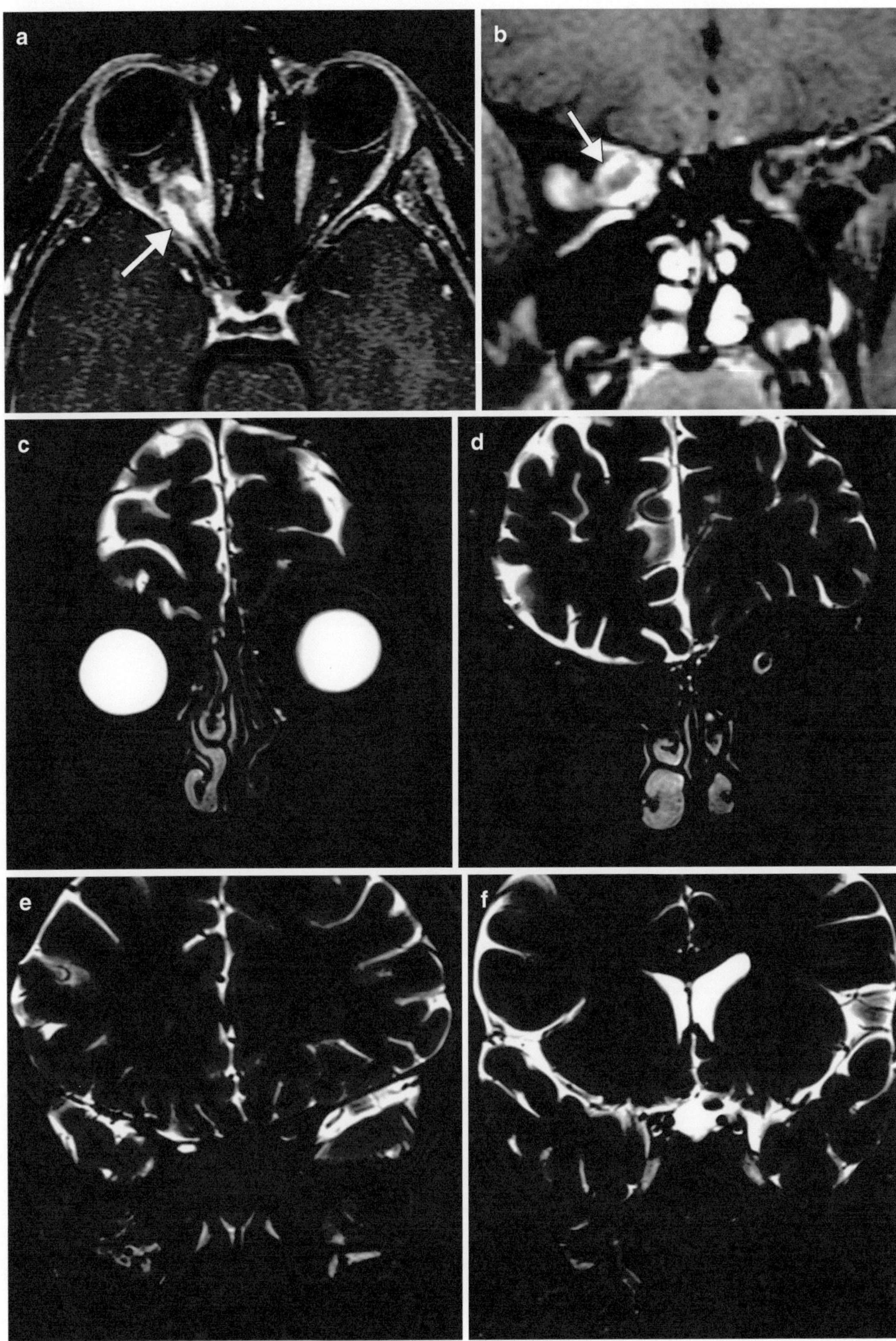

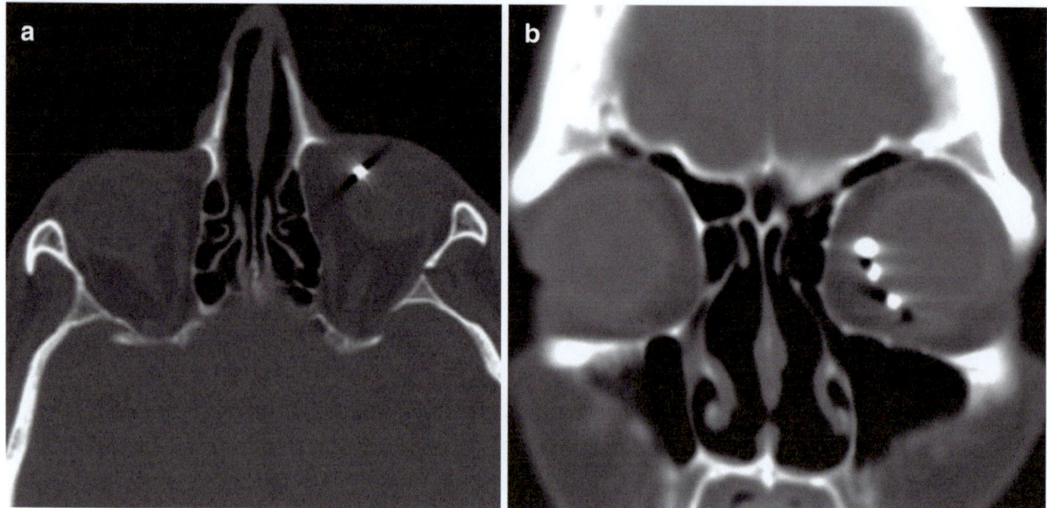

Fig. 8.21 Tantalum rings. Axial (**a**) and coronal (**b**) CT images show several punctate hyperattenuating tantalum rings attached to the inferomedial aspect of the left globe

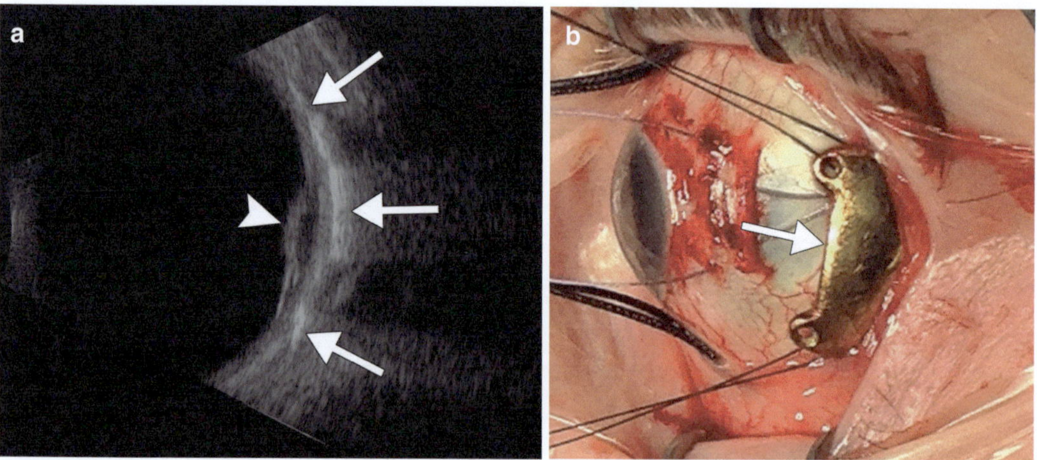

Fig. 8.22 Brachytherapy plaque. The patient has a history of choroidal melanoma. B-mode ultrasound (**a**) demonstrates the echogenic brachytherapy plaque positioned alongside the globe (*arrows*) and the intraocular tumor (*arrowhead*). Intraoperative photograph (**b**) of the brachytherapy plaque in situ (Courtesy of Arun Singh MD)

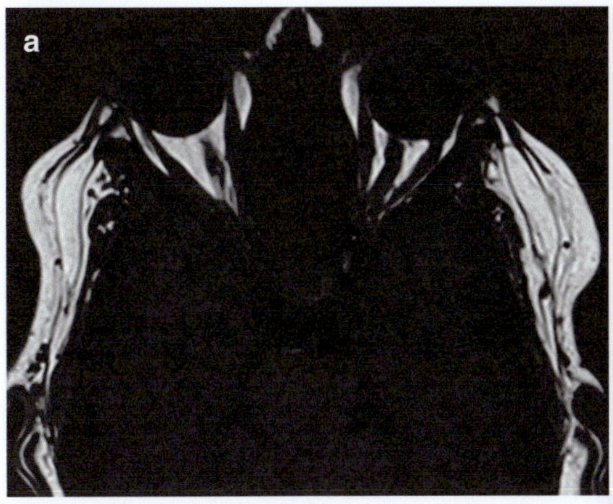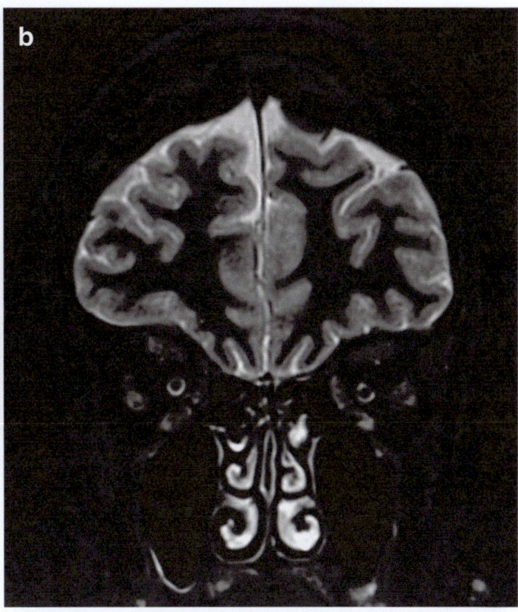

Fig. 8.23 The patient has a history of widespread metastatic breast cancer (non-scirrhous type) with left inferior and lateral rectus muscle orbital metastases treated with radiation. Axial T1-weighted (**a**) and coronal fat-suppressed T2-weighted (**b**) MR images show left enophthalmos due to diffusely reduced orbital fat content and asymmetric left extraocular muscle atrophy, mainly involving the inferior and lateral rectus muscles. There is also a heterogeneous appearance of the calvarial bone marrow, which reflects the presence of widespread bone metastases (Courtesy of Juan Small MD)

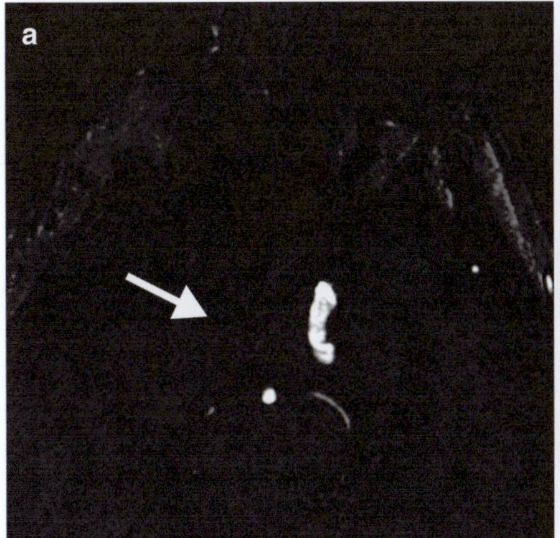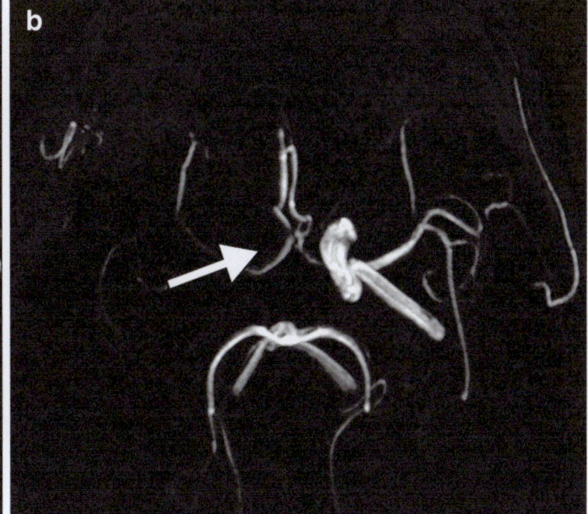

Fig. 8.24 Radiation-induced vasculopathy. The patient has a history of bilateral retinoblastoma during childhood, which was treated on the right side with radiation and orbital exenteration and on the left side with enucleation. The patient recently presented with right-sided facial pain. Axial (**a**) and MIP (**b**) time-of-flight MRA images show absence of flow-related enhancement within the right internal carotid artery (*arrows*)

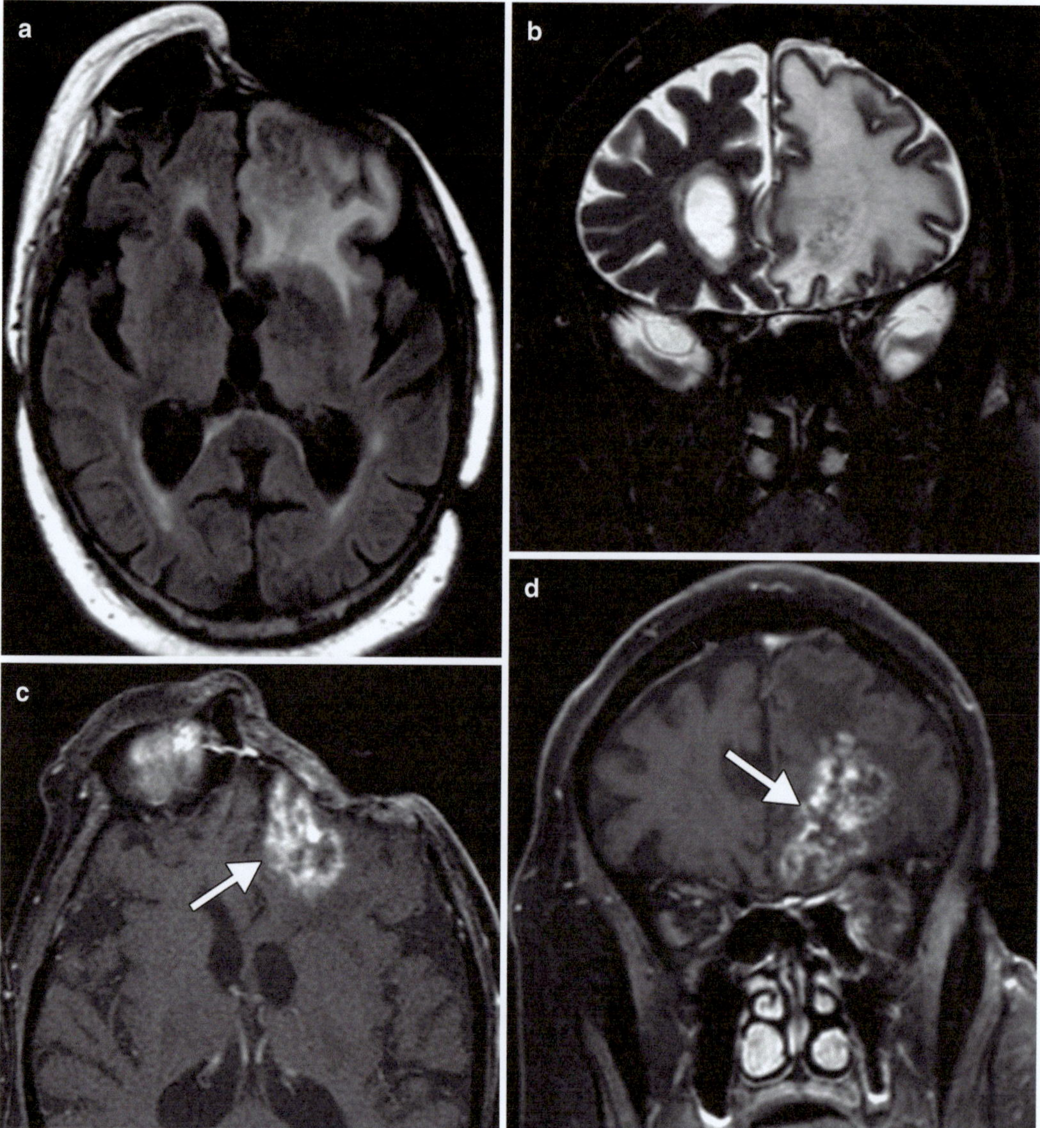

Fig. 8.25 Radiation necrosis of the brain. The patient has a history of a left orbital malignancy treated with radiation approximately 2 years earlier. Axial FLAIR (**a**), coronal fat-suppressed T2-weighted (**b**), and axial (**c**) and coronal (**d**) post-contrast fat-suppressed T1-weighted MR images show confluent vasogenic edema with areas of enhancement (*arrows*) that suggest a "soap bubble" appearance in the left frontal lobe, on the side of the orbital exenteration and within the field of the radiation

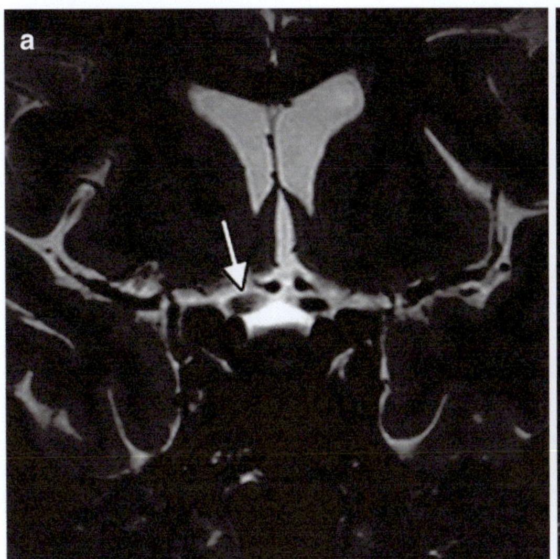
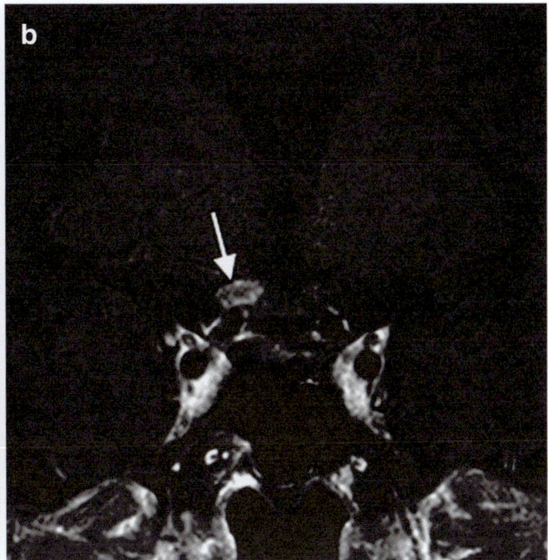

Fig. 8.26 Radiation-induced optic neuropathy. Coronal T2-weighted (**a**) and post-contrast fat-suppressed T1-weighted (**b**) MR images show a swollen and enhancing right optic nerve (*arrows*) in a patient who underwent radiotherapy to the right orbit approximately 2 years before

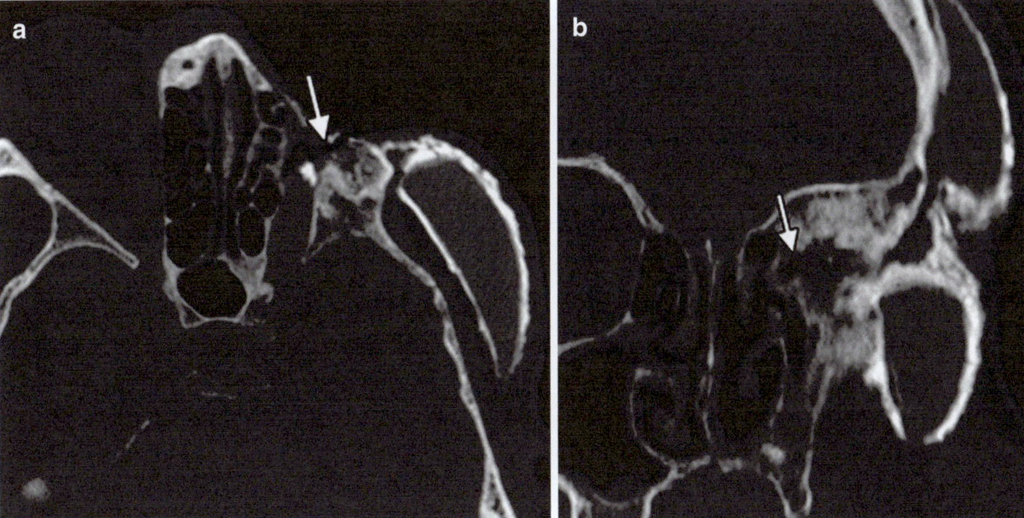

Fig. 8.27 Osteoradionecrosis. The patient underwent external beam radiation therapy and enucleation surgery for retinoblastoma and presented with a wound defect. Axial (**a**) and coronal (**b**) CT images show a soft tissue defect (*arrow*) overlying exposed bone, which displays mixed lucent and sclerotic appearance consistent with osteoradionecrosis

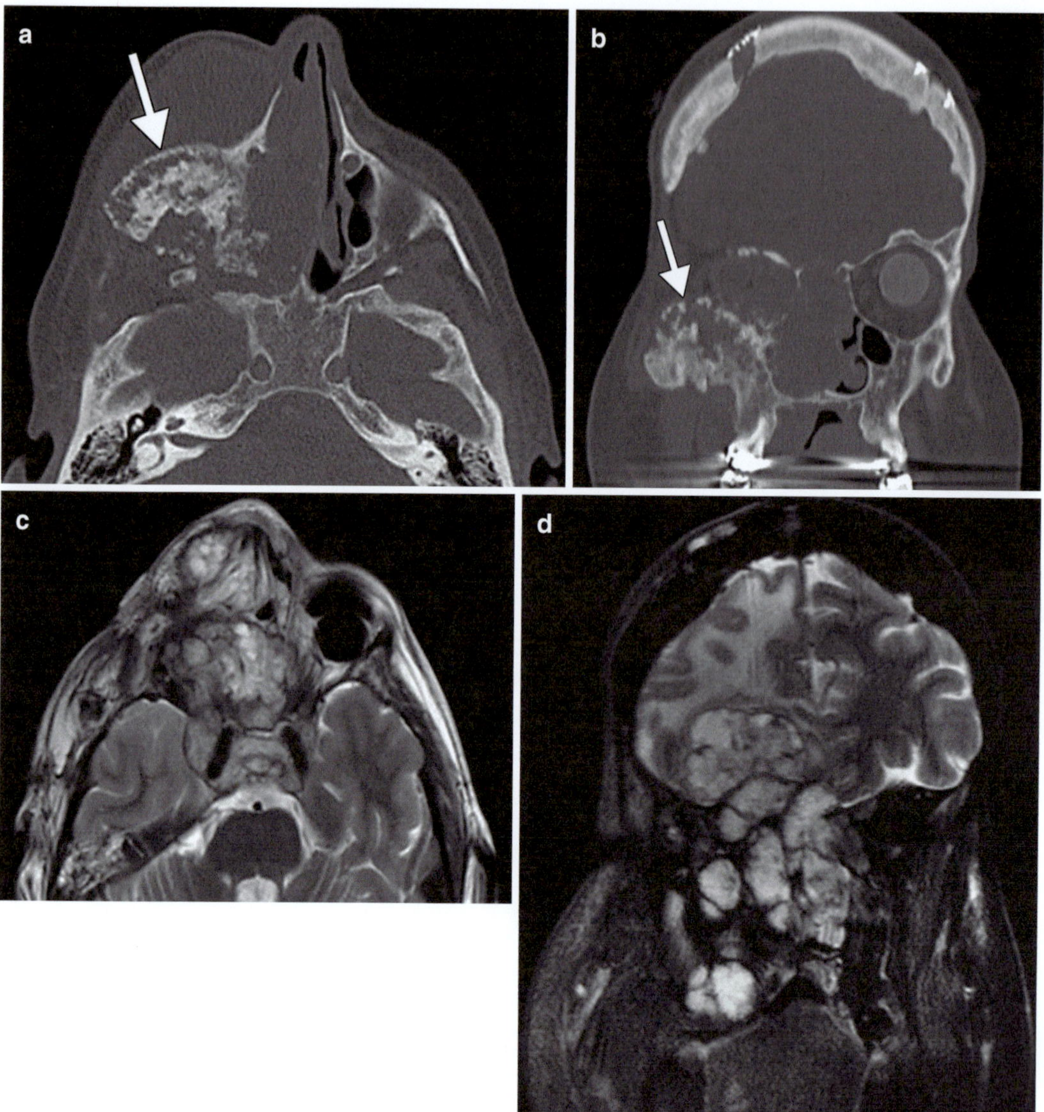

Fig. 8.28 Radiation-induced osteosarcoma. The patient has a history of retinoblastoma treated with enucleation and radiation many years prior. Axial (**a**) and coronal (**b**) CT images show a large mass involving the right maxilla and orbit containing both soft tissue and mineralized components (*arrows*). Postoperative findings reveal bilateral enucleations with a nonporous spherical orbital implant and ocular prosthesis on the left. Axial and coronal T2-weighted (**c**, **d**) and axial and coronal (**e**, **f**) post-contrast fat-suppressed T1-weighted MR images show a heterogeneously enhancing lobulated mass extending intracranially

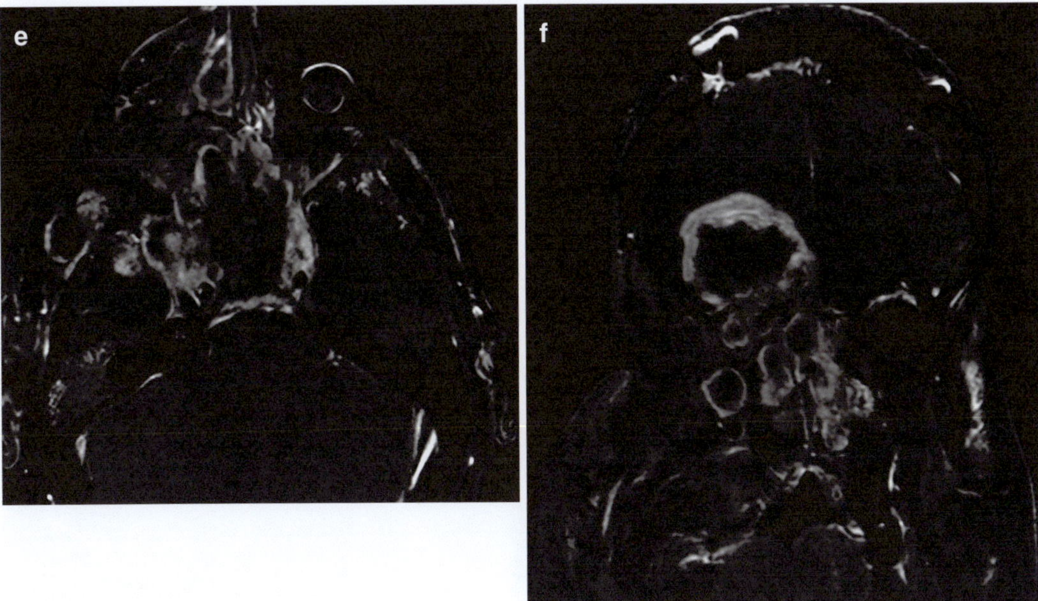

Fig. 8.28 (continued)

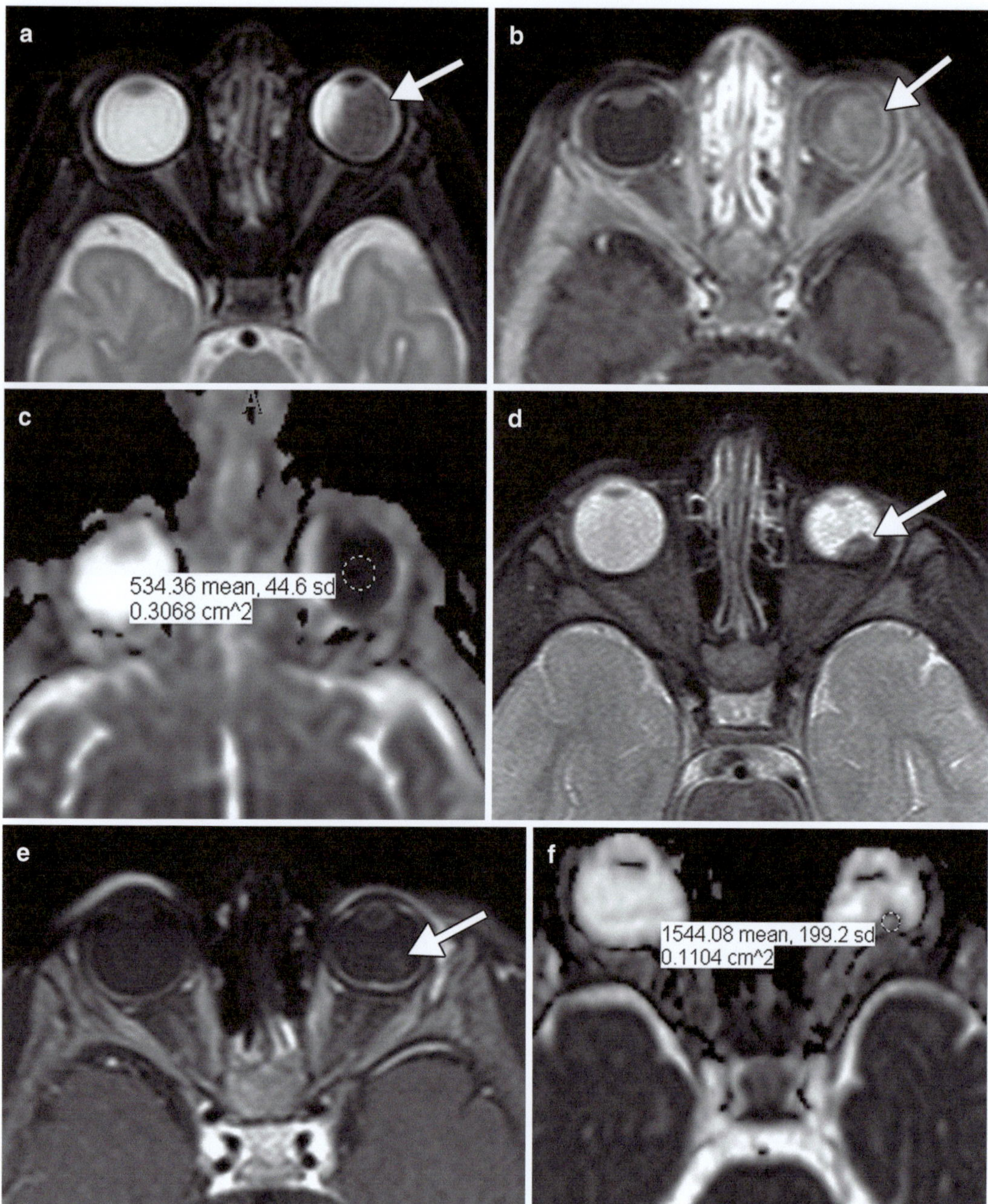

Fig. 8.29 Treatment response. Pretreatment axial T2-weighted (**a**) and post-contrast T1-weighted (**b**) images and ADC map (**c**) show a T2 hypointense, enhancing intraocular mass (*arrows*) with markedly reduced ADC. Following the administration of chemotherapy, the corresponding MR images (**d**–**f**) show interval decrease in size and enhancement of the tumor (*arrows*), as well as increased diffusivity (regions of interest are drawn over the tumor for reference)

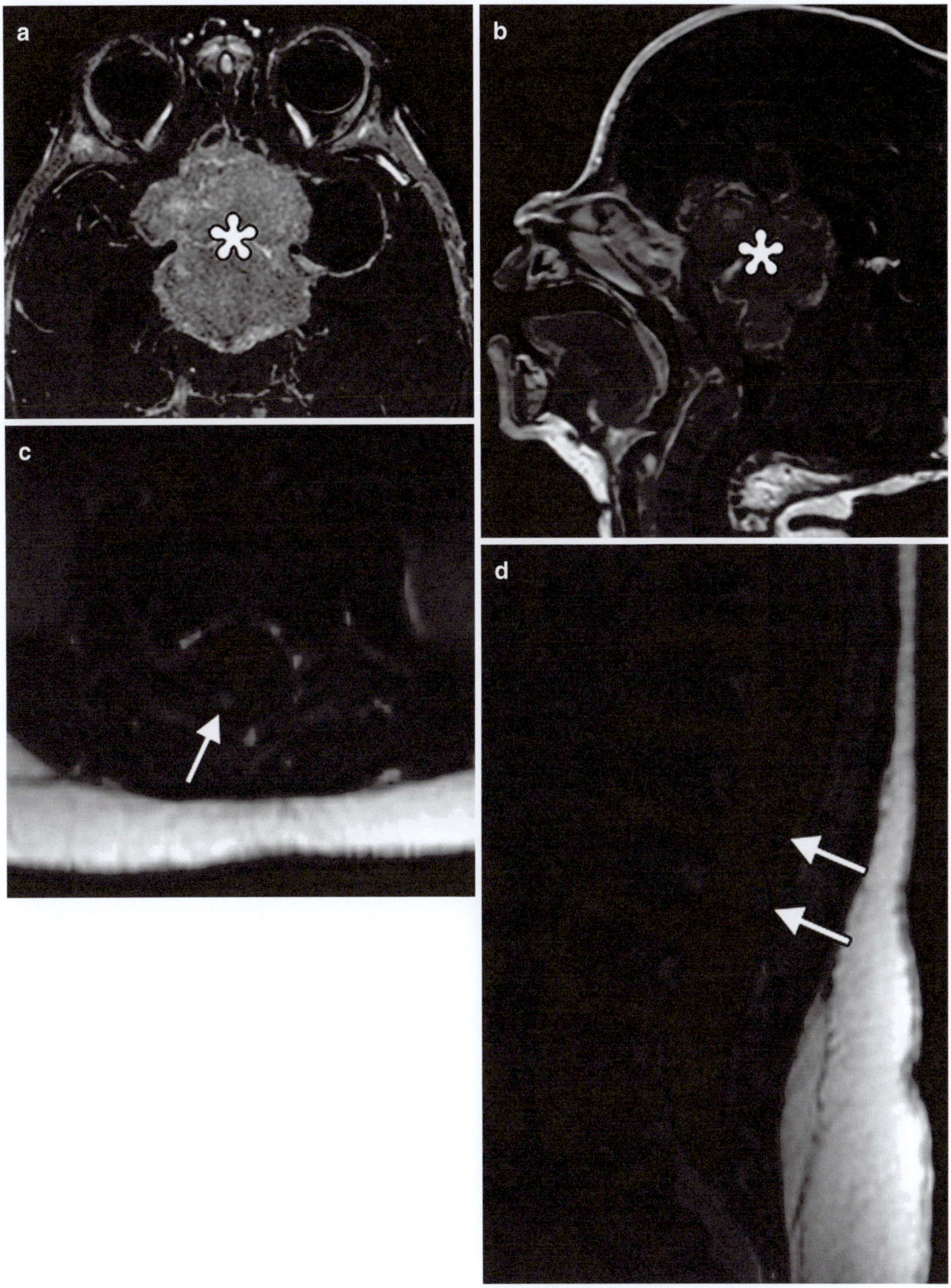

Fig. 8.30 Trilateral retinoblastoma and drop metastases. The patient is status post chemotherapy for ocular retinoblastoma and subsequently developed a suprasellar mass and spine drop metastases. Axial (**a**) and sagittal (**b**) post-contrast T1-weighted MR images of the brain show an enhancing bulky suprasellar mass (*). Axial (**c**) and sagittal (**d**) post-contrast T1-weighted MR images of the spine show numerous enhancing nodules along the cauda equina (*arrows*)

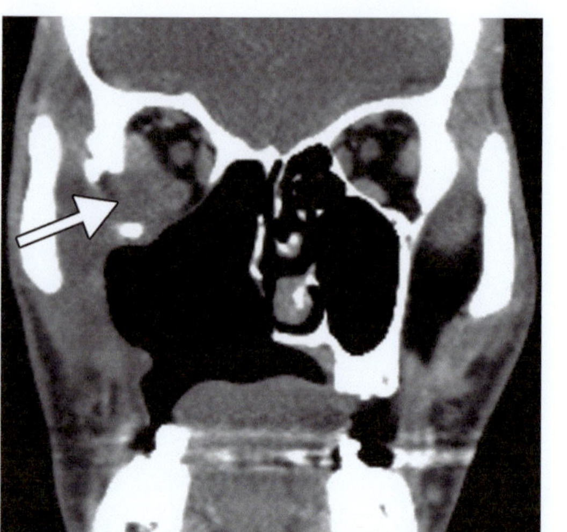

Fig. 8.31 Recurrent sinonasal tumor involving the orbit. The patient has a history of sinonasal squamous cell carcinoma status post maxillectomy with orbit preservation and status post adjuvant radiation and chemotherapy. Coronal CT image shows tumor (*arrow*) that extends into the right intraconal space where it encases the inferior and lateral rectus muscles

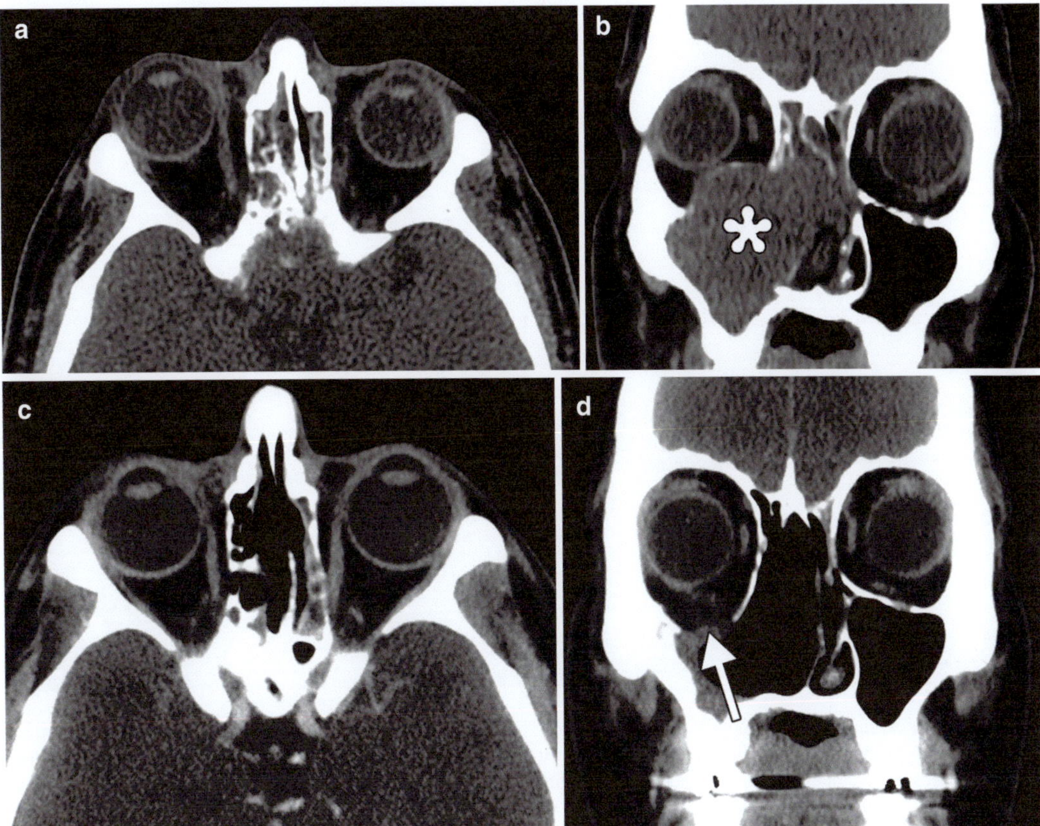

Fig. 8.32 Enophthalmos following sinonasal melanoma resection. Preoperative axial (**a**) and coronal (**b**) CT images show right hyperglobus related to extension of the right maxillary sinus tumor (*) into the extraconal orbit via a defect in the orbital floor. Postoperative axial (**c**) and coronal (**d**) CT images show interval tumor resection with new right enophthalmos associated with sagging of orbital contents through the persistent defect in the right orbital floor (*arrow*)

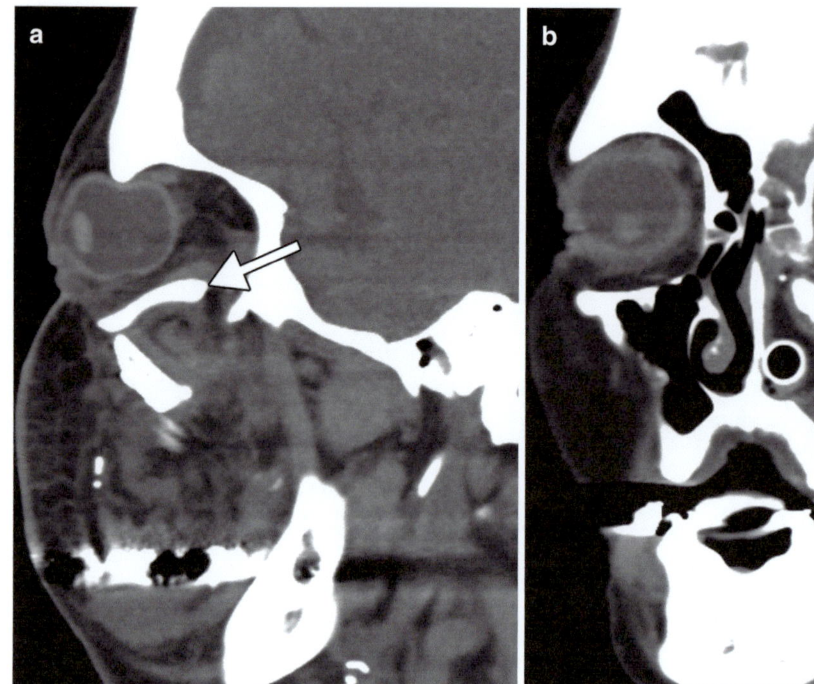

Fig. 8.33 Strabismus and globe compression after maxillectomy. The patient presented with ocular dysmotility following recent maxillectomy with myocutaneous flap and left orbital floor bone graft reconstruction. Sagittal (**a**) and coronal (**b**) CT images show compression of the globe due to superior displacement of an orbital floor bone graft (*arrows*) secondary to a swollen left maxillary sinus myocutaneous flap with hemorrhage

Further Reading

Abramson DH, Ellsworth RM, Kitchin FD, Tung G. Second Nonocular tumors in retinoblastoma survivors. Are they radiation induced? Ophthalmology. 1984;91(11):1351–5.

Alberti W. Acute and late side effects of radiotherapy for ocular disease: an overview. Front Radiat Ther Oncol. 1997;30:281–6.

Alhilali L, Reynods AR, Fakhran S. Osteoradionecrosis after radiation therapy for head and neck cancer: differentiation from recurrent disease with CT and PET/CT imaging. AJNR Am J Neuroradiol. 2014;35(7):1405–11.

Almond MC, Cheng AG, Schiedler V, Sires BS, Most SP, Jian-Amadi A. Decompression of the orbital apex: an alternate approach to surgical excision for radiographically benign orbital apex tumors. Arch Otolaryngol Head Neck Surg. 2009;135(10):1015–8.

Augsburger JJ. Diagnostic biopsy of selected Intraocular tumors. Am J Ophthalmol. 2005;140:1094–5.

Brady LW, Shields J, Augusburger J, et al. Complications from radiation therapy to the eye. Front Radiat Ther Oncol. 1989;23:238–50.

Cassady JR, Sagerman RH, Tretter P, Ellsworth RM. Radiation therapy in retinoblastoma. An analysis of 230 cases. Radiology. 1969;93(2):405–9.

Chan W, Poh E, Bartholomeusz D, Selva D. Novel use of positron emission tomography/computed tomography in the diagnosis of infected porous orbital implant. Clin Experiment Ophthalmol. 2011;39(7):704–5.

Christmas NJ, Gordon CD, Murray TG, Tse D, Johnson T, Garonzik S, O'Brien JM. Intraorbital implants after enucleation and their complications, a 10 year review. Arch Ophthalmol. 1998;116:1199–203.

Croce A, Moretti A, D'Agostino L, Zingariello P. Orbital exenteration in elderly patients: personal experience. Acta Otorhinolaryngol Ital. 2008;28(4):193–9.

Danesh-Meyer HV. Radiation-induced optic neuropathy. J Clin Neurosci. 2008;15(2):95–100.

De Potter P, Duprez T, Cosnard G. Postcontrast magnetic resonance imaging assessment of porous polyethylene orbital implant (Medpor). Ophthalmology. 2000;107(9):1656–60.

Eddleman CS, Liu JK. Optic nerve sheath meningioma: current diagnosis and treatment. Neurosurg Focus. 2007;23(5):E4.

Eide N, Walaas L. Fine-needle aspiration biopsy and other biopsies in suspected intraocular malignant disease: a review. Acta Ophthalmologica. 2009;83:588–601.

El-Sawy T, Frank SJ, Hanna E, Sniegowski M, Lai SY, Nasser QJ, Myers J, Esmaeli B. Multidisciplinary management of lacrimal sac/nasolacrimal duct carcinomas. Ophthal Plast Reconstr Surg. 2013;29(6):454–7.

Finger PT. Radiation therapy for orbital tumors: concepts, current use, and ophthalmic radiation side effects. Surv Ophthalmol. 2009;54(5):545–68.

Graue GF, Finger PT. Physiologic positron emission tomography/CT imaging of an integrated orbital implant. Ophthal Plast Reconstr Surg. 2012;28(1):e4–6.

Hadad G, Bassagasteguy L, Carrau RL, Mataza JC, Kassam A, Snyderman CH, Mintz A. A novel reconstructive technique after endoscopic expanded endonasal approaches: vascular pedicle nasoseptal flap. Laryngoscope. 2006;116(10):1882–6.

Helms HA, Zeiger Jr HE, Callahan A. Complications following enucleation and Implantation of Multiple Glass Spheres in the Orbit. Ophthal Plast Reconst Surg. 1987;3:87–9.

Hui JI, Murray TG. Radioactive plaque therapy. Int Ophthalmol Clin. 2006;46(1):51–68.

Jamison A, Gregory ME, Lyall DA, Kemp EG. Visual outcomes following orbital biopsy. Orbit. 2013;32(5):304–8.

Kim JW, Kathpalia V, Dunkel IJ, Wong RK, Riedel E, Abramson DH. Orbital recurrence of retinoblastoma following enucleation. Br J Ophthalmol. 2009;93(4):463–7. Epub 2008 Aug 29.

Lemon JC, Kiat-amnuay S, Gettleman L, Martin JW, Chambers MS. Facial prosthetic rehabilitation: preprosthetic surgical techniques and biomaterials. Curr Opin Oto laryngol Head Neck Surg. 2005;13(4):255–62.

Lessell S. Friendly fire: neurogenic visual loss from radiation therapy. J Neuroophthalmol. 2004;24(3):243–50.

Liu JK, Forman S, Moorthy CR, Benzil DL. Update on treatment modalities for optic nerve sheath meningiomas. Neurosurg Focus. 2003;14(5):e7.

Locatelli M, Carrabba G, Guastella C, Gaini SM, Spagnoli D. Endoscopic endonasal removal of a cavernous hemangioma of the orbital apex. Surg Neurol Int. 2011;2:58.

López F, Suárez C, Carnero S, Martín C, Camporro D, Llorente JL. Free flaps in orbital exenteration: a safe and effective method for reconstruction. Eur Arch Otorhinolaryngol. 2013;270(6):1947–52.

Makimoto Y, Yamamoto S, Takano H, Motoori K, Ueda T, Kazama T, Kaneoya K, Shimofusa R, Uno T, Ito H, Hanazawa T, Okamoto Y, Hayasaki K. Imaging findings of radiation-induced sarcoma of the head and neck. Br J Radiol. 2007;80(958):790–7.

Margalit NS, Lesser JB, Moche J, Sen C. Meningiomas involving the optic nerve: technical aspects and outcomes for a series of 50 patients. Neurosurgery. 2003;53(3):523–32; discussion 532–3.

Menderes A, Yilmaz M, Vayvada H, Demirdover C, Barutçu A. Reverse temporalis muscle flap for the reconstruction of orbital exenteration defects. Ann Plast Surg. 2002;48(5):521–6; discussion 526–7.

Morioka T, Matsushima T, Ikezaki K, Nagata S, Ohta M, Hasuo K, Fukui M. Intracranial adenoid cystic carcinoma mimicking meningioma: report of two cases. Neuroradiology. 1993;35(6):462–5.

Mullins ME, Barest GD, Schaefer PW, Hochberg FH, Gonzalez RG, Lev MH. Radiation necrosis versus glioma recurrence: conventional MR imaging clues to diagnosis. AJNR Am J Neuroradiol. 2005;26(8):1967–72.

Nassab RS, Thomas SS, Murray D. Orbital exenteration for advanced periorbital skin cancers: 20 years experience. J Plast Reconstr Aesthet Surg. 2007;60(10):1103–9.

Nishino M, Jagannathan JP, Ramaiya NH, Van den Abbeele AD. Revised RECIST guideline version 1.1: what oncologists want to know and what radiologists need to know. AJR Am J Roentgenol. 2010;195(2):281–9.

Offiah C, Hall E. Post-treatment imaging appearances in head and neck cancer patients. Clin Radiol. 2011;66(1):13–24.

Ozdemir H, Yücel C, Aytekin C, Onal B, Ataman A, Ozsunar Y, Işik S. Intraocular tumors. The value of spectral and color Doppler sonography. Clin Imaging. 1997;21(2):77–81.

Padula GD, McCormick B, Abramson DH. Brain necrosis after enucleation, external beam cobalt radiotherapy, and systemic chemotherapy for retinoblastoma. Arch Ophthalmol. 2002;120(1):98–9.

Pereira PR, Odashiro AN, Lim LA, Miyamoto C, Blanco PL, Odashiro M, Maloney S, De Souza DF, Burnier Jr MN. Current and emerging treatment options for uveal melanoma. Clin Ophthalmol. 2013;7:1669–82. Epub 2013 Aug 22.

Peter NM, Laitt R, Leatherbarrow B. Osteoradionecrosis of the exenterated orbit. Orbit. 2014;33(3):220–2.

Pinheiro-Neto CD, Snyderman CH. Nasoseptal flap. Adv Oto rhino laryngol. 2013;74:42–55.

Potter PD, Shields CL, Shields JA, Flanders AE. The role of magnetic resonance imaging in children with intraocular tumors and simulating lesions. Ophthalmology. 1996;103(11):1774–83.

Provenzale JM, Gururangan S, Klintworth G. Trilateral retinoblastoma: clinical and radiologic progression. AJR Am J Roentgenol. 2004;183(2):505–11.

Rahman I, Cook AE, Leatherbarrow B. Orbital exenteration: a 13 year Manchester experience. Br J Ophthalmol. 2005;89:1335–40.

Remulla HD, Rubin PA, Shore JW, et al. Complications of Porous Spherical Orbital Implants. Ophthalmology. 1995;102:586–93.

Rousseau P, Flamant F, Quintana E, Voute PA, Gentet JC. Primary chemotherapy in rhabdomyosarcomas and other malignant mesenchymal tumors of the orbit: results of the International Society of Pediatric Oncology MMT 84 Study. J Clin Oncol. 1994;12(3):516–21.

Saito N, Nadgir RN, Nakahira M, Takahashi M, Uchino A, Kimura F, Truong MT, Sakai O. Posttreatment CT and MR imaging in head and neck cancer: what the radiologist needs to know. Radiographics. 2012;32(5):1261–82; discussion 1282–4.

Sepahdari AR, Aakalu VK, Setabutr P, Shiehmorteza M, Naheedy JH, Mafee MF. Indeterminate orbital masses: restricted diffusion at MR imaging with echo-planar diffusion-weighted imaging predicts malignancy. Radiology. 2010;256(2):554–64.

Silva MM, Goldman S, Keating G, Marymont MA, Kalapurakal J, Tomita T. Optic pathway hypothalamic gliomas in children under three years of age: the role of chemotherapy. Pediatr Neurosurg. 2000;33(3):151–8.

Stannard C, Sauerwein W, Maree G, Lecuona K. Radiotherapy for ocular tumours. Eye (Lond). 2013; 27(2):119–27.

Tyers AG. Orbital exenteration for invasive skin tumours. Eye. 2006;20:1165–70.

Wang C, Roberts KB, Bindra RS, Chiang VL, Yu JB. Delayed cerebral vasculopathy following cranial radiation therapy for pediatric tumors. Pediatr Neurol. 2014;50(6):549–56.

Yun JY, Kang SJ, Kim JW, Kim YH, Sun H. Osteoplastic reconstruction of post-enucleatic microorbitalism. Arch Plast Surg. 2012;39(4):333–7.